Kitchen Cures

Revolutionize Your Health with Foods That Heal

Peggy Kotsopoulos

PINTAIL

PINTAIL
a member of Penguin Group (USA)

Published by the Penguin Group
Penguin Group (Canada), 90 Eglinton Avenue East, Suite 700, Toronto,
    Ontario, Canada, M4P 2Y3

Penguin Group (USA) Inc., 375 Hudson Street, New York,
    New York 10014, U.S.A.
Penguin Books Ltd, 80 Strand, London WC2R 0RL, England
Penguin Ireland, 25 St Stephen's Green, Dublin 2, Ireland
    (a division of Penguin Books Ltd)
Penguin Group (Australia), 707 Collins Street, Melbourne, Victoria 3008,
    Australia (a division of Pearson Australia Group Pty Ltd)
Penguin Books India Pvt Ltd, 11 Community Centre, Panchsheel Park,
    New Delhi – 110 017, India
Penguin Group (NZ), 67 Apollo Drive, Rosedale, Auckland 0632,
    New Zealand (a division of Pearson New Zealand Ltd)
Penguin Books (South Africa) (Pty) Ltd, 24 Sturdee Avenue, Rosebank,
    Johannesburg 2196, South Africa

Penguin Books Ltd, Registered Offices: 80 Strand, London
    WC2R 0RL, England

First published in Penguin paperback by Penguin Canada, 2013

Published in this edition, 2013

1 2 3 4 5 6 7 8 9 10 (RRD)

Manufactured in the U.S.A.

ISBN 978-0-14-318884-1

Visit the Penguin US website at **www.penguin.com**

ALWAYS LEARNING   PEARSON

*To Melissa and Anjelica, my sisters
and lifelong besties, whose giggles, presence
and love make the best cure-alls ever*

Also by Peggy Kotsopoulos
Must Have Been Something I Ate

contents

Introduction

We all know her—the perky, annoying chick who bounces into work in the morning. It's barely 7:30 A.M. and she's already finished a workout, walked her dog, and made all her meals for the day. All this, and she still looks more put together than a cover model for Marc Jacobs. Seriously. What gives? Was she just born this way? Or does she know something we don't?

Chances are, the secret to her success is actually very simple: it's something she ate. How you look and feel is a direct reflection of what you eat, and more important, what you assimilate. It affects pretty much everything, even things you wouldn't think of right away. Like, how about those tiny bumps on the back of your arm? The luster in your hair? Or the fact that you're just too damn tired to even think of having sex? The answer: yes, yes, and *yes*—all of these things have to do with what you eat. Food shapes the way you think, the way you process information, the clarity of your ideas and thoughts, your mood, your energy, your waist size, your libido, your skin, and your metabolism. It's all about food! And that's a good thing, because who doesn't love food?

My passion for food started pretty much when I was born. I grew up in a Greek household, so I really had no choice. My life revolved around food! We weren't even done eating breakfast and my mother was already working on our next meal. But my *awareness* of how food made me feel began around the ripe old age of five. Even then, I knew that if I ate a burger I'd be sluggish and lethargic and wouldn't have the energy

1

to play. Whereas if I ate a pint of strawberries, my face would get these vibrant little tingles and I'd be filled with energy. Gut instinct? Maybe. But about 10 years later, it all started to make even more sense.

At age 15 I was hit by a car that was going 80 kilometers per hour on impact. I was broken into pieces. After hours of surgery and some serious complications, the doctors didn't think I'd survive. But I knew I would. I believed this so firmly that I was out of the hospital in two and a half weeks. They called me "miracle child." But it wasn't a miracle. It was a choice I made while lying in that hospital bed, knowing I still had so much to live for and to experience. And I wanted to live life to the fullest! This realization is what caused me to look long and hard at what I was eating and how food nourishes both the body and the soul. I remembered how those strawberries used to make my face tingle, and decided that this was how I wanted to feel every day! If we can make the choice to live in a state of optimal health—spiritually, emotionally, and physically—why wouldn't we?

There's no excuse for not feeling your best. Yes, we all have occasional off days when we'd rather hide under an oversized pair of aviators and a fedora hat and pretend that real life isn't out there waiting for us. But if you've ever felt you could use just a bit more energy and be less scatterbrained, or if you've ever thought your skin could be brighter or you could stand to lose a few pounds, *you absolutely can*. Every day. And it's not about major life changes like giving up your favorite things, running away to some boot camp, or signing up for a reality TV weight-loss show. It's about making little changes that can collectively add up to something ginormous—completely transforming how you look and feel.

For those of you who have read *Must Have Been Something I Ate*, I have taken your advice and added more sections on bone health, pain and inflammation, and memory, and tackled health topics such as menopause and heart health. And since beauty was a hot topic for most of you, I've totally expanded the beauty section into four new chapters and have provided DIY products for your entire body in the Kitchen Beautician chapters. Plus, I've added more nutritious and delicious recipes! So you get the same go-to resource guide in a new, expanded edition, with a lot more goodness!

Because food affects, well, everything, I've divided this book into five parts—so you can quickly find the info that will help you the most. Part 1 takes a look at the impact of what we eat on how we feel—how the right foods can boost our energy levels, reduce our stress levels, help us get more zzz's, rev up our sex drive, sharpen our memory, and even combat depression. In Part 2 I explain how food affects how we look, including combating those muffin tops and thunder thighs! Part 3 is all about beauty and which foods to eat to keep you looking smokin' hot. Plus it gives you tools to create your own DIY spa, right out of your kitchen! Part 4 explores the nutrients and foods that contribute to our immune and digestive health, and how food pertains to such ailments as bone degeneration, inflammation, and heart problems. And it even contains tips for combating psycho-chick PMS moments and mentalpause! Finally, in Part 5 I give you plenty of delish drink, appetizer, soup, salad, entrée, and dessert recipes to put everything you've learned into practice so you don't have to think so much.

Before we bite right into how food affects our minds and bodies, here are some key principles to remember.

1. You don't have to give up your favorite foods.

You know that ooey-gooey lasagna smothered in four types of cheese and baked to perfection in a chunky tomato sauce? Maybe not the best choice you could make. But that doesn't mean you have to give it up cold turkey forever. Imagine thinking you could never have a piece of lasagna for the rest of your life ... ever. Chances are you'd suffer from some serious separation anxiety, feel miserable, and in the end, fail. Don't go cold turkey on anything. Instead, start not by focusing on what you need to give up, but by adding *more*.

That's right, just add more real, nutrient-dense whole foods to your diet and make small changes to the ingredients you use regularly. Begin by using only half the cheese, replacing the white refined noodles with brown rice noodles or even thinly sliced strips of eggplant or summer squash, and throwing some spinach or sunflower sprouts into the mix. Or just have a small piece of the real thing—and make the other half of your meal a peppery arugula salad (topped with candied walnuts, freshly julienned pear, and crispy sunflower sprouts, sprinkled with creamy hemp seeds and a citrus olive oil drizzle). Doable? I think so. It's about making those small changes. If you're at a fast-food joint, nix the fries in your combo for a side salad. Try sprouted-grain bread instead of whole wheat. Substitute kelp noodles for refined noodles in an Asian stir fry. Trade in chocolate-covered peanuts for cocoa-kissed Savi Seeds. Top your meals with some sunflower sprouts.

Once you start adding more goodness to your diet, you'll start feeling fabulous. Your energy will improve, your complexion will get clearer, and your eyes will be brighter. As for the not-so-good stuff? You'll find that you don't really want it anymore, and it'll naturally fall off your radar, like that multicolored jersey dress that was so last season. And if you really want it—go ahead! Just be conscious of how you feel, and trust me, in time you'll be craving more of that arugula salad instead.

2. Nourish your spirit.

Sometimes it doesn't matter how well you eat. If you're in a bad head space or are overly stressed, you won't absorb nutrients, vitamins in your body will be depleted, and antioxidants just won't be able to keep up.

I spent nearly 10 years in the investment world before delving wholeheartedly into my passion for nutrition. At the time, I thought I was the healthiest person around. I was a strict raw-food vegan, worked out like a crazy chick, and thought I was at the top of my game. Until I went down to the Hippocrates Health Institute in West Palm Beach and had a blood cell analysis done, that is. The results nearly killed me. Or, more accurately, I nearly killed me. "*What?*" I remember gasping. My antioxidant levels were at a mere 27 percent; I thought they'd be at almost 100 percent! At first I didn't get it—I thought I was doing everything right. That's when it hit me: I wasn't being true to myself. I was in a job that didn't fulfill my purpose and I wasn't living in alignment with my own core values. My body was stressed. Although I didn't think I was stressed, internally my body and mind were completely depleted. Only when I let go of everything that didn't truly matter to me did my health pick up.

In order to achieve full health, we need to let go of things that have no meaning for us or that don't serve our life purpose. Once we do that, we free up space in our own energy field, allowing that space to be suffused with fulfillment, purpose, ultimate happiness, and health! And all the goodness we consume from the food we eat will nourish us completely. If you're not there yet, don't worry—what you eat, as you'll see in this book, may just help you get there. When you eat clean, it quiets your stomach. When you have a quiet stomach, you have a quiet mind, and when you have a quiet mind, you can listen to your heart—and your heart speaks the truth.

3. Practice mindful eating.

I know, I know, we're all busy. Eating on the go—whether it's in your car, at your desk, or while running to the gym—is pretty much the norm. We all do it. But keep in mind that when you eat in such a hurried (and harried) manner, you're not in an optimal state to digest food and assimilate nutrients. As powerful as your body is, even superwoman can run into issues. Ask yourself why you're eating. Are you truly hungry, or just bored, stressed, or low on energy? You need to make sure you're eating the right foods to get you going, and the right foods for how you feel. If you're tired, eat energy-boosting foods. If you're depressed, eat mood-boosting happy foods. If you're bored … then get your ass moving and hit the gym or go for a run!

Food is energy: it nourishes our cells and our souls. Practice conscious eating. Know where your food is coming from and who's preparing it. "Comfort" food doesn't have to be something that's high in calories and fat—it can be something that's made with love. So go ahead, enjoy a pint of strawberries and feel your face tingle!

4. Reach for real food.

If it came out of a box, bag or wrapper, chances are you're not giving yourself the absolute best nutrients your body deserves. Whenever possible, reach for real, fresh whole foods. Choosing mostly whole foods—ideally plant-based and unrefined—means that you are fueling your body with nutrient-rich, age-defying, disease-busting goodness. Shop the outside aisles of the grocery store or, better yet, hit the farmer's market. Choose whole foods in a wide range of colors, flavors and textures to add variety and balance to your life.

And remember, this doesn't mean you need to spend hours in the kitchen. Whole-food eating can be as simple as grabbing an apple for a snack rather than that sugar-laden granola bar. Plus, some great companies out there are making strides in convenient natural health foods. Have you tried the Vega One chocolate almond bar? Um, YUM. Check out the Resources section on page 337 for details on my faves.

Emotional Eating

The foods I talk about in this book are functional foods that contain key nutrients required to balance any nutritional deficiency that's making you feel a certain way, whether you're stressed, depressed, or just feel like you're dragging your butt. Emotional eating is something totally different. Many of us are emotional eaters. We tend to reach for comfort food in the hope that it'll fill an emotional void—which doesn't really work.

Cookie-Dough Ice Cream

So you got bad news, are in a deep funk, and feel like the only thing in the world that could bring you the smallest shred of joy right now is the tub of Ben & Jerry's sitting in your freezer. Or, if it's not in your freezer, you'll go to any length to find it at whatever sad little 24-hour food market is open at 2 A.M. Finally, sitting in your pajama bottoms and worn-out college sweatshirt, you plunge your oversized spoon into the tub, bring the sugary frozen cream to your lips, and—bam! The dark clouds part, the sun shines through, and you can hear the birds singing again. Or maybe that's just severe brain freeze. Either way, it's working.

Is there *really* something in that tub of cookie-dough ice cream that can get you out of your funk?

If you're the type who can't get food in your face fast enough when feeling blue, emotional, heartbroken, overwhelmed, stressed, or anxious (even when it's good stress/anxiety), then you, my friend, are an emotional eater. You might even be the type who, when working on a project, feels that your brain simply cannot function unless you're munching on something, *anything*, regardless of the huge meal you just ate. And sometimes you feel like you can't control it. You know you're not hungry (you're probably even full), and you try to talk yourself out of what you're about to do as you journey toward the fridge, but this supernatural force keeps driving you onward and takes over as you begin to scavenge for something to satiate that hunger for ... wait a minute. What are you hungry for? I'd bet that 99.9 percent of the time it's not cookie-dough ice cream, or that jar of almond butter, or whatever your "comfort food" is. It's something deeper. It's something we try to bury with food.

The Skinny on Comfort Food

Let's for a moment think of ourselves as energetic beings, with our energy divided into these two parts:

1. Physical energy Our bodies, including our digestive system, organs, hair—everything we can touch or feel.
2. Nonphysical energy. Our mental/emotional/spiritual selves, our mind, our thoughts—the things we can't touch.

For illustration purposes, let's say that 100 percent of our energy is always divided between the physical and nonphysical, whether the ratio is 90/10, 60/40, 50/50, or whatever. When we eat a big, rich meal, a huge amount of energy is allocated to our physical being. Think of all the work your body has to go through internally to digest that food, break things down, and process its nutrients. And think about what happens to your energy levels—you might feel exhausted. That's because your body is running a full-on factory inside. So let's say this takes up 80 percent of your entire energy bank. That means that only 20 percent is left to feel.

Now let's flip things around. Imagine you're doing a juice cleanse or a fast. Your body isn't working so hard internally now, is it? Your digestive system doesn't require all that energy, so your ratio shifts to something like 50 percent physical, 50 percent emotional/mental, or maybe even 40/60. What happens here? We start to FEEL! I know, right? Crazy. Emotions, stresses we don't want to deal with, feelings we don't know *how* to deal with, and even great things like dreams, aspirations, our true passions and desires—they all come bubbling up into our consciousness. But even when it's good, it can scare the heck out of us! So what do we do? We eat to bury those feelings and shift our energy back to a ratio where we feel most comfortable, narrowing the energetic space of emotion and widening the energetic space of processing food.

This is why when people do cleanses and fasts, a lot of emotional stuff that's been buried away begins to surface. It becomes not just a cleanse of the body, but a cleanse of the mind and emotions too.

I went through this before I left my investment career. A few years before I made the switch, I was on a raw-food diet. Toward the end it got fairly intense, and I don't mean cashew-cream and avocado-pudding intense. I mean that pretty much all I ate those last few months were organic greens, veggies, sprouts, algaes, and sea veggies. I wouldn't eat a nut, seed, or grain unless it was sprouted, and green-juice cleanses were a part of my life at least one full day a week (sometimes all week). Still, it was a cleanse with a silver lining: it gave me a serious case of emotional disgorge. It initiated the most provoking, challenging, uncomfortable, life-changing time I'd ever experienced. And because I was barely eating, I had no freakin' clue what to do, except to just deal. So I became an emotional spitfire. I was forced to let go of what was "secure" and familiar but unfulfilling (including my career and relationships) and venture into the land of the unknown. It was simultaneously terrifying and exhilarating. When people asked me what I was going to do, my response was "I don't know, but I know it'll be *wonderful!*"

So for me, as for many of you, food is a tool for dealing with emotions and feelings. You can use it against yourself by burying your emotions, or you can use it positively by eating only when you're hungry and in a way that nourishes your body, mind, and entire being. Those days of crazy cleansing (while maybe not the best thing for my body at the time) helped me get to where I am today. They forced me to listen to my heart and not to bury things. It wasn't easy. What I had to learn (and what I'm still learning) is how to find that calm. How to shift energy into action. How to listen without fear. How to turn the unknown into excitement and desire.

What *Really* Fulfills

I'm not telling you to do a crazy cleanse, nor am I telling you to quit your job or leave your spouse. All I'm saying is that when you're stressed, anxious, sad, or feeling like a train wreck, put down the cookie-dough ice cream and reach for something that will truly fulfill you.

Here are some of my favorite things to fill up on:

1. Love. Fill up that space with an abundance of love. Friendships, family, lovers, crushes—people who make you happy. People who fill you up with joy when you're around them. Fill up on hugs and kisses and laughter. Fill up on THEM.

2. Passion. Irene Cara totally had it right in "Flashdance" when she sang "Take your passion, and make it happen." As a kid, that was my anthem. 'Kay, maybe it still is (but only when I run). Do the things you love to do, and do them often. It doesn't have to be a huge change in your life. (Although it could be.) All you have to do is start small by focusing on the things you're good at, the things that come easily and naturally to you. Fill up on your own passions. What a feeling!

3. Words. When things surface—an emotion, a memory, a desire—write them down! It gets them out of your head and into the universe. Record your dreams, thoughts, inspirations, and gratitudes. You'll be amazed at how powerful words can be. A great teacher once taught me that journaling is the window to your soul and to the manifestation of your dreams. She was right. Dream big.

4. Gratitude. It takes just a few minutes to acknowledge and appreciate what you have and what's around you. Doing so can immediately shift your perspective and put you into a happy place. In fact, research suggests that expressing gratitude can boost happiness by 25 percent![1] What are you grateful for?

This, of course, is just part of the equation for feeling and looking your best, but it's an important part. You have to get a handle on your relationship with food before you can really harness its power to change the way you look, live, and feel. Once you do that, though, a door opens, and suddenly you're driving your own destiny. That's where the rest of this book comes into play. I hope you enjoy it and use it well!

With gratitude,
Peggy

PART 1
The Food–Mood Connection

Explore the foodie connection to higher energy,
less stress, deeper sleep, better sex, a better mood,
increased happiness, and a sharper mind!

Our lives are permeated by choice. It feels as though every minute there's a decision to be made: *Do I stay in bed for an extra five minutes or get up right away? Do I go to the gym or take another rest day? Should I make my lunch or buy it?* And what you choose to eat each day is probably among the most important decisions you make. What you eat directly impacts your thoughts, your actions, your mood, and your psyche. What you eat is what you think, and what you think is what you become.

Let's look at how exactly food can affect your mind and mood.

How Our Mind Works

What we eat can affect more than just our waistline; it directly affects our brain. The brain is made up of about 100 billion neurons—nerve cells that transmit information by electrical or chemical signaling. The chemical messengers that deliver communication from one neuron to another are called neurotransmitters. The space between neurons is called a synapse, which is where neurotransmitters swim in order to send and receive information.

Here's the kicker: these neurotransmitters are partly responsible for our happiness, sadness, stress response, anger, energy, sex drive, and overall mood and feeling. And they're made up of amino acids we get *through our food*. As well, certain vitamins, minerals, and nutrients are essential in the conversion of amino acids to neurotransmitters. Therefore, different foods have the ability to affect mood by altering the levels of neurotransmitters in the brain. Certain foods can either increase or suppress the messenger activity happening between the brain's billions of neurons.

Each neurotransmitter has its own specific receptor cell that it fits into and unlocks, kind of like a key, for communication to occur. In order for the message to get across, the neurotransmitter must bind onto a receptor cell, and one that fits.

How does this work? Think of the neurotransmitter as a plug, and the receptor cells as an electrical outlet. Now, imagine you're at the gym: you've just finished your workout, you've showered, and now you need to blow-dry your hair. You go to plug in your blow dryer, and to your luck, you have tons of options. You can plug it in by the big mirror, small mirror, full-length mirror, close to your friends, away from your friends—anywhere you want because there are outlets everywhere. So you're happy, and you leave the gym with a fabulous blowout. But what if there were no electrical outlets, or the only ones left were two-prong outlets and your blow dryer has a three-prong plug? You'd need to pack away that blow dryer and walk out with your mop-head wet hair wrapped under a hoodie, not feeling so glam.

The same thing can happen to neurotransmitters. Once they're released, if they don't bind onto a receptor cell or if they don't fit, communication is lost.

Here are examples of the kinds of neurotransmitters and how they affect your mood:

Amino Acid	Neurotransmitter	Function
Tyrosine	Dopamine	Increases motivation, drive, sense of reward, and pleasure.
Tryptophan	Serotonin	Makes you happy! Boosts mood and fights depression.
Glutamine	Melatonin	Helps you relax and sleep.
Glutamine	GABA	Calms and relaxes without stimulating.
Choline	Acetylcholine	Improves mental clarity and alertness.

The brain isn't the only organ that has neurotransmitter receptors. Immune cells, blood cells, and tissues also have receptors, and there's a lot of chitchat going on between the brain, immune system, endocrine system, and nervous system.

In short, everything is connected—and everything is affected by what you eat!

1. Get Energized

It's the crack of dawn, and the piercing sound of your alarm clock causes more pain than running around town in five-inch stilettos that are half a size too small. "Just five more minutes!" Or at least that's what you tell yourself as you hit snooze repeatedly for the next hour and a half. Then, when finally realizing you're oh-so-late, you fly out of bed, down two cups of coffee, and attempt to regain some consciousness and sensibility as you try to put yourself together and bolt out the door. Oops, didn't make the gym *again* this morning, but it's okay, you'll get there after work. Yep, that's what you'll do. After all, you're feeling pretty pumped at the moment from all the adrenaline kicking through your body as you race to get to your morning meeting on time.

But that high was extremely short-lived, and now you need to physically hold your eyelids open with the back of your pen as you sit through never-ending dialogue about … oh, it doesn't matter, you're not paying attention anyway. So you pretend to take notes to force yourself from literally falling asleep in your seat. But it's not working. Your head is getting heavy, you have no clue what anyone is talking about, and you just pray you won't start snoring or you're totally screwed. Thank goodness for lunch to get you chipper again. And because you're going to the gym after work, you figure you can afford a few extra carbs. And maybe another coffee, just because, well, it's been *that* kind of day.

Now it's 3 P.M. and you're counting down the minutes until you can reunite with your pillow. Your soft, comfy, luxurious, bamboo-threaded pillow. Yep, that's where you're headed straight after work. What? The gym? Dang. Not happening. You feel guilty for all of 30 seconds as you contemplate the idea, but then you convince yourself that you're just too darn tired. So you figure you'll just skip dinner in lieu of working out, get a good night's sleep, and will for sure get up early the next morning and hit the gym when you're more energized.

And the vicious cycle continues. The only exercise you get is lugging that gym bag around with you every day with the intention of doing some kind of physical activity. But you just don't ... have ... the energy. Sound familiar?

Food, literally, is your fuel. It's what drives you, motivates you, and gives you that extra pep in your step. But as they say, if you put crapola in you get crapola out. The quality of your energy, vibrancy, and *life* is a direct reflection of what you put in your chomper and assimilate. Those refined carbs, sugar fixes, and caffeine-induced energy drinks only set you up to fail. They might jack you up temporarily, but will have you crashing before you even start whatever it was you needed the energy to do. They don't fix the core problem. And about that skipping meals business ... also fail.

Key Nutrients for Boosting Energy

Now, you might already be eating well and working out, but you may still find that you're not on your A-game. Here are some key nutrients that will have you putting the Energizer Bunny up for some stiff competition.

Tyrosine

Tyrosine is a non-essential amino acid, meaning your body produces it on its own (via phenylalanine, another amino acid). However, it can also be obtained directly through diet. The reason this amino acid is so fab is that it's a precursor to the neurotransmitter dopamine, which is responsible for motivation and drive. It's what gives us that "get up and go" feeling. You know, the one we're typically lacking when we'd rather stay in bed all day? (Unless of course you're staying in bed for other reasons related to dopamine—see page 47, wink, wink.) Studies show that supplementing with tyrosine improves mental and physical endurance, especially during times of stress.

Iron

Iron deficiency is a significant cause of fatigue, low energy, and anemia, especially in premenopausal women. Without enough iron, your body can't produce enough hemoglobin, which is a type of protein in red blood cells that enables them to carry oxygen throughout your body, giving it energy. The more oxygen getting to your cells, the more energetic and vibrant you'll be!

HEME IRON (ANIMAL PRODUCTS)

Heme iron, derived from hemoglobin, is the most absorbable form of iron. It comes from such animal sources as clams, red meat, pork, chicken, and fish.

NON-HEME IRON (PLANT-BASED FOODS, DAIRY, AND EGGS)

The majority of dietary iron comes from non-heme sources. Unfortunately, it's not absorbed as well as heme iron is. But no need to fret—pairing up these foods with vitamin C helps things along. For example, adding lemon juice (a source of vitamin C) to chickpeas (a source of iron) or eating hummus with raw red peppers (an excellent source of vitamin C) will increase the absorption of iron.

Additional plant-based sources of iron:

- Blackstrap molasses
- Spinach
- Raisins
- Prunes
- Sea veggies (kelp, dulse, nori)
- Chlorella

Try the following combos to maximize iron absorption:

Iron	with	Vitamin C
Hummus		Red peppers
Lentils		Parsley and lemon
Quinoa		Black currants
Oatmeal		Strawberries
Spinach		Garlic

Calcium, tannins (found in wine and tea), and phytates (found in legumes and whole grains) decrease iron absorption. But legumes and grains are also rich in iron, and so to reduce the amount of phytic acids that try to burst the iron bubble, soak and sprout these grains and legumes before cooking. Iron: 1, Phytates: 0.

TIP
Try to consume calcium and iron at different times of the day to ensure maximum absorption of each.

B Vitamins

B vitamins, dubbed the "energy" vitamins, are essential for mental and physical health and vitality—they're a pick-me-up for both mind and body! They help convert carbs, proteins, and fats into usable energy. While all B vitamins are essential and work together synergistically, B12 is probably the most important when it comes to boosting energy levels. B12, also known as cobalamine, is required for the production of red blood cells. It helps your body use iron, supports the immune system, and is used in the treatment and prevention of many diseases and mental health disorders. Unfortunately, getting enough B12 is one area where most people fall short.

Many North Americans are B12-deficient. Although vitamin B12 is difficult to obtain from plant-based sources, that doesn't let omnivores get off scot-free! It all depends on the state of your intestinal health, your stomach's ability to produce what's known as "intrinsic factor," and reabsorption. B12 is a bacteria-synthesizing vitamin and is made solely out of microorganisms. Your body actually manufactures B12 through its own good bacteria, and much of it can be stored in the liver. As a result, most B12 deficiencies are due to the body's inability to perform in these key areas:

- The stomach needs to produce enough intrinsic factor, which is a protein released by the stomach lining that then latches onto B12 to help your body to absorb it.
- The stomach must produce enough hydrochloric acid (HCl) to pull out the B12 from your food (see Chapter 15 for more info on HCl), so if you have digestive issues this may be a problem.

•B12 is excreted from the bile and reabsorbed. A deficiency could result from lack of reabsorption.

Although algae appear to be rich in vitamin B12, it's in a fake analog form and is not a reliable source of B12. Because B12 analogs are structurally similar to vitamin B12, they can compete for absorption and don't satisfy dietary needs.

Top Energy-Boosting Foods

What you eat can help you wake up feeling all bright-eyed and bushy-tailed, even before your alarm goes off! Imagine that.

Some energy-dense foods:

- Quinoa
- Beans and legumes
- Nuts and seeds
- Apples
- Berries
- Green tea
- Yerba maté
- Maca
- Almonds
- Hemp seeds
- Kombucha
- Kale
- Broccoli
- Bananas

Chlorella

Chlorella is a green, single-celled, freshwater-grown algae, and is one of the highest sources of chlorophyll in the world. It also boasts an amazing concentration of protein, vitamins, minerals, and those precious trace minerals for optimal health. Its rich chlorophyll content increases the number of red blood cells in your body, which help deliver oxygen to your cells. The more oxygen to your cells, the more nutrients will be absorbed, and the more energy you'll have. Chlorophyll also boosts immune function, reduces inflammation, and promotes alkalinity. And the more alkaline your body is, the healthier and more vibrant you'll look and feel.

DID YOU KNOW?

Chlorella contains up to 5 times more chlorophyll than wheat grass, up to 10 times more than spirulina, up to 12 times more than barley, and up to 50 times more than alfalfa (depending on species and grade).

An amazing chlorella phenomenon is the Chlorella Growth Factor (CGF), which means that this little microscopic alga spreads faster than a run in your tights. Seriously. It literally quadruples itself every 20 to 24 hours, making it the fastest-growing plant in the world! And now why would you want to ingest that? This jacked-up superfood increases tissue building and repair (helping you look and feel fab), multiplies the "good" active bacterial culture in your intestines (improving digestion and assimilation of nutrients and energy), and supercharges white blood cell activity. All of this boosts your immune system, health, and vitality. Feeling pumped already? Yep. Thought so.

But wait. There's more.

Chlorella is one of the highest food sources of RNA, a nucleic acid similar to DNA and an essential component of all life forms. It regulates gene expression, synthesizes proteins, and helps DNA copy and express genetic material. Dr. Benjamin S. Frank, who pioneered the research behind RNA therapy, concluded that supplementing with foods rich in RNA increases energy and endurance, improves oxygen utilization, boosts the immune system, detoxifies and repairs cell damage, and counteracts the effects of aging.[2] Frank suggested that nucleic acids significantly increase cellular energy and rejuvenation. The greatest benefits are seen with those who are ill, have compromised immune systems, or have undergone chemotherapy.

> ## TIP
> Chlorella's rich chlorophyll content not only boosts energy, but also gives you fresher breath than a Tic Tac!

The CGF is made up of these nucleic acids (RNA/DNA) in addition to proteins, peptides, polysaccharides, beta glucans, sulfur, and manganese, which are found in the nucleus of the cell. This forms the core of chlorella's medicinal properties. Therefore, the higher the CGF, the better it is.

But we can't stop there! Chlorella is also rich in protein. At 60 percent, chlorella has 12 times more digestible protein than beef. This helps balance blood-sugar levels and ward off hunger and carb/sugar cravings. Protein also provides sustainable energy so that you don't experience those crazy spikes and dips that have you raiding the vending machine mid-afternoon.

See what I mean? Chlorella rocks. It's rich in energy-boosting and stress-busting B vitamins, especially B1, B2, and B6, in addition to antioxidant-rich vitamins A, C, and E. Chlorella has strong detoxification properties and helps remove heavy metals, pesticides, and other toxins from the body—including alcohol! Plus, the high protein content will balance out your blood-sugar levels, if you just so happened to indulge.

DID YOU KNOW?

Chlorella makes a great hangover remedy—taking it before and after a night of drinking helps cleanse alcohol from your liver.

HOW TO USE

To really boost energy, swap out your morning java for chlorella. It will have you feeling so energized you'll be fist-pumping all the way to work. 'Kay, maybe not exactly, but over time, you'll notice a *huge* difference in energy levels. For optimal health, two to three grams per day is suggested. It can be taken any time of the day with or without food; however, it's best to take it in the morning, so that it can boost your energy levels all day long. Make sure to get chlorella that's had the cell wall broken or cracked to ensure absorption and digestibility. Because of its detox properties, you may initially experience such symptoms as nausea, acne, or flu-like feelings if your system is heavily polluted. You can get it in tablets (the easiest, most convenient, and palatable form), or you can get it in powder form and add it to smoothies or juices.

Sunflower Sprouts

Sunflower sprouts are "micro-greens" sprouted from the sunflower seed and harvested in the beginning stages of their growth. This is when the plants are the most nutrient-dense, bio-available, and enzyme-rich. These crisp, fresh-tasting sprouts are rich in protein, vitamins (including B and D), and phytonutrients, which help protect against disease.

When sprouting, the nutritional profile of sunflower sprouts can increase anywhere from 100 to 600 percent, making sprouts superior to any other leafy (macro) green. They're higher in chlorophyll than any macro green, increasing the number of red blood cells that deliver oxygen to your cells. They also have amazing detoxification properties. These sprouts are extremely alkalizing, with several healing properties. Benefits include blood purification, cancer prevention, improved circulation, and strengthened immune system. Eat these raw and as close to harvest as possible for maximum nutritional benefit!

Sunflower sprouts are one of the most enzyme-rich foods around. Enzymes are the catalysts of all life: they spark the electrical conduit for every chemical reaction that occurs in our body. They help repair skin, recover from illnesses, heal wounds, and digest food. We're actually born with a full bank of enzymes, but over time, stresses from our environment, nutritionally void food, and negative thoughts deplete their numbers, and the aging process and cellular degradation occur. This is why eating foods rich in enzymes is so important—they add to our "bank." And raw, plant-based foods are the only natural source.

TIP
Soak all seeds, grains, and legumes 8 to 12 hours before consuming or cooking. This process activates enzymes and pre-digests macronutrients (carbs, proteins, and fats), allowing your body to more easily assimilate the nutrients.

HOW TO USE
Do not cook these! It's important to eat them raw, as cooking will destroy the precious nutrients and enzymes that make these sprouts so powerful. Sunflower sprouts make a great base or addition to a salad. They can be added to sandwiches and wraps, sprinkled on soups, or rolled into sushi rolls. Juicing sunflower sprouts provides great detoxification as well as blood- and liver-cleansing benefits. Juice or blend with cucumber, apple, lemon, and ginger for a refreshing and cleansing cocktail.

Sea Veggies

Sea veggies are just that—veggies grown in the sea. Varieties include arame, nori, kelp, wakame, and dulse. Just like land-grown veggies, sea veggies are über-high in vitamins, minerals, and phytonutrients. They're also laced with beneficial trace minerals difficult to get from any other food source. Your body needs minerals to create energy-producing reactions in your cells, and sea veggies are loaded with them! As well, they're among the highest plant-based sources of iron, and because they're rich in vitamin C, the iron's bioavailability is increased.

Sea veggies are also rich in the amino acid tyrosine, a precursor to dopamine production. Dopamine is the neurotransmitter that stimulates drive, lighting the fire under your butt to get moving when you're feeling lazy. It's known to rev up the brain, which can help you feel more alert and focused. Who couldn't benefit from that?

In addition, sea veggies have exceptionally high iodine content. Iodine is essential for thyroid function. Your thyroid must absorb sufficient amounts of iodine from your blood in order to manufacture and distribute hormones throughout your body. If the thyroid is sluggish and not functioning optimally, your metabolism slows and fatigue and lethargy kick in—which means you feel lazy, and maybe even fat. By incorporating sea veggies into your diet, especially kelp, which has the highest iodine content, you can ensure you'll feel fab.

Here's how sea veggies rank in the hierarchy of greens, based on nutrient density and chlorophyll levels.

Good	Better	Best	Bestest!
MACRO GREENS	MICRO GREENS	SEA VEGGIES	SEA ALGAES
Dark leafy greens: • Kale • Spinach • Collards • Mustard greens	Sprouts: • Sunflower sprouts • Pea sprouts • Buckwheat sprouts • Broccoli sprouts • Sprouted legumes	• Kelp • Dulse • Nori • Wakame • Arame • Hijiki	• Chlorella • Spirulina • AFA

HOW TO USE

Sea veggies typically come dried and can be rehydrated in water for about five minutes. Arame and wakame are great additions to salads or soups, or sprinkled over steamed veggies. They also make a great salad on their own, drizzled with some sesame oil. As well, they add a nice saltiness to dishes. Nori, which is a great snack in itself, is typically used to roll up veggies or maki rolls. Kelp and dulse also come in granules, and although they look like pepper, they taste like salt. So they make a great salt substitute—just sprinkle the granules on top of your food for a great mineral boost. My favorite way to eat dulse is in a DLT—a dulse, lettuce, and tomato sandwich—with a little avocado for good measure.

Clams

Here's another nutrient-rich sea creature. Although not a plant, clams boast the highest concentration of heme iron, which is the most bio-available form of iron. Iron deficiency is a significant cause of fatigue, low energy, and anemia, especially in women. Without enough iron, your body can't produce enough hemoglobin, which means your red blood cells can't carry enough oxygen to your body. And oxygen equals energy! At roughly 23 milligrams of iron per three-ounce serving, clams are one of the highest food sources of this energy-boosting nutrient.

Clams are also an excellent source of vitamin B12: they can give you over seven times the recommended daily amount. B12 is essential to boosting energy levels and mental concentration, and aids in the absorption of iron and the production of red blood cells. Clams' iron-B12 combo is a surefire way to boost energy.

Bonus! Clams are also rich in protein, helping balance blood-sugar levels and provide sustainable energy to last throughout the day.

HOW TO USE
Purchase live, fresh clams that are "clammed" tightly shut. Once they've been cooked, discard the clams that don't open, as they were dead prior to cooking. You can add them to your favorite pasta dish, or they taste delish on their own in a tomato or herbed white wine sauce.

Water

The most common cause of fatigue is dehydration. If there isn't enough fluid in your body, blood volume can drop. As a result, your body (and heart) must work harder to supply your cells with oxygen and nutrients. Poor hydration results in mental fogginess, poor short-term memory, dizziness, and fatigue.

TIP
How much water should you drink every day? A good rule of thumb is to drink half your body weight in ounces. So if you weigh 130 pounds, you need 65 ounces of water a day—just over eight cups. If you want more energy in your day, drink up!

Coconut

Coconut really is one of the most perfect foods. The fleshy meat is loaded with protein, fiber, and figure-friendly, energy-boosting fats, while the water inside is loaded with energy-boosting, hydrating electrolytes. In other words, every single part of the coconut provides energy benefits. Here's the rundown:

COCONUT MEAT	This is the flesh of the coconut. It's high in protein, fiber, and fat, which are your blood sugar's (and waistline's) BFFs. They help keep you fuller longer and your blood sugar in check, thereby keeping energy levels stable and going strong. Young coconuts contain a soft, gel-like meat, whereas the meat of mature coconuts is hard and fibrous. Health benefits tend to be richer in the young coconut.
COCONUT OIL	Coconut oil and coconut butter are actually the same thing. Many refer to the oil as butter, since it remains solid at room temperature, but at the slightest heat it will turn into its liquid form. Although the majority of the oil found in the coconut is a saturated fat, it's a medium-chain fatty acid, which makes it easily absorbed by the small intestine. Because it doesn't require the full digestive process, it converts to fuel faster than any other fat, making it an amazing energy source. Try a tablespoon of it before your workouts and you'll be amazed at the energy and endurance it provides. Plus it helps to improve the absorption of omega-3 fatty acids, which are essential for optimal health and well-being. Coconut oil is a stable fat and has a high smoking point, making it great for cooking. Use coconut oil when sautéing, roasting, or frying for a healthier alternative to other oils. It's also great added to smoothies (improving flavor and silkiness) as well as to many desserts. Just replace the oil or butter with coconut oil. And don't worry about weight gain. Several studies have linked the intake of coconut oil to weight loss![3]
COCONUT CREAM/ COCONUT MANNA	Sometimes you might find coconut cream (also called coconut manna). It's like a thick, fibrous version of coconut oil, but unlike the oil it doesn't dissolve into a clearish liquid. The cream is typically made from coconut oil blended with coconut meat, or derived from tougher, more fibrous mature coconuts. This makes it a thicker spread, and so it's great for baking or smothered on sprouted-grain toast in the morning. It's loaded with energy-boosting protein, fiber, and fat!
COCONUT WATER	Coconut water comes from the inside of a young coconut. It takes about nine months to fill a young coconut with water, and it's purified through its fibers. Coconut water is nature's best sports energy drink. It's an exceptional source of electrolytes, similar to our own blood plasma, which makes for immediate hydration and nutrient absorption. It's great to keep you energized and hydrated during any workout, run, soccer game, or any time of the day! If you're feeling sluggish, sipping on coconut water might just be the trick to get you from empty to energized. (Plus, it makes an amazing hangover remedy.)

COCONUT KEIFER	Coconut keifer is a great probiotic and digestive tonic. It's basically coconut water with a probiotic culture added to it. Proper digestion and assimilation of nutrients is required for optimal energy levels. If food doesn't get digested or absorbed properly, it can totally bog you down. It also helps with getting rid of belly bloat!
COCONUT MILK	Coconut milk is made by blending coconut meat with coconut water. With its rich, creamy consistency, the milk makes a great dairy alternative. Choose the unsweetened variety, as it's lower in calories and sugar. The sweetened variety can be used as a treat or in baked goods.
COCONUT YOGURT	This is coconut milk with probiotic culture added to it—a great alternative for those who want the benefits of a probiotic yogurt but are avoiding dairy or soy.
COCONUT SUGAR	Coconut sugar is a natural sugar derived directly from the sap of the coconut tree's flower blossoms, so it doesn't come from the coconut itself. It's low on the glycemic index—much lower than cane sugar (35 GI vs. 68 GI)—so it will keep blood-sugar levels (and energy levels) much more stable. It's rich in minerals (magnesium, potassium, and zinc) and vitamins B and C. And it tastes DELICIOUS! Kind of like the top of a crème brûlée: yum.
COCONUT FLOUR	Coconut flour is dried coconut meat, defatted and finely ground into a powder. It's super high in fiber, containing 58 percent dietary fiber. Fiber is essential for weight loss, as it promotes a feeling of fullness. Coconut flour is also gluten-free/wheat-free, so you won't get bloated. The remainder consists of coconut oil (which makes up about 15 percent), water, protein, and carbs. It also contains the lowest digestible carb count of any other flour. And it can replace regular flour in baked goods—although, since it breaks down easily when cooking, it's best to add a binding agent like ground chia or eggs.

2. Stress Case

Whether you're about to give a huge presentation, are worried about finances, have just sprained an ankle, have had too many drinks, feel overwhelmed with life, have lost your job, have started a new job, are trying to balance a career, children, and a spouse, or are just pulling your hair out trying to squeeze into a pair of jeans that you *swear* fit you just last week, you've met with stress.

Physiological Responses to Stress

All types of stress—even if its cause is something we made up in our heads—generate a physiological response. At the onset of stress, your brain triggers your adrenal glands, which sit on top of your kidneys, causing them to release the stress hormones adrenaline and cortisol. Adrenaline speeds up heart rate, increases blood pressure, and boosts energy. Cortisol, which is the primary stress hormone, shifts energy away from the digestive and immune systems to prepare for an "alarmed" state, increasing blood-sugar levels and the brain's uptake of glucose.

Some stress is great. If you're about to run a race, those stress hormones pumping through you might just give you the edge to run that much faster. It's the "fight or flight" response that revs up your body and makes it work hard. But the key here is that it's finite. The race eventually ends and, in the process, you burn off all the elevated sugar and fat that were released as a response to stress through physical exertion. Your blood pressure drops, your heart rate slows, and your body returns to its normal state.

The problem occurs when stress is chronic and ongoing, when one stress follows another. Day-to-day demands, worry, tension, and poor lifestyle habits cause your adrenals to fire constantly, and cortisol levels are released in excess.

Excess Cortisol

Here are some of the chronic effects of excess cortisol:

- Leads to weight gain (especially belly fat!), obesity, and inability to burn fat
- Interferes with the neurotransmitter serotonin, which can lead to clinical depression, anxiety disorders, and insomnia
- Can cause mental clutter, poor concentration, and impaired memory function
- Breaks down collagen and speeds up the aging process
- Increases blood pressure, blood clotting, and cholesterol levels
- Suppresses the immune system and the function of pathogen-fighting T-cells
- Increases the risk of heart attack, stroke, and kidney disease
- Promotes insulin resistance, which leads to additional belly fat
- Increases levels of estrogen, which also leads to weight gain and mood swings
- Increases cravings

Basically, in time, it'll make you fat. And the end result: more stress.

Food Cravings

Why do we crave certain foods when we're stressed? Take a look at what our cravings are really telling us:

FATS	Bad saturated and trans fats can numb the receptors in the brain that regulate emotional responses.
CARBS AND SUGARS	Carbohydrates help release serotonin, a neurotransmitter in our brain that makes us feel happy and relaxed. But refined carbs and sugars cause blood-sugar imbalances and lead to greater feelings of stress, anxiety, and depression.
SALT	Stress depletes our body of precious minerals and throws off our sodium/potassium balance. Cortisol is also a natural diuretic, which can lead to dehydration, which can lead to salt cravings.

(Continued)

CHOCOLATE	Chocolate releases endorphins, which alleviate pain, and—if it's raw or extremely dark chocolate—may contain magnesium, which helps alleviate tension.

What you eat absolutely makes a difference to how your body deals with stress. The problem is that when we're stressed and reach for the *wrong* types of food—foods that are nutritionally void and high in refined carbs, sugar, fats, or caffeine—our stress is exacerbated. These foods actually *cause* stress. They worsen the symptoms and issues at hand. Caffeine and sugar stimulate the nervous system, increasing agitation and nervousness. High-fat foods are difficult for your body to break down and digest, while foods that are just flat-out nutritionally void cause your body added stress, as they don't supply it with the precious nutrients it needs to function optimally.

Happy Hour

What about alcohol? A few glasses of wine are sure to take the edge off after a crazy day … right? Actually, they can. Alcohol increases the production of GABA, the neurotransmitter responsible for feelings of calm and relaxation. GABA is what squashes nervousness in social situations after a few drinks. It alleviates tension and keeps you from being uptight. Perfect remedy for a first date or dinner with the in-laws, right? Maybe not so much.

The GABA kick via alcohol consumption is relatively short-lived. Once GABA plummets, it'll have you feeling *blah*. So chances are you'll reach for another drink, and the vicious cycle will continue. It then goes on to interrupt your sleep and cause further stress, irritability, and agitation. As for tranquilizers, such as Valium or Ativan, they're highly addictive and can lead to further anxiety in the long run.

Key Stress-Busting Nutrients

For all you stress cases and type-A personalities out there, here are some of the nutrients your body needs to relax naturally.

GABA

GABA is an amino acid and neurotransmitter that helps us chill. It's an "inhibitory" neurotransmitter (vs. its "excitatory" dopamine counterpart). It promotes a feeling of calm and relaxation, and shuts off excess adrenaline. It helps manage stress and improve mental focus—balancing out all those crazy thoughts. The best way to increase GABA production naturally and healthfully is through food. A precursor to GABA production is the amino acid glutamine. Hence, foods rich in glutamic acids (or glutamate) help increase GABA production.

Foods rich in glutamic acids:

- Seaweed (kombu)
- Cabbage
- Soy
- Parsley
- Spinach
- Sesame seeds
- Sunflower seeds
- Cod
- Tomatoes

Adaptogens

Adaptogens are nutrients found in herbs that increase the body's ability to resist and adapt to stress. They can help alleviate anxiety, stress, and trauma by restoring the body's natural balance and homeostasis.

Adaptogen sources:

- Maca
- Ginseng
- Relora
- Holy basil
- Licorice
- Rhodiola
- Ashwagandha
- Schizandra berries

Vitamin B6

B vitamins are stress-busting—especially B6, B12, folic acid, and niacin—and are essential in the production of neurotransmitters. But while B6 is the most important for reducing stress, it's also the first to be depleted in its presence. A lack of B6 could lead to depression due to its inability to produce the feel-good neurotransmitter serotonin. And because B vitamins are water soluble, they don't hang around in your body very long—so it's critical to ingest them throughout the day.

Foods rich in vitamin B6:

- Fatty fish (tuna)
- Red and green peppers
- Cod
- Hazelnuts
- Cashew nuts
- Potatoes
- Spinach
- Bananas
- Turnip greens
- Garlic
- Cauliflower

Vitamin C

Vitamin C is a powerful antioxidant. Not only does it help protect against oxidative stress and free-radical damage caused by physical stress, but it can also help curb the large spikes in cortisol caused by mental stress. In one study, rats that weren't given vitamin C while undergoing stress experienced three times the level of cortisol of those not supplemented with vitamin C.[4]

Foods rich in vitamin C:

- Kakadu plums
- Camu camu
- Guava
- Black currants
- Red peppers
- Parsley
- Kiwis
- Broccoli

Calcium and Magnesium

Deficiencies in these important minerals can aggravate anxiety and tension. (In fact, magnesium is one of the most common mineral deficiencies.) Calcium and magnesium have calming effects on the body and nervous system, helping to relax nerves and muscles, alleviate muscle cramping and headaches, and even help you fall asleep. If supplementing, it's best to take before bed.

Foods rich in calcium and magnesium:

- Kale
- Broccoli
- Sesame seeds/Tahini
- Almonds
- Maca
- Sacha inchi seeds

TIP

Omega-3 fatty acids also help alleviate anxiety and depression.

Foods That Help You Chill
Holy Basil

Next time you're stuck in holy traffic, you might want to reach for some holy basil! Holy basil (also known as tulsi) is an herbal plant that's native to India but now cultivated all over the world. Oh, and by the way, it tastes nothing like the regular basil you're used to, so here's a word of advice—don't put it in pasta dishes! It's been used historically in Ayurvedic medicine to reduce fever, strengthen the immune system, calm nerves, and act as an anti-inflammatory and antioxidant. However, more recent studies have shown that holy basil has the ability to lower cortisol and blood-sugar levels—that is, help our bodies cope with stress!

Holy basil is an adaptogen, meaning it doesn't directly affect your mood, but it does help your body respond to stress, anxiety, trauma, and depression by normalizing neurotransmitter levels in the brain. Research has shown that ursolic acid and the triterpenoic acids, both found in holy basil, effectively improve the body's response to stress and reduce the amount of cortisol released during stress. Ursolic acid also has anti-cancer and anti-tumor properties—can't beat that! Additional compounds demonstrate anti-stress effects by normalizing blood-sugar and cortisol levels and reducing the enlargement of the adrenal glands. And compared with ginseng, another adaptogenic herb, holy basil exhibits greater anti-stress properties, with a higher margin of safety.

Researchers at the Dr. B.C. Roy Institute of Post Graduate Medical Education and Research in India screened 35 subjects with generalized anxiety disorder (GAD) in a clinical investigation. Each subject was given 500 milligrams of holy basil twice a day. After 60 days, it was observed that the severity of GAD, associated stress, and depression was significantly reduced in the subjects.[5]

Holy basil also contains various other therapeutic compounds, such as rosmarinic acid, which has anti-inflammatory properties and can help reduce inflammation of the adrenal glands. Holy basil also has strong antioxidant properties, which helps protect your body from the free-radical damage associated with stress. In addition, it contains oleanolic acids, which have strong anti-tumor and antiviral (including anti-HIV) properties.

HOW TO USE

Holy basil has a spicy, clove-like flavor and is not traditionally used in cooking (except in Thai cooking for hot stir fries and curries). It's mainly used in North America as a supplement—typically as a soft gel containing standardized holy basil leaf extract in an oil base (look for supercritical extract). You can also find it as whole dried-leaf capsules, in a tea form (tulsi tea), or as seed oil.

Raw Chocolate

Who doesn't feel good after eating chocolate? It releases the same feel-good endorphins that suppress pain and stress, and gives the same euphoric feeling you get from having sex or going for a run. But it's the *raw* chocolate (aka cacao) where all the good stuff is stored—so step away from the vending machines! Raw chocolate is rich in antioxidants, minerals, and stress-alleviating compounds, giving you a guilt-free boost.

Cacao contains a compound called phenylethylamine (PEA), which promotes a happy, elated feeling and alleviates stress and depression. They call it the "love molecule," as it raises your pulse and gives you the same feeling you get while falling in love. In addition, pure, raw chocolate is one of the highest sources of magnesium, which is essential in reducing muscle tension, calming the nerves, and promoting relaxation. Chocolate also contains a neurotransmitter known as anandamide that has the ability to alter dopamine levels in the brain, causing a sense of peace and relaxation. And it gets even better—cacao is rich in B vitamins, which help the body cope with stress. So if you're looking to de-stress and relax, a piece of raw chocolate should do the trick!

DID YOU KNOW?

Chocolate is the number-one craved food in the world; an oft-cited survey even suggested that 50 percent of women would rather eat chocolate than have sex!

Stress can have a profound negative impact on your heart, including elevated blood pressure and increased risk of heart attack. But cacao can help counter the negative effects of stress on heart health. A team of researchers at the University of Adelaide in Australia found that for those with high blood pressure, the flavonols found in chocolate reduced blood pressure to a similar degree as 30 minutes of physical activity![6] This could reduce the risk of a cardiovascular event by 20 percent over five years.

Cacao also has an exceptionally high ORAC value, which is the measurement of antioxidant activity. It trumps blueberries and pomegranates in antioxidant levels, making it an amazingly delicious way to prevent against oxidative stress, free-radical damage, and disease.

Passionflower

I know what you're thinking—shouldn't *passion*flower be in the chapter on sex? Despite its name, passionflower is primarily known as a calming herb. It grows in many parts of the world, but is native to North, Central, and South America. Passionflower has been used for years to treat anxiety, stress, insomnia, and nervousness. The second half of its name is also misleading: the actual medicinal benefits are found in the stem and root of the plant, not in the flower itself. It's used as an herbal remedy in a tea form or as a liquid extract or capsule.

Passionflower has mild sedative and tranquilizing effects that can calm nerves and reduce anxiety, and is without addictive properties. A study in the *Journal of Clinical Pharmacy and Therapeutics* indicated that passionflower was just as effective as the prescription medication oxazepam in the treatment of GAD, and did not have any of the side effects such as impaired job performance.[7] Out of the 36 subjects with GAD, half were given 45 drops of passionflower extract per day, and the other half were given 30 milligrams of oxazepam per day. After the four-week trial, there was no significant difference between the two groups. The study also determined that passionflower increases levels of the neurotransmitter GABA, which helps with calm and relaxation.

Chrysin, a flavonoid compound found in passionflower, has anti-anxiety effects. It's also a powerful antioxidant and anti-inflammatory that helps to protect against disease and the aging process. In particular, it inhibits COX-2 and 5-lipoxygenase enzymes, which play a role in inflammation and pain and in Alzheimer's disease. As well, this flavonoid has libido-boosting properties, as it can inhibit the conversion of testosterone to estrogen. So maybe there's some passion in this flower after all! Researchers in India reported that when chrysin was combined with benzoflavone moiety (BZF), it increased the sexual function of aging rats.[8] Hmm. Perhaps the anti-anxiety effects knocked out performance anxiety?

Sweet Potato

When you're totally maxed out and in search of some good comfort food to feed your soul, look no further than the sweet and starchy sweet potato. This delish root veg is jam-packed with stress-busting nutrients, including vitamin B6, vitamin C, antioxidant beta-carotene, and calcium.

Carbohydrates get a bad rap, but they can, in fact, help chill you out. Studies show that carbs can reduce stress levels, improve mental performance, and help mitigate stress-induced depression. They increase serotonin levels in the brain, our feel-good neurotransmitter, and promote a feeling of calmness. This is why we tend to reach for carbs when we're feeling overwhelmed: they make us feel better physiologically. However, the issue lies in the type of carb consumed. Simple, refined carbs such as breads, sugars, and white pasta may make us feel better temporarily, but the effects are extremely short-lived. Then they leave us feeling bloated, fat, depressed, and even more stressed, so we continue to eat more simple carbs, and the vicious cycle continues.

On the other hand, complex carbohydrates such as sweet potatoes, quinoa, and oats are slow-releasing carbs that keep us more satiated and feeling less anxious for longer periods of time. When we're stressed, our cortisol levels are elevated and our blood-glucose levels increase, which means ongoing stress can totally muck up blood-sugar levels. But sweet potatoes actually help balance blood-sugar levels, making them a great stress antidote. They increase blood levels of a hormone called adiponectin, which regulates the metabolism of insulin; contain phytic acids, which lower blood glucose levels; and also contain caiapo (found in white sweet potatoes), which Austrian researchers indicate improves metabolic control by lowering insulin resistance in type 2 diabetics.[9] So, energy levels will be balanced, cravings controlled, and anxiety levels managed. Sweet!

Sweet potatoes are a rich source of B vitamins, especially B5 and B6, which support and calm the nervous system and play a key role in the production of neurotransmitters. And they're rich in antioxidant vitamins A (beta carotene) and C, which are essential for protecting the body from the free-radical damage caused by stress. Vitamin C also keeps your immune system in check, which tends to suffer during stressful times. Because vitamin C and the B vitamins are water soluble, they don't last very long in your body and need to be replenished frequently, especially during times of stress. And sweet potatoes, particularly the purple varieties, are high in anthocyanins—a powerful antioxidant that combats the effects of stress, aging, and cognitive decline. They also contain calcium and magnesium, two important minerals for calming and relaxing muscles and nerves.

TIP

Cooking sweet potatoes lowers their glycemic index—which is a good thing, because they taste WAY better that way!

Fats increase the absorption of beta carotene, so eat sweet potatoes with a little drizzle of extra virgin olive oil, hemp seed oil, or even coconut butter … YUM!

Almonds

Misery loves company. If you feel like you're going nuts, you might as well start adding them to your diet! These bite-size gems are the perfect snack food for those times when you feel like crawling under a rock. Almonds are fantastic stress relievers; they're packed with essential vitamins, minerals, and nutrients that support mental health and help you achieve a calm, cool mind.

Almonds are a great source of many B vitamins, which are essential for smooth nervous system function. They're especially high in vitamin B2, which helps produce anti-stress hormones, including serotonin—our all-time "happy" neurotransmitter. Almonds also have tons of magnesium. High levels of magnesium support a relaxed and body and promote nervous-system health. Magnesium also activates many mes required for energy production in the body, which is key when stress is high and immune function is low. As B vitamins and magnesium are both involved in the production of serotonin, they can further help regulate mood and relieve stress.

As well, almonds contain high levels of zinc, which is crucial for the immune system, an area that often takes a beating when you're stressed. For this reason, zinc has been shown to fight the negative effects of stress and anxiety. Vitamin E, also found in almonds, is an antioxidant that destroys free radicals related to stress, resulting in a reduction of oxidative stress that translates to reduced stress in the body. Finally, almonds contain omega-3 fatty acids, which are essential for proper brain function and lower levels of the stress hormone cortisol, reducing feelings of stress and anxiety in the body and mind.

HOW TO USE

With all these positive health effects, it's easy to want to overload on these highly nutritious goodies, but it's important to keep in mind that these little guys are still high in calories and fat (even if it's the good kind). As with everything, they should be consumed in moderation. A couple of tablespoons two or three times a week is more than enough to get that desired calming effect. Be sure to eat almonds raw, not roasted, as roasting depletes many of the nutritional benefits.

The skin of almonds contains enzyme inhibitors that keep almonds in a dormant state. Since almonds are a living food, these enzyme inhibitors are what prevent them from growing just by sitting on your counter. But they can also make it difficult for them to be broken down in your body. That's why it's best to soak almonds in water for 8 to 12 hours before eating. The enzyme inhibitors are released during the soaking process and the nut begins to germinate. Many of the fats are released (making it a slightly lower-calorie nut), and the macronutrients (proteins and fats) are broken down into a pre-digestible form, making it easier to digest and assimilate the nutrients. Once the almonds are done soaking, give them a good rinse and munch away! If you miss the crunch (and if you're stressed, chances are you LOVE the crunch), just lightly toast them at a super-low temperature to maintain the nutritional benefits.

Relora

Although Relora was introduced as a natural health product in the last decade, the herbs that make it up have been used traditionally for centuries. Relora is an entirely natural dietary supplement that helps combat the effects of stress on the body. Not only does this wonder supplement help alleviate stress, it also counteracts stress-related eating, promotes healthy weight loss, and has amazing anti-aging benefits, which mean fewer things to be stressed about!

Relora is a combination of two active herbal plant extracts commonly used in traditional Chinese medicine—*Magnolia officinalis* and *Phellodendron amurense.* Those in the alternative medicine field as well as in the medical community have praised it for its efficacy. Relora works by quieting the functioning of the endocrine organs (like the adrenal and pituitary glands), lessening the effect that stress has on the body. The active ingredients in Relora bind to receptor target sites in the central nervous system that are associated with stress and anxiety. Studies have shown much success with diet and stress levels while supplementing with Relora. It not only moderates hormone levels, but also seems to limit an individual's *perceived* level of stress. As a dietary aid, Relora inhibits the production of cortisol, an excess of which can prevent weight loss. And although it's non-drowsy in nature, it has also proven effective for those suffering from stress-related insomnia.

If the stress-busting, weight-loss benefits aren't enough to get you running for some Relora, it also has amazing anti-aging benefits! Relora naturally increases DHEA, which is our body's anti-aging, anti-stress hormone. It's like our rock star hormone, and with it kicking full throttle in our bodies, it helps reduce body fat, increase lean muscle, and keep us youthful! Studies show that the benefits of using Relora can be seen as quickly as two weeks![10]

HOW TO USE

Relora is non–habit forming and can be taken by anyone trying to relieve stress or lose weight in a healthy way. However, it should be used in conjunction with an exercise plan and a fresh, whole-food diet for best results. If you're taking Relora for stress, anxiety, or other mood disorders, it should be part of a complete wellness plan. It's also best to consume it on an empty stomach and prior to going to bed.

Stress-Busting Practices

Adding real, nutrient-dense, stress-reducing foods to your diet is key. But of course that's not all you can do to help alleviate stress; here are other actions you can take:

1. Exercise, practice yoga, meditate.
2. Hang out with friends. **Yes, some quality bonding time with your pals is one of the most powerful ways to reduce stress and boost your health. Just as good as, if not better than, exercise!**
3. Get some good shut-eye. **Sleep helps regulate cortisol levels.**
4. Journal. **Get all that crap out of your head (and body) and onto paper.**
5. Think happy thoughts. **Most of the stress in our life is perceived stress—things *we* create in our head. Change the way you look at and think about things. Find a new perspective. Always think in the positive. Shiny, happy thoughts!**
6. Take a deep breath.
7. Laugh out loud!

3. Counting Sheep

Count sheep? Who the heck has time for that when there are much more important things to think about, like how to face your boss tomorrow knowing that you didn't hit your deadline on time but that you still need to leave work early to take your kid to soccer practice. Regardless of what's keeping you up at night—relationships, work stress, financial matters, family—getting enough sleep is totally underrated.

What Promotes Sleepiness

Tick-tock, people, tick-tock. Whether we like it or not, our bodies operate on an internal clock. Not the "Holy crap, I'm getting old!" clock, but the circadian clock, and it's constantly ticking. Circadian rhythms tell our body when it's time to sleep and when it's time to wake—and unfortunately there's no snooze button. It's totally influenced by our environment. When night falls, darkness triggers the production of melatonin. Melatonin, secreted by the pineal gland in the brain, is a hormone and antioxidant responsible for sleep. The darker it becomes, the more melatonin is secreted; as it becomes lighter, melatonin decreases. But since we're living in an age of fluorescent lights, city lights, computer screens, and PVRs, we totally mess up our body's innate ability to sleep soundly.

So, what do you need to do to get some good shut-eye?

1. Sleep in complete darkness. Yes, that means no sleeping with your BlackBerry or television. Even the light from your alarm clock can prevent you from getting your beauty sleep. The blue light emitted from your television, digital clocks, and media devices interferes with melatonin production. If you do need an alarm clock, opt for one with red lights, as red has a more calming effect on the brain. Even better, invest in one that gradually wakes you up with light or soft sounds.

2. Don't eat before bed. Contrary to popular opinion, eating before bed will *not* result in weight gain, but it *will* disrupt your sleep. Lying down post-nosh will lead to indigestion, leaving you wrestling with your sheets.

3. Avoid stimulating foods. These include not only caffeine but also alcohol. Even though we're convinced that a glass (or four) of red wine will knock us out at night, its effects won't last very long and will keep us up most of the night.

4. Cool down. If the room temperature is too high (over 70°F, or 21°C), it may prevent you from getting your best sleep. Body temperature typically drops when you fall asleep, so a cooler room temperature is more aligned to your body's own innate sleep temperature.

5. Sleep or have sex. Those are the only two things you should be doing in your bed. Period.

Why You Need Your Sleep

Need to lie on your bed just to squeeze into your skinny jeans? Get more shut-eye during the night and you'll be sliding into them like a pair of cashmere gloves. It's been found that women who sleep fewer than seven hours a night are likely to gain more weight than those who get seven-plus hours of sleep.[11] If that's not enough reason to hit the hay, sleep deprivation also causes extreme stress on your body. Not only will it make you all moody, it also affects your concentration, memory, and reaction time, depletes your body of nutrients such as zinc, and pretty much sucks dry *all* vitamin C. As well, sleep deprivation can elevate blood pressure and increase your risk of diabetes and cancer. For example, studies show that women who do shift work have higher incidences of breast cancer.[12]

Melatonin, which is produced during sleep, slows down estrogen levels. If we're not sleeping well, melatonin production is reduced and excess estrogen, which is linked to breast cancer, is kickin' full throttle. But it's not limited to just "the girls." Since melatonin is also an antioxidant, a decrease in production means less juice to give cancer-causing free-radical damage a kick in the ass. Research also shows that melatonin can stop the growth of cancer cells dead in their tracks for many cancers, including colorectal, prostate, and liver, whereas a decrease in melatonin can rapidly accelerate tumor growth.[13] Not cool.

It's when we're sound asleep that our body is the most efficient and working the hardest to heal and repair itself from the day's abuses: cortisol levels are restored, cells are regenerated, human growth hormone (HGH) is secreted, fat is burned, and the liver detoxes—just to name a few. So the more sleep hours you sacrifice, the more you're missing out on being your best self.

Sleep and Weight Loss (or Weight Gain)

As noted above, lack of sleep wreaks havoc on your metabolism and has negative physiological effects that promote weight gain. And if that's not enough incentive to get good shut-eye, try this on for size: sleep promotes more FAT burned when trying to lose weight.

If you're eating clean, exercising, and trying to lose weight, lack of sleep can impede your efforts. A study conducted at the University of Chicago suggests that lack of sleep reduces weight loss efforts by 55 percent. In addition, of those who slept less, only 25 percent of their weight loss came from fat—the rest came from loss of muscle and water (not good)—whereas those who slept more lost more actual fat.[14]

Sleep also regulates your hunger hormone. When you compromise on sleep, your body produces more ghrelin (the hormone that triggers hunger) and less leptin (the hormone that tells you to stop eating). Adequate levels of sleep (seven to eight hours) regulate your hunger hormones, whereas five hours or less promote a hormonal imbalance. Think about it: if you're tired, you tend to reach for food to fuel your energy, and tend to be hungrier thanks to ghrelin. But higher ghrelin levels are also associated with reduced energy expenditure and reduced fat oxidization. That, coupled with the decrease of leptin that tells you to stop eating, is a weight-gain nightmare.

And the lack-of-sleep depletion of vitamin C we talked about? This also leads to weight gain. Vitamin C is such an important vitamin in helping to manage stress, support your immune system, slow down aging, boost mood, and lose weight. In fact, studies show that upping the intake of vitamin C before a workout promotes more calories burned, and that a vitamin C deficiency can be correlated to weight *gain*.[15]

Sleepy-Time Foods
Tart Cherries

Our precious antioxidant/neurotransmitter melatonin not only is produced by our pineal gland, but also can be found in high concentrations in some plant-based foods—in particular, the tart (aka sour) cherries in your favorite cherry pie. The two main varieties are Montmorency, which are bright red sour cherries, and Balaton, which are darker in color and have more of a sweet/sour taste. Although all varieties of tart cherries contain the highest plant-based source of readily absorbable dietary melatonin, Montmorency cherries contain six times more than the Balaton variety. A study conducted by the University of Rochester Medical Center concluded that the consumption of tart cherry juice significantly reduces the severity of insomnia and the "wake periods" after sleep onset.[16] So although it won't necessarily get you to sleep quicker, once you fall asleep, it'll keep you there.

In addition to all this sleep-enhancing goodness, these delish little morsels contain a decent dose of anthocyanins, which can reduce oxidative stress, inhibit the growth of cancer cells, and help prevent diseases such as atherosclerosis, diabetes, and Alzheimer's disease.

DID YOU KNOW?

For all you athletic types, research suggests that tart cherry juice makes a phenomenal sports recovery drink. The antioxidant, anti-inflammatory properties help reduce muscle damage, inflammation, pain, and the oxidative stress associated with endurance training. The juice also helps speed up the recovery of muscle function. In a study published in the *Journal of the International Society of Sports Nutrition,* researchers at Oregon Health and Science University's Department of Medicine suggested that ingesting tart cherry juice for seven days prior to and during a strenuous running event can minimize post-run muscle pain.[17] Less pain, better sleep—and better health all around!

HOW TO USE

Tart cherries can be consumed as a concentrated juice, in supplement powder form, or by eating the cherries on their own. (You can find them whole, frozen, or dried at most major health food stores.) For maximum sleep benefit, drinking one or two eight-ounce glasses of the juice daily or eating approximately 20 to 25 whole cherries should do the trick. When eating the cherries whole, please don't go for the can of pie filling! Those cherries have been cooked to death, are completely devoid of any nutritional benefit, and are laced with fat-causing sugar. Trust me—a week of that and you won't be happy, just fat and probably sleep-deprived.

Valerian Root

Valerian is a perennial plant that's native to Europe and Asia but now grows in North America too. Known for its sedative properties, it's used in the treatment of insomnia and anxiety. Who needs to count sheep? Valerian's sedative effects speed up the initial falling-asleep process. While it may not necessarily improve the quality of sleep as tart cherries do, it makes the process of getting there a little less painful.

The variety of components found in valerian root work together to make it happen. GABA, our relaxing neurotransmitter, is typically present in valerian root extract. However, it's not necessarily the GABA in the extract that causes the sedation, as it's difficult for GABA to cross the blood-brain barrier. Instead, valerian increases the release of GABA from the brain's nerve endings and prevents GABA's reabsorption into the synaptic cleft. Studies show that, rather than working as a one-shot sleeping aid, valerian root's efficacy has a cumulative effect, happening over time with daily use. The fact that valerian helps to reduce anxiety contributes to its sleep-inducing effect. You know those nights when you're bone-tired and yet you lie awake for hours while your mind goes round and round about all the stuff that's stressing you out? The less stressed and anxious we are, especially at bedtime, the quicker we'll fall asleep, and valerian is a great combo stress-buster and sleep-inducer.

HOW TO USE

Valerian can be consumed as a tea or herbal tincture, in which the oil is extracted from the dried root. Research shows that approximately 600 to 1,000 milligrams of the extract should be consumed for it to work effectively. If greater amounts are taken, some report a feeling of drowsiness in the morning—not what we're going for here! Just add some drops of valerian extract to passionflower or chamomile tea, which also has calming effects, for a soothing bedtime drink. Keep in mind that valerian root extract smells and tastes, well, pretty much nasty. It's very pungent. Best thing to do is add the drops in a glass with one or two ounces of water and take it down like a shot of tequila. And you may need the lemon wedge chaser. FYI.

Chamomile

Chamomile has been used for years as a natural sleep aid. Its calming effects not only help combat insomnia, but also help alleviate anxiety, even in small doses. What's great about this delicious, fragrant flower is that the results are quick. So if you're an immediate-gratification kinda gal or guy, this is for you!

Unlike many other natural sleep aids, you don't need to ingest chamomile for weeks on end to reap the benefits. One cup of tea 45 minutes before bed should have you sleeping soundly! Chrysin, the active flavonoid component found in chamomile, is the goddess chemical that makes this baby chill you out and promote sleepiness. Research shows that chamomile can significantly reduce the time it takes to fall asleep, exhibiting almost hypnotic effects. Not only will its beauty-sleep-promoting properties make you look all fresh, rejuvenated, bright-eyed and bushy-tailed in the morning, but its antioxidant, anti-inflammatory, and antiseptic properties reduce puffiness, skin inflammations, and irritations such as acne, rashes, psoriasis, and eczema. Plus, it has cell-regenerating properties, which, coupled with the cell-regenerating benefits of sleep, means you'll be looking sexy hot forever.

Another reason we don't get good-quality sleep at night is indigestion. As great as our intentions are to go to sleep on an empty stomach, without eating *anything* three hours before bed, don't even pretend you never hover in front of an open fridge, wearing your PJs and trying to decide what you're going to nosh on right before jumping in the sack. It happens. And you know what else happens? Indigestion and poor-quality sleep. Here's where chamomile comes to the rescue. Not only will it help you sleep better, it's an awesome remedy for intestinal health and indigestion too. No, it won't solve the problem of eating right before bed. Your body can't easily digest food while lying horizontally, and you just won't sleep well. But if you replace that bedtime snack with a cup of chamomile tea, you'll help alleviate any discomfort, heartburn, or indigestion from foods eaten earlier in the day.

HOW TO USE

Chamomile is best consumed as a tea before bed, or anytime during the day to promote relaxation. Steep two or three tablespoons in one cup of boiling water for 5 to 10 minutes. You can also add a couple of drops of passionflower for additional anti-anxiety and sleep-promoting benefits. Other options are to add two milliliters of chamomile extract to a cup of warm water, drizzle drops of chamomile essential oil on your pillow, or add a sachet of the dried flower under your pillow at night. You can also use the tea topically as skin toner and to alleviate skin irritations.

Lemon Balm

Lemon balm is a wonderfully fresh, fragrant herb that can help replace your stress head with clear, happy thoughts. This calming herb is very similar to mint, and belongs to the same family. Native to the Mediterranean region of Europe and now grown in many parts of the world, lemon balm not only is a culinary ingredient but also has antibacterial, antiviral, and mild sedative properties. Studies show that lemon balm's anti-anxiety properties work best as a sleep aid when combined with other sleep-inducing herbs, such as valerian, chamomile, or hops. Lemon balm also contains the chemical compound eugenol, which helps calm muscle spasms and promote relaxation.

HOW TO USE

Lemon balm smells and tastes amazing, so use it whenever you can! It can be included in many dishes as a fresh or dry herb, and can add a nice twist as a mint replacement. To get the most bang out of this dainty little herb, the dried herb can be steeped into a tea, or the extract can be added to hot water or another variety of herbal tea, such as chamomile or passionflower. Soon you'll be drifting off and putting your anxiety to rest!

Oats

Yes, that's right. Your healthy breakfast staple can help put you to sleep. This complex carbohydrate is also rich in protein, in particular tryptophan (the same amino acid found in turkey that makes us sleepy after Thanksgiving dinner). Tryptophan is an essential (meaning you must get it from food) amino acid that, in the presence of vitamin B6 and magnesium, is responsible for the production of serotonin, our feel-good neurotransmitter. Not only does serotonin help alleviate depression (see Chapter 5), it also regulates the onset of sleep and is a precursor to melatonin production.

Oats contain the dynamic duo of tryptophan and its faithful sidekick, carbs. Here's how it works. Amino acids don't play well together—they're like a rowdy bunch of children screaming "Pick me! Pick me!" They compete for uptake into the bloodstream during the digestive process, with tryptophan being just one of these amino acids trying to get your attention. So that's where carbs come in, giving tryptophan the edge. Carbs trigger the release of insulin, which pushes all the large neutral branch-chained amino acids directly into muscle cells—except for tryptophan, leaving it all by its lonesome. But that's a good thing. Insulin pushes out all the competition, giving tryptophan a clear playing field to quickly cross the blood-brain barrier, get converted to serotonin, and then be metabolized into melatonin—which makes you feel oh-so-peaceful and relaxed, blissfully oblivious to the amino acid bullying that just went on in your body. So, regarding your turkey dinner ... it isn't just the turkey that gives you food coma, it's all the carbs you consume alongside it that really knock you out!

Oats are a high source of vitamin B6, which is essential for the conversion of tryptophan into serotonin. B vitamins also help reduce stress and support the adrenal glands. And, no surprise here, oats are rich in fiber, giving a feeling of fullness without all the extra calories. They're also great for digestive health, they keep you regular, and they help lower cholesterol levels.

HOW TO USE

Cook up some steel-cut oats and sprinkle with cinnamon. You can have them for breakfast or make yourself a small serving a few hours before bed as a relaxing snack. Try slicing up some apples and baking them with a little bit of water, cinnamon, and oats. They also make great cookies and are perfect in muffins (especially in my Chill-Out Cherry Almond Muffins; check out the recipe on page 324). You can stir oats into yogurt instead of granola, or even use oats in soup—a different take on your traditional mushroom barley!

4. Get Your Sex On

Let's talk about sex. Can you believe that nearly 40 percent of us complain of having a low sex drive? Isn't that insane? Crazy! But if you skipped straight to this chapter, then maybe you *can* believe it. Low libido is the most common sexual issue among women and men. And yet healthy, regular sex is essential for optimal health and for your relationship with your partner. Fortunately, I have some secrets that can help you get in the mood.

Why Sex Is So Important for Your Health

If you want to achieve optimum health, then get busy in the bedroom! And no, once a month—or even once a week—does not cut it. I'm talking frequent sex. The benefits reach far beyond euphoria. Not only do regular romps increase your self-confidence and emotional connection, but having sex more than once a week can also boost your immune system. Research shows that those who have frequent, safe sex have higher levels of the antibody immunoglobulin A (IgA), which helps prevent colds. Sex can also boost cardiovascular health. So don't worry about giving someone a heart attack in the sack. Get wild and crazy. For men, having sex twice or more a week (compared with less than once a month) can lower blood pressure and cut the risk of heart attack by HALF. As well, having frequent ejaculations (more than 21 per month) significantly cuts the risk of prostate cancer. Got a headache? That's no excuse. Having sex may actually help alleviate the pain—and the same goes for joint pain, muscle pain, and PMS. Basically, as endorphins are increased, our levels of pain decrease. Win-win.

Nutrients to Put You in the Mood

If all these health benefits still aren't enough motivation for you to get your sex on, you're not alone. In an iVillage survey of 2,000 women, 63 percent said they'd rather sleep, watch a movie, or read than have sex.[19] Seriously, people, that's almost two-thirds of women! A good chunk of men also suffer from sexual problems such as erectile dysfunction or premature ejaculation. What's the cause? Work and family demands, everyday stress, certain medications, and health issues can cause sexual desire to plummet faster than a sinking ship, leaving you and your partner frustrated. But before you go running out the door to grab a prescription for Cialis, first check out these key libido-boosting nutrients to help get you in the mood.

Zinc

One of the many causes of low sex drive in both men and women is a decline in testosterone, the most important libido-boosting sex hormone. A poor diet high in saturated fats, caffeine, and alcohol can result in this. On the flip side, a healthy diet and lifestyle can help balance hormones and naturally boost testosterone, whetting your appetite for sex. One of the most important testosterone-boosting nutrients is zinc. Zinc is essential for testosterone production and sperm production, and it blocks the enzyme that converts testosterone into estrogen. Low levels of zinc correlate to erectile and sexual dysfunction.

Foods high in zinc:

- Oysters (lobster, crab)
- Wheat germ
- Sesame seeds
- Roasted pumpkin seeds
- Crimini mushrooms
- Spinach
- Summer squash
- Cocoa powder
- Miso
- Maple syrup

Tyrosine

Tyrosine stimulates the production of dopamine, the neurotransmitter responsible for pleasure and arousal. It's the core of our sexual drive and motivation. Tyrosine stimulates our reward center, guilty pleasures, and desires. It drives and motivates us to do things. The pleasure/reward associated with sex is typically driven by dopamine; hence, low levels of dopamine can weaken our desire to have sex. But foods rich in the amino acid tyrosine can stimulate dopamine production, as tyrosine converts to dopamine in the brain. Tyrosine can be obtained through food, or it can be manufactured in the body as the result of the conversion of the amino acid phenylalanine.

Foods rich in tyrosine:

- Soy
- Fish
- Peanuts
- Oats

- Almonds
- Lima beans
- Avocados
- Bananas

- Pumpkin seeds
- Sesame seeds

Heart-Healthy Nutrients

Here's the deal. If you want to enjoy sex, you need blood flowing to your genitals, pronto. In women, an increase in genital blood flow induces vaginal swelling and spurs the lubrication process. In men, blood vessels in the penis dilate, fill with blood, and cause an erection. Now, what do you think happens if there's a buildup of plaque in the arteries? Blood wouldn't flow freely, now, would it? A reduction in blood flow means less blood pumping to the genitals. Therefore, high cholesterol is directly correlated to erectile dysfunction. So if all the other reasons to embrace a heart-healthy diet aren't enough motivation, maybe an improved sex life will be! Omega-3s play a star role here, as they lower blood triglyceride levels by 25 to 45 percent, and also boost dopamine levels in the brain's pleasure center. Here are some other nutrients that can get your blood flowing:

L-arginine is an essential amino acid that stimulates the release of nitric oxide from the walls of blood vessels, dilating the blood vessels and improving blood flow. Pretty much the same deal as Viagra.

Vitamin B3 (niacin) is essential for circulation and improved blood flow, especially to your extremities. It also increases the skin's sensitivity to touch. Fun times!

Vitamin B6 helps with the conversion of neurotransmitters and increases blood flow, meaning it can help boost dopamine levels, transitioning you from disinterested damsel to purring sex kitten.

Vitamin E aids in the production of sex hormones, supplies the genitals with oxygen, and protects against free-radical damage.

Selenium is a mineral essential for a man's sex drive and sperm production. Half the selenium in a man's body is found in his testicles. Toss him a couple to keep him pumped (literally).

Foods high in selenium:
- Brazil nuts
- Tuna
- Oysters
- Crimini mushrooms
- Mustard seeds
- Barley
- Oats

Sexy Foods

Maca

Maca is known as "nature's Viagra," so if you want a natural way to increase your libido, this is the superfood for you! A little bit of maca in your system and you'll be raring to go.

While touted for its sex-enhancing properties, maca does much more than increase libido. This powerhouse Peruvian herb is packed with nutrients and has been used for centuries to boost energy, improve memory and concentration, overcome anemia, and fight depression. Those ancient Peruvians knew what they were talking about! Maca is an adaptogen, meaning it helps restore balance within the entire body system. One of nature's greatest aphrodisiacs, maca is known to increase sex drive, stamina, performance, and frequency. It also increases erectile function and sperm count in men as well as ovarian function in women, enhancing fertility. It does this by improving overall health, vitality, energy, and balance, naturally increasing libido.

One of the best qualities of maca is its ability to support the body's endocrine system. Maca on its own doesn't contain hormones, nor does it actually change blood-hormone levels when ingested. Rather, it restores the endocrine system through the hypothalamus–pituitary axis by improving communication between the brain and the pituitary gland, as well as the adrenals. This ensures proper hormone balancing and secretion within the body by transmitting the hormone's message.

For example, let's say you have a craving for vanilla ice cream and you ask your man to get some for you, but (like most men) he isn't really listening. So one of two things happens: either he doesn't bring you ice cream at all (because he wasn't listening) or he brings you chocolate instead. You don't get what you want and you're not happy. Fail. But if you both took maca there'd be great communication between the two of you, he'd get your message clearly and would bring you vanilla ice cream, and all would be good! Maca just improves the pituitary glands' "listening skills" to send and receive the correct info, without changing blood-hormone levels. Too bad maca doesn't work on relationships! From a speaking-and-listening perspective, that is. On the sex front, it's got your back.

> ### TIP
> Got milk? No need when maca trumps milk gram for gram in the amount of calcium.

The maca root is also a rich source of energy-dense complex carbohydrates and packs in more than 10 percent protein, including 19 amino acids. As well, it's super-high in B vitamins (particularly B1 and B2, which help boost energy and manage stress, respectively), vitamins C and E, and a plethora of minerals, including significant amounts of iron (more than most red meats, beans, seeds, and nuts), potassium, magnesium, zinc, iodine, and calcium. Finally, maca is a significant source of dietary fiber and essential fatty acids. How sexy is that?

Maca's medicinal use dates back to Incan civilization as early as 1600 BCE; Peruvians still use it as both a food and an herbal remedy to heighten fertility, mood, and endurance. While the long list of benefits is impressive, here are a few really worth noting:

- Increases energy, stamina, and athletic performance
- Improves memory, concentration, and mental alertness
- Alleviates depression and enhances mood
- Reduces symptoms of menopause and PMS
- Balances endocrine system, hormones, and thyroid function
- Natural aphrodisiac
- Enhances sexual function in both men and women
- Concentrated source of iron helps fight anemia (higher than most red meats!)
- High in calcium and magnesium, both essential for bone health

Pumpkin Seeds

These delicious seeds, sometimes called pepitas, are rich in B vitamins, vitamin E, zinc, and essential fatty acids, including oleic acids, omega-6, and the anti-inflammatory, antioxidant omega-3.

For men, these seeds help support prostate health due to their high magnesium and zinc properties. As men age, their levels of zinc tend to decline, which can lead to testosterone deficiency, erectile dysfunction, and enlargement of the prostate. Zinc can help reduce prostate inflammation and is essential in building seminal fluid and increasing sperm count. Plus, pumpkin seeds are rich in phytosterols, which contribute to prostate health. They've also been praised for their cholesterol-lowering properties. And as we know, the higher the cholesterol, the weaker the erection.

In women, these nutrient-rich seeds help build hormones, activate sexual organs, and increase sexual fluid secretions. They also contain the amino acid myosin, which is essential for muscle contractions. So to reap the benefits of good sex, you might want to ensure those muscles are in good working order for the big O.

HOW TO USE

Pumpkin seeds should be eaten raw (not roasted) to maintain their health benefits. They can be eaten on their own as a crunchy snack, combined with other nuts and seeds, added to trail mix, topped on salads, cereals, and oatmeal, or sprinkled on soups for added texture and crunch. You can also enjoy their health benefits by drizzling pumpkin seed oil on veggies or using raw pumpkin seed butter as a spread. Soaking the raw seeds for 8 to 12 hours prior to eating makes them easier to digest. They can then be dehydrated to restore crunch, while still maintaining their nutritional benefits.

TIP

Researchers at Chicago's Smell and Taste Treatment Research Center found that the smell of pumpkin pie increases men's penile blood flow by 40 percent—making it a great libido booster![20]

Garlic

Although garlic may seem the antithesis of sexiness, pop back a few mints, suck on some cinnamon sticks, and spice up your sex life with this potent bad boy. Yep, garlic will get your blood flowing in all the right places. It contains allicin, the sulfur-based organic compound that gives garlic its funky aroma. Well, start to love it, because it's allicin that increases blood flow to sexual organs. It does this by increasing nitric oxide, a chemical gas used by blood vessel walls to trigger the arteries and surrounding muscles to relax. The more nitric oxide, the wider the blood vessels become and the more blood flow increases, causing a sexual response in both males and females. Viagra knocks off this process through its chemically created blue pill that enhances nitric oxide pathways in the penis, triggering an erection.

In addition, garlic helps prevent blood platelets from building up and forming artery-clogging blood clots, which assists the whole blood-flow process. Garlic is also a great natural antibiotic, has antibacterial and antifungal properties, and can help protect against some cancers.

HOW TO USE

Minced, chopped, crushed, smashed. That's how allicin is formed and becomes effective. When alliin, the preceding compound in garlic, is combined with the garlic's own enzyme (alliinase), it converts to allicin. The only way the enzymes can break down alliin into allicin is through this manual chopping process, or through some serious chewing. On its own, alliin doesn't contain any beneficial health properties; it must be converted into allicin to be effective. It takes some time for this process to occur, so after you've minced your garlic, let it sit a few minutes to allow the magic to happen. It's best to eat garlic raw, as heat destroys allicin. Cooking garlic whole can kill the enzymes before allicin is formed, making it pretty much worthless. Add some minced, raw garlic to salad dressings, or mix with extra virgin olive oil and drizzle over steamed veggies ... perhaps some asparagus!

DID YOU KNOW?

A study published in the *Journal of Nutrition* concluded that garlic, coupled with an increase in dietary protein, increases testicular testosterone (the sex hormone).[21]

Asparagus

Asparagus is super-high in vitamin E, which is essential for a healthy sex drive. Vitamin E helps increase vaginal lubrication and can help boost energy and stamina.

Its powerful antioxidant properties help protect sex cell membranes and oxygen-rich blood flow to the genitals from free-radical damage. It also aids in the dilation of blood vessels, increasing blood and oxygen flow.

Asparagus is high in niacin (vitamin B3), which helps enlarge blood vessels and produce sex hormones. In addition, niacin is required for histamine production, an absolute necessity for orgasm. It also increases the skin's sensitivity to touch and produces that "sexual flush," making the whole experience much more pleasurable. Asparagus is a good source of vitamin B6, which ignites our feel-good transmitters; zinc, which enhances libido-boosting testosterone; and selenium, which helps increase sperm count. It's also rich in antioxidant, immune-boosting, beautifying vitamin C, keeping us at the top of our game.

> ## HOW TO USE
> Asparagus is super versatile, whether you're looking for a snack or an addition to a great meal. Try it raw, chopping it into your fave salad or dipping it into hummus. Steam some up and toss with hemp or olive oil, sea salt, and a squeeze of lemon. Or throw it into your next stir fry or soup.

Walnuts

Walnuts have been around for more than 2,000 years. In Roman times they were commonly used as an aphrodisiac, and you'll be happy to hear they're still used for that purpose today. Throughout history, these nutritious nuts have been linked to love and fertility, and for good reason.

Walnuts are very high in a wide range of nutrients that support not only sexual and reproductive health but also the health of many other body systems. Besides being high in protein and a great source of beneficial fiber, walnuts are associated with sex and love. They're a good source of folic acid, an important nutrient for women who are trying to conceive. They also contain L-arginine, which, apart from being an essential amino acid, helps men attain erection and maintain stamina in bed. It's an equal opportunity nutrient—it increases libido and intensifies sexual sensation in women, too.

Walnuts and walnut oil are a great source of omega-3 fatty acids. Diets that include these healthy fats stimulate the fire necessary to sustain a healthy sex life. Healthy fats are essential for lovers because they're necessary for the production of many sex hormones. And walnuts also contain zinc. Both zinc and omega-3s are great for the sexual health of men, supporting heart and blood circulation; research shows that walnuts are directly linked to helping some men maintain erections. In fact, walnuts can increase sex drive so substantially that in recent years they've been used in an alternative form of Viagra.

L-tyrosine, the precursor to dopamine, is another amino acid found in walnuts that helps boost your sex drive. Dopamine is the neurotransmitter that will get you begging for it! It stimulates drive, motivation, and the brain's reward/pleasure center. But that's not all: walnuts are rich in vitamin E, which not only helps balance your hormones, naturally stimulating your libido, but also makes your skin super soft, inviting it to be touched!

HOW TO USE

Like all other nuts, walnuts are best enjoyed raw. And feel free to throw them wherever you like—enjoy them alone as a snack, ground into a piecrust, tossed into a salad, stirred into yogurt, blended into smoothies, and mixed into breakfast cereals. Walnut oil makes not only a great salad dressing, but also a skin moisturizer ... and an edible massage oil! These nuts are calorie-dense, so consume only a small handful a couple of times a week to reap the rewards of a healthy and happy sex life.

5. Don't Worry, Be Happy

It's estimated that within the next 10 years depression will become the second most common health problem in the world, with women being affected almost twice as much as men. Most of us occasionally feel sad or down, whether through the loss of a loved one, the end of a relationship, or losing a job. But for many, this overall feeling of sadness can last beyond weeks. It can be debilitating, affecting work performance, relationships, and social interactions. It can create a feeling of hopelessness, pessimism, low self-esteem, and withdrawal. And it can cause fatigue, exhaustion, and a lack of motivation to do anything.

Unfortunately, many people who feel this way think it's the norm. That it's uncontrollable. That it's just "how they are." This is not the case! You don't need to feel that way. Depression is not just a "feeling" of unhappiness. It's an ailment that affects the mind, just as the flu or arthritis affects the body. And, like the flu, it can be prevented and treated. If you think you're struggling with something more serious than everyday blues, it's best to consult your health practitioner or psychotherapist, as he or she can best help you. Depression *is* treatable. You *can* feel your absolute best every day. And what you put into your body *does* make a significant difference.

Nutritional Factors That Put You in a Funk
Sugar, Alcohol, and Caffeine

Depression isn't just in the mind—it involves the whole body. And many nutritional factors can trigger or compound depression. Stimulants such as sugar, alcohol, and caffeine can create blood-sugar imbalances, which can lead to depression. Too much caffeine can deplete the body of vitamin B6, the crucial nutrient required for the production of our "happy" transmitter, serotonin. As well, blood-sugar imbalance (and lactose intolerance) prevents the absorption of tryptophan in the intestine, which impedes the production of dopamine and serotonin. So when life throws you lemons and you'd rather use them as a twist to accompany your big bottle of Grey Goose—or perhaps just bury yourself in that triple-layer chocolate fudge cake and grande caramel macchiato—it may not help so much. Sure, we might feel fabulous for a whole nanosecond (or two) while all that sugar, alcohol, and caffeine shocks our system, but once we come off that high we'll feel even worse.

Allergies and Food Sensitivities

Allergies and food sensitivities can also play a major role in depression. Food allergies promote inflammation, alter hormones and brain chemicals, and can lead to both schizophrenia and one of its main symptoms, depression. In fact, in a study conducted by allergy expert Dr. William Philpott involving 52 patients with schizophrenia, 64 percent adversely reacted to wheat, 50 percent to cow's milk, 75 percent to tobacco, and 30 percent to petrochemical hydrocarbons.[22] Many allergies and food intolerances are due to artificial food dyes and pesticides, so eating natural, organic food as much as possible is essential for your physical *and* mental health!

Nutritional Deficiencies

Another factor that can lead to depression is nutritional deficiency. Diets high in refined sugar, processed foods, pesticides, preservatives, and additives have all been linked to depression. But it's not just the bad stuff you're adding in that's making you depressed—it's also the good stuff you're keeping out! When we fill our stomachs with foods that are nutritionally void, there's no room left for all the healthy foods our bodies and minds crave. And depriving your body of the essential nutrients it needs for optimal health will certainly have a negative impact on your mental health.

Eat Your Antidepressants: Serotonin

Serotonin is our feel-good neurotransmitter. Although all serotonin is produced in the brain, about 20 percent resides in the central nervous system, where its role is to help regulate mood, sleep, and appetite. It also plays a star role in helping combat depression and stimulating a feeling of overall well-being, which is why it's known as the happiness hormone. The remaining 80 percent is found in the gut (where it helps regulate intestinal activity) and in blood platelets. Depression is largely associated with a serotonin deficiency. If there aren't enough serotonin neurotransmitters being sent and received, depression can strike.

> **DID YOU KNOW?**
> Men synthesize 52 percent more serotonin than women, which is one of the reasons why more women become depressed than men.

Tryptophan, an amino acid found in foods such as sacha inchi seeds, eggs, beans, oats, chicken, and turkey, is the precursor to serotonin production. With the help of vitamin B6, vitamin C, and zinc, tryptophan is converted to a chemical called 5-HTP, which crosses the blood-brain barrier and converts to serotonin. Tryptophan and 5-HTP are the *only* precursors to serotonin production. Antidepressants don't manufacture serotonin; they only block its reuptake from the "sending" neuron so that it's not reabsorbed. This increases serotonin circulation in the synapse (the space between neurons) so that it can be more readily picked up by a receptor site. That's why these antidepressants are called selective serotonin reuptake inhibitors (SSRIs); they include Prozac, Zoloft, Paxil, Celexa, Lexapro, and Luvox.

Other antidepressants focus on the neurotransmitters dopamine and epinephrine, which, although also linked with depression, are mainly associated with lack of motivation and energy. Serotonin, in contrast, is associated with mood.

Again, none of these medications actually *manufacture* serotonin, but rather maintain what's already there through the foods you eat. Only by changing your diet or supplementing with 5-HTP can you actually increase serotonin production. Plus, many people can't tolerate antidepressants due to their laundry list of side effects, such as anxiety, sexual dysfunction, and weight loss or weight gain, just to name a few.

Key Nutrients That Alleviate and Prevent Depression
Omega-3 Fatty Acids

With 60 percent of the brain made up of fat, we need fat for our brains to function optimally. But it's the *type* of fat that's critical. Just as trans fats are bad for your heart, the same holds true for your mind. Unhealthy fats like saturated and trans fats won't only build up plaque in your arteries, they'll also congest the brain. A third of brain fat is made up of polyunsaturated fatty acids (PUFAs), which are in turn made up of omega-3 fatty acids and omega-6 fatty acids. Good sources of omega-3s include cold-water oily fish, algae, nuts, and seeds such as flax, sacha inchi, and chia.

The optimal ratio in our diet is two parts omega-6s to one part omega-3s. However, today's North American diet has shifted the ratio to more like 20 to 1. This significantly skewed ratio causes inflammation, allergies, cognitive issues, and a whole host of other problems. Omega-6 fatty acids promote inflammation, whereas omega-3 fatty acids reduce inflammation. This is why we need to add more omega-3s to our diet and make a conscious effort to reduce the amount of omega-6s consumed.

Foods rich in omega-3:
- Wild salmon
- Mackerel
- Herring
- Anchovies
- Algae
- Sacha inchi seeds
- Chia seeds
- Flax
- Walnuts
- Soybeans

Foods rich in omega-6:
- Vegetable oil
- Palm oil
- Sunflower oil
- Safflower oil
- Canola oil
- Soybean oil
- Corn oil

Omega-3 fatty acids are *the* most important fat for your brain and for alleviating depression. A Harvard study showed that omega-3 fatty acids are an effective alternative to drug therapies in treating depression, and when complemented with traditional drug therapies can increase their efficacy.[23] A meta-analysis found that omega-3s had significant effects in treating depression, bipolar depression, and ADHD.[24]

Omega-3 fatty acids (especially DHA) stabilize the brain's cell membranes, making them more fluid and making communication across the synapses more effective. For example, imagine you're a messenger (neurotransmitter) trying to send a gift of happiness to your neighbor. However, there's a river separating your house from your neighbor's. Now, if this river is crystal clear and free flowing, you can get across it, no problem. But if it's all swamplike, thick and nasty, it might take you a bit longer to cross. Omega-3 fatty acids are fluid-like fats that assist in the transduction of neurotransmitters from one neuron to another. The lack of omega-3s can cause communication breakdown to occur—the message gets stuck in the swamp, so to speak. Omega-3s also help increase your brain's neuronal connections and the number of feel-good serotonin receptor sites.

B Vitamins

B vitamins are like a whole family of superstars, just waiting to kick into action and boot your depression to the curb. B1 (thiamine) fuels the brain with glucose for energy and is required for nerve stimulation. A deficiency in B3 (niacin) is linked to both depression and anxiety, and B3 is used by health professionals in the treatment of schizophrenia. Vitamin B6, required for the production of serotonin and other neurotransmitters, is essential in regulating mood. B12 is also needed for the production of serotonin and other neurotransmitters, and is essential for the nervous system to function properly. A strong link exists between depression and B12 deficiency.

Folate

Folic acid isn't just for women who are pregnant; folate deficiency is common in those with depression. Folate is another nutrient required for the production of serotonin—so if you're lacking in folate, you're probably lacking in serotonin, which we know can lead to depression.

Foods rich in folate:

- Spinach
- Broccoli
- Lentils
- Asparagus
- Bananas

Foods That Fight Depression
Fish Oil and/or Cold-Water Oily Fish (Wild Salmon)

EPA and DHA are derivatives of omega-3 fatty acids and can be found naturally in oily fish such as salmon, tuna, halibut, herring, and cod. When choosing a fish oil, keep in mind that it should contain significantly more EPA than DHA, with no less than 1,000 milligrams of EPA per day for adults and 500 to 600 milligrams of EPA per day for children. EPA and DHA can also be converted in the body from ALA (alpha-linolenic acids), which are found in plant-based sources such as nuts and seeds. However, the conversion rate from ALA to EPA and DHA in humans is fairly low, which is why direct, fish-based sources of EPA and DHA are most effective for the treatment of depression. For example, someone who eats fish once every two weeks would get the same amount of EPA as someone who consumes over three tablespoons of flaxseed oil (a source of ALA) every day. Getting your EPA and DHA from a direct source is by far the more effective method.

HOW TO USE

Look for a fish oil with at least 1,000 milligrams of EPA per daily dosage. Be sure to purchase oil in capsule form instead of liquid. Liquid fish oils become rancid very quickly—they're fine until they're opened, but after that they oxidize rapidly, even if kept in the fridge. They're extremely sensitive to light, heat, and oxygen, so every time you open and close the bottle, the exposure to oxygen will damage the oil. And make sure you're using pharmaceutical-grade oil—if not, you may be ingesting more than you bargained for, including such contaminants as heavy metals! Not so good for the brain.

TIP

Fish oil is also phenomenal for cardiovascular health. It lowers triglycerides by 25 to 45 percent and also raises HDL, a good cholesterol, by 5 to 15 percent.

Sacha Inchi Seeds

Although sometimes known as an Inca peanut, there's nuttin' nutty about this seed. Yep, that's right, sacha inchi is a seed, not a nut, and can also go by the names Savi Seed, sacha peanut, mountain peanut, and *Plukenetia volubilis* (for the grown-up, scientific types). The seeds are found in the plush, star-shaped green fruit of the semiperennial, shrub-like, viney sacha inchi plant that grows deep within the Peruvian Amazon rainforest. The incubation combination of intense sunlight and mineral-rich soil contributes to its superior nutritional density.

Sacha inchi seeds are in fact one of the most nutrient-dense seeds around, especially when it comes to brain health. At approximately 48 percent, they contain the highest plant-based source of omega-3 fatty acids in the world! And even with the relatively low conversion of plant sources, these seeds contain such a concentrated amount that they still come out on top. Omega-3 fatty acids help improve cognitive functioning and fight depression by enhancing the reception of our lovely mood-lifting neurotransmitter serotonin. In addition, they're significant in helping lower bad cholesterol, thereby improving overall heart health. Sacha inchi seeds have strong anti-inflammatory properties, which helps ward off pain and disease. The seeds are also high in fiber, which binds onto cholesterol (helping your body eliminate it), helps improve digestive health, increases satiety, and helps balance blood-sugar levels, which is paramount in combating depression.

And, at almost 28 percent, these seeds are extremely high in digestible protein. Ounce for ounce, they trump any meat source—and most other seeds! And why should this make you happy (literally)? For every gram of protein, sacha inchi seeds have 29 milligrams of serotonin-making tryptophan. What's important here is the ratio of tryptophan to total protein. Remember, amino acids compete, so the greater the ratio of tryptophan as a percentage of protein, the more clout it has relative to the other amino acids, increasing its magic-making odds.

To put things into perspective, check out the chart on the facing page.

	Total Protein	Total Tryptophan	% Tryptophan
	PER 100 GRAMS	PER 100 GRAMS	IN PROTEIN
SACHA INCHI SEEDS	28	0.812	2.90
EGG WHITES	81.1	0.998	1.23
TURKEY	21.89	0.243	1.11
SESAME SEEDS	17	0.370	2.17
MILK	3.22	0.080	2.34
SPIRULINA	57.47	0.930	1.62

We usually associate tryptophan with turkey, right? But not only do sacha inchi seeds have more total protein ounce for ounce, they have over three times the amount of tryptophan. Plus, the ratio of tryptophan as a percentage of total protein significantly trumps the big bird.

In addition to its happiness-boosting properties, the seed's rich protein content combined with the anti-inflammatory omega-3 make it ideal for aiding quick muscle recovery and growth. It's also high in iodine, which is good for thyroid function and metabolism, and high in the antioxidant vitamins A and E, which are great for improving skin and hair.

DID YOU KNOW?

The tiny amount of sweetness that hugs these scrumptious sacha inchi seeds helps increase the rate at which tryptophan enters the blood-brain barrier, speeding up the rate of serotonin production and ultimate happiness. That's right, jump for joy ... it has that effect!

Saffron

Saffron, an aromatic spice native to Southwestern Asia, is a culinary staple in many Middle Eastern and Indian delish dishes. It comes from the dried stigma of the *Crocus sativus* (saffron crocus) flower, which is a lily-like perennial. While its high price tag may incline us to savor the spice in small quantities, we may be getting more bang for our buck than we could have imagined.

Studies show that saffron works just as effectively as Prozac (an SSRI) in treating mild to moderate depression—without the side effects. Researchers at the Tehran University of Medical Sciences found that during an eight-week trial involving 40 depressed patients, 30 milligrams of saffron extract per day worked as well as 20 milligrams of Prozac per day.[25] In another six-week study, 30 milligrams of saffron per day was compared with 100 milligrams of imipramine, a tricyclic antidepressant. Out of 30 depressed patients, both treatments provided similar relief; however, those who took saffron didn't have the associated side effects such as dry mouth and sedation.[26]

TIP

Soaking saffron before use helps to activate its mood-boosting properties.

Crocin and safranal, chemical compounds found in saffron, are reported to relieve depression by raising serotonin and other mood-enhancing chemicals in the brain. Crocin is a carotenoid antioxidant that gives saffron its orange color, while safranal gives the spice its distinctive aroma. In addition to saffron's ability to bust you out of a rut, it has anti-cancer, anti-mutagenic, and antioxidant properties, helping to prevent disease. Persians have used it for years to help alleviate stomach aches, vomiting, inflammation, and PMS symptoms—which can benefit everyone! Recent research also suggests it can help boost memory. It might be worth it to break the bank and invest in some saffron—who says money can't buy happiness?

Brazil Nuts

As the name suggests, these rich and creamy nuts are native to Brazil, as well as other South American countries like Bolivia, Venezuela, Colombia, and Peru. The trees can grow to 200 feet tall, and it isn't until they're about 12 years old that they start to produce fruit. And since these fruits are more high-maintenance than a Hollywood star, they'll bloom only in the most pristine growing conditions. (Trees that grow in the ghetto part of the rainforest get no love—the pollinating bees just don't fly there.) The Brazil nut fruit resembles the fuzzy brown coconut in shape and size and houses 8 to 24 Brazil nuts.

Brazil nuts' mood-boosting properties are highly attributable to their rich selenium content. Selenium is a trace mineral and antioxidant essential for combating depression, and at roughly 100 micrograms per nut, these nuts contain the richest known source. Low selenium levels in one's diet can lead to irritability, depression, and fatigue. In a U.K. study, 50 subjects received either 100 micrograms of selenium or a placebo every day over a five-week period. The selenium intake was associated with heightened mood and lower feelings of depression, anxiety, and fatigue.[27]

In addition, selenium is required for the synthesis and metabolism of thyroid hormones, which can also tamper with your mood. Those suffering from a sluggish thyroid (see Chapter 8) tend to suffer from feelings of depression and fatigue as well. Thyroid disease can interrupt neurotransmitter receptor cells in the brain, preventing the feel-good chemicals from latching on. Selenium actively increases thyroid hormone T3 (triiodothyronine) by kick-starting the conversion of T4 (thyroxine), boosting metabolism and mood, and helping alleviate symptoms of thyroid disease. Selenium will make you feel good in other ways, too. It's known to boost libido, which can get you out of the dumps and into the sack. It also can help prevent cancer, especially those of the breast and prostate.

Brazil nuts are rich in vitamin B1 (thiamin), which helps stabilize blood-sugar levels by converting blood sugar to energy. You know how cranky and tired you get when your blood sugar plummets? The B1 in Brazil nuts helps prevent these feelings of depression and fatigue. It's also essential in the production of the neurotransmitter acetylcholine, which boosts mood and improves memory. As well, Brazil nuts are a rich source of the antioxidant vitamin E and contribute to heart health with their mono-unsaturated fats. Their higher, healthy fat content also increases satiety, keeping you fuller longer. And if you're feeling full, you're less likely to reach for those chocolate chip cookies as a pick-me-up!

Spinach

Everybody knows that eating your vegetables is an important part of any healthy diet, but dark leafy greens like spinach really up the ante in their benefits to health, and to the nervous system in particular.

Spinach is packed with B vitamins, which are essential for balancing mood and keeping the nervous system in check. Low levels of folate (or B9) are directly linked to depression. In fact, folate is critical for stable moods and proper nervous system function—making it a great remedy for wild mood swings associated with PMS or other times when we feel like we're going a little crazy.

Dark leafy greens such as spinach, kale, collard greens, and broccoli are also high in magnesium, calcium, potassium, and vitamin C. These nutrients are all essential for proper nervous function and are depleted when stress is high—which is just when you need them the most! Magnesium is crucial for a healthy nervous system, and spinach provides lots of it, with just one cup containing about half of the recommended daily intake. Magnesium relaxes the body and the muscles; a deficiency of this calming nutrient is believed to be one of the causes of depression. Magnesium is involved in hundreds of important metabolic functions, and a large portion of current Western society is believed to be deficient. So get munching on those leafy greens, people!

Spinach and other leafy greens also contain tryptophan, which converts to serotonin in the body, enabling us to feel happy. Tryptophan can be obtained only through diet, and leafy greens like spinach are some of the best whole-food sources.

HOW TO USE
Spinach is best consumed either raw or lightly steamed, as other methods of cooking can drain key nutrients, including those that are essential for mood support. Have a crisp spinach salad for lunch or even blend some leaves into your smoothie—you won't taste the greens, but your body will feel them!

A Note on Happiness

Happiness is deliberate. I often get asked what Kool-Aid I'm drinking for being so happy all the time. Yes, I am happy, but there's no Kool-Aid. I'm *genuinely* happy because I choose to be. Happiness is a fully conscious effort and a choice I make every single day. I'm grateful for so many things and am surrounded by the most amazing people. And I always go back to this place of gratitude no matter what pops up trying to burst my happy bubble. Of course there are moments I want to burst into tears or scream at the top of my lungs, but those are few and far between, and I get out of that place as fast as I possibly can. I don't want to stay there because it totally SUCKS! Happiness is more fun.

If something happens that makes me upset, I acknowledge it, and if it's worthy I decide for what period of time I'll allow myself to be upset. Sometimes it's a minute, sometimes it's a full day. Once my time period is up, I force myself to snap out of it and put on a happy smile. Even if you feel you'd much rather stay in bed all day, listening to sappy songs and basking in misery, sometimes you just need to get up, turn that frown upside down, and *pretend*. The reality is, even faking it can boost your mood so fast that it quickly becomes genuine happiness and reality. The more happiness you put out there, the more happiness you'll get back. It's the law of the universe.

Smiles are contagious, hugs are therapy, and laughter really *is* the best medicine. Get out and put on that happy face!

6. Brain Drain

Where are my keys? I'm late for my date, but I can't leave because I can't find my keys! I've checked 12 different purses, the front table, the kitchen table, every cupboard, the bedroom, and the bathroom—twice—but they're nowhere to be found!

Maybe I left them somewhere … yes, that's what I did. I must have left them at the restaurant last night, and someone else must have taken them by accident. Except that's not possible because I used them to drive home and get back into the house. What's wrong with me? Why can't I find my darn keys! Now my heart is starting to race. Where can they be? I mean, they can't just pick up and walk away on their own, right? Never mind. I'll just leave my front door unlocked and take a cab since I have no more time to spare and even two more seconds of this stress would cause my essential oil–scented zinc ricinoleate deodorant to surrender to sweat stains—not exactly charming. But just as I run out the house and close the door behind me, I hear a telltale jangling singing along to the door slamming shut. I look back, and there they are, my glittery set of keys dangling off the door lock. And it hits me: when I unlocked the door last night, I forgot to take them out of the lock!

Now how many times has something like this happened to you? Yes, meditation and being "present," clear-minded, and focused has a ton to do with it, we know, but have you ever walked into a room and completely forgotten what you came in there for? Or bumped into someone on the street whom you've met repeatedly but still can't remember her name? Or tried to find that word on the tip of your tongue but it just won't come out? Or walked laps around a parking lot not having a clue where your car is? Yep—you've had a brain fart!

How to Make a Memory

We've all made excuses. "I haven't had my coffee yet." "I'm not a morning person." "I was abducted by aliens last night and it really ruined my REM sleep." Whatever your favorite explanation for memory lapses, blown deadlines, or conversational faux pas may be, at some point or another, you have to level with yourself. Yes, rough days happen to everyone now and then. But are you having more off days than on? Like most bad habits, cloudy thinking creeps up on us without our noticing until it's simply part of who we are and how we think. And it's time to change it.

The Personal Assistant

The all-important hippocampus is responsible for storing and filing long-term memories as well as spatial navigation. It's the part of the brain associated with personal experiences, stories, memories, and the emotions attached to them. It's the continual gatherer of information, and it allows us to use this information to problem-solve and make everyday decisions in life. For example, you know better than to eat that entire bag of cookies, because the last time you did, it made you sick. So just looking at the bag triggers a memory. The hippocampus decides what memories you'll keep and stores them safely in there.

Acetylcholine is the key neurotransmitter responsible for memory. Its main role is to pull those memories from your brain's hippocampus for recall. It's like having a personal assistant. Let's say you worked on a bunch of documents. You created all these documents (just as you create a memory through images, sounds, etc.), but they needed to be filed away for later use. So you gave them to your assistant to organize them into a system. Since your assistant manages this filing system, he holds the key and knows where everything is; if you ask him to pull a file, he can easily do so. But if he decides not to show up for work one day and you need that file? You are in deep kimchi. You have no idea where he keeps things and have no way of getting to that file without him, leaving you totally S.O.L.

The same thing happens within your brain. Even if you already have a memory stored in your brain cells, if you don't have enough circulating acetylcholine, you won't be able to pull that memory from your files.

Why Our Brains Go from Sharp to Sludge
Stress

Both chronic and short-term (two- to four-hour) stress can have an ill effect on your memory. Memories are stored in several different brain cells in your hippocampus. The more brain cells it used in creating that memory—for example, you saw the hot stove (visual) and felt the burn (tactile)—the more brain cells it will occupy. These brain cells are all linked together by dendrites, which are stimulated by new information. However, the stress hormone cortisol causes dendrites to shrivel up, making new memories difficult to form and store.[28] Even the corticotropin-releasing hormones, which are activated by acute, short-term stress, have the same effect.

Low Acetylcholine

Poor memory might also be the result of low levels of acetylcholine, a neurotransmitter responsible for memory, which is stored in the brain's hippocampus. People suffering from Alzheimer's generally have low levels of acetylcholine; similarly, when you don't have enough circulating acetylcholine, you'll have trouble recalling the info stored in your hippocampus.

> **DID YOU KNOW?**
> According to a Finnish study, those who were living with a life partner during midlife were less likely to show cognitive impairment.[29] So if you're middle-aged and single, for brain's sake, shack up!

Sugar Sugar

Just as sugar sucks for your body, it sucks for your mind. It causes blood-sugar imbalances and brain fog, disrupts concentration, and promotes inflammation. This inflammation is a main contributor to the formation of amyloid plaques in your brain, which slows down communication and can ultimately cause Alzheimer's. A recent study conducted by researchers at UCLA found that a high intake of fructose damages the connection between brain cells, altering your brain's ability to learn and retain information. In other words, sugar can make you stupid.[30] In addition, refined sugar depletes your body of precious vitamins and minerals (namely B vitamins) essential for producing the neurotransmitters that send and receive information. If that isn't enough reason to nix your afternoon pastry fix, research at Massachusetts Institute of Technology confirms an inverse correlation between refined carbs and IQ.[31] The higher the intake of refined carbs, the lower the IQ. The lower the amount of sugar and refined carbs, the smarter you become!

Inflammation

Chronic inflammation is closely linked to memory decline and many cognitive disorders. Several studies suggest that inflammation in the brain is the underlying cause of aging and neurodegenerative diseases like Alzheimer's. Alzheimer's, the most common form of dementia, causes damage to the memory-storing hippocampus. For ways to help prevent and treat inflammation, see Chapter 17, as well as the foods listed below.

> **TIP**
> Chronic pain, smoking, lack of sleep, lack of exercise, food allergies, and heavy metals can all impair brain function and hinder memory.

Brain-Boosting Nutrients

So how can you boost your acetylcholine levels, banish brain fog, and spiffy up your memory? It all starts with these key nutrients.

DMAE

DMAE is converted to choline in the liver. Choline on its own can't pass the blood-brain barrier because it's a charged molecule. But since it's a precursor to the neurotransmitter acetylcholine, once it's converted into acetylcholine, it can enter the brain. Alzheimer's decreases levels of acetylcholine in the brain, so DMAE may help to increase acetylcholine levels through this pathway and thus improve memory. And since your brain is so smart, you might as well be a pretty face too: DMAE is also great for the skin and helps to even skin tone.

> **TIP**
> Sources of DMAE include anchovies, sardines, and wild salmon.

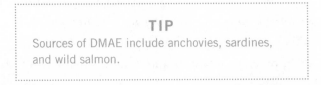

Phospholipids

Your brain loves fat. And when it comes to boosting IQ, it has a mega love affair with phospholipids: the smarty-pants of fat. They help make up the insulation that forms around a nerve and allows information to transmit quickly in the brain, keeping you sharp. There are two types of phospholipids essential for the job:

1. Phosphatidylcholine (PC). PC is a precursor for the memory neurotransmitter acetylcholine, which acts as your lackey—or to be "PC," your personal assistant—pulling stored memories from the brain. Sources include eggs, salmon, scallops, cauliflower, broccoli, Swiss chard, collard greens, and asparagus.

2. Phosphatidylserine (PS). This memory-molecule plays a key role in the cells' receptor sites, helping to boost communication between brain cells and hence providing memory-boosting power. The majority of PS is found in organ meats, but modest amounts are found in other food sources, such as white beans, peanuts, beets, and rice.

> **TIP**
>
> Supplementing with PS can be beneficial for those who have learning difficulties or age-related memory decline.

B Vitamins

B vitamins not only provide mental energy and help boost mood but also are essential for keeping your memory in tip-top shape. While all B vitamins work synergistically, some stand out when it comes to memory: B5 (pantothenic acid) helps convert choline into the powerful neurotransmitter acetylcholine; B9 (folic acid) can protect the brain from aging; B12 keeps brain cells healthy (a deficiency can lead to brain fog); and B3 (niacin) can provide memory-enhancing properties.

Sources of B vitamins:

- Sweet potatoes
- Leafy greens
- Whole grains (quinoa, oats, amaranth)
- Almonds
- Lentils/Legumes
- Asparagus
- Bananas

Zinc

Zinc is an important mineral, and part of the team that helps to encode and store memories in the brain. Plus, zinc assists in the conversion of proteins to neurotransmitters. Low zinc can lead to learning difficulties and long-term complications, such as dementia.

Foods high in zinc:

- Oysters (lobster, crab)
- Wheat germ
- Sesame seeds
- Roasted pumpkin seeds
- Crimini mushrooms
- Spinach
- Summer squash
- Cocoa powder
- Miso
- Maple syrup

DID YOU KNOW?
Can't remember your dreams from last night? That might be a sign you're deficient in zinc.

Vitamin C

Vitamin C is a powerful antioxidant that can prevent oxidative damage to brain cells, impairing memory and function. And like zinc, vitamin C plays an important role in the production of neurotransmitters, which can affect our memory and mood.

Foods rich in vitamin C:

- Camu camu
- Guava
- Black currants
- Red peppers
- Parsley
- Kiwis
- Broccoli
- Strawberries

Superfoods for Your Brain

Everyone loves a hero. And while these foods may not come with a cape and mask, they work wonders for your brain.

Turmeric

Multitasking is one of those qualities that bosses love in their employees, and that we love in our foods. Just as your boss would love it if you were able to reply to emails while simultaneously putting the finishing touches on your PowerPoint presentation and picking up coffee for the entire office, we love turmeric because it does everything from reducing inflammation to clearing up our heads.

Turmeric is a root veggie that belongs to the ginger family, but most of us know it best in its powdered form as a bright yellow spice. Its active flavonoid, curcumin, helps reduce injury-related inflammation and can be just as effective as anti-inflammatory drugs like cortisone. It also alleviates symptoms associated with rheumatoid arthritis and inflammatory bowel disease. And if that weren't enough, curcumin is an amazing antioxidant that protects against free-radical damage and helps prevent tumor formation. It even stimulates liver function.

But I've saved the best for last. Recent research suggests curcumin has neuroprotective properties that may be beneficial in slowing down the progression of neurodegenerative diseases like dementia and Alzheimer's. It does this by reducing the number of amyloid plaques—protein deposits—in the brain. The buildup of these plaques is an inevitable degenerative process that happens to ALL of us as we age, gunking up our brains and decreasing our memory and learning abilities. Studies show that turmeric can reduce the number of these plaques by HALF. Curcumin has also been shown to inhibit the cell death of neurons in mice with Alzheimer's, significantly improving their memory ability.

And remember that neurotransmitter acetylcholine? Well, curcumin has an acetylcholinesterase inhibitory effect. In normal parlance, that means it increases the concentration of acetylcholine in the brain, which enhances memory and is a good thing for everyone.

DID YOU KNOW?

There's a reason why turmeric is the darling of the nutritional world. This sunny little spice packs a lot of punch in the benefits department. In addition to its memory-enhancing qualities, turmeric has anti-inflammatory, antioxidant, anti-cancer, and antimicrobial properties.

Eggs

There's a reason why eggs are a breakfast staple. Egg yolks are one of the richest sources of phosphatidylcholine, which is a precursor to acetylcholine production. For optimal mental function, one to two eggs per day can boost memory. The choline found in eggs can also reduce inflammation, which causes age-related memory decline.

Eggs are especially important for mamas and mamas-to-be. New research suggests that consuming eggs during pregnancy and feeding them to babies (when permitted) can enhance a child's lifelong memory. Why? Eggs' high levels of choline theoretically optimize the birth and death rate of nerve cells in the hippocampus.

But eggs have more to recommend them than phosphatidyl choline. They also have high levels of tryptophan, which promotes the synthesis of serotonin and results in better long-term memory—and long-term happiness.[32]

Sunflower Lecithin

Who doesn't love sunflowers? In case anyone wants to send me some, they're my absolute FAVORITE! They're relentlessly cheerful and their seeds are loaded with phosphatidylcholine, that same precursor to acetylcholine production we love in eggs. And when taken as a daily supplement, sunflower lecithin has been shown to improve memory in the elderly. In fact, it's been found to reduce the incidence of memory lapse in just a few weeks.[33] Studies also suggest that it may help treat verbal memory loss associated with multiple sclerosis.[34]

TIP

Try adding sunflower lecithin in powder form to homemade pancakes, smoothies, or baked goods for memory-boosting brainpower.

Rosemary

Want a quick way to improve your mental acuity *and* add some green to your office? Then get a rosemary plant. Just inhaling its aroma increases blood flow to the brain and makes for a stimulating effect on the mind. Studies show that smelling rosemary improves cognition, memory, alertness, and even performance in speed and accuracy tests.

If it can do all this when you breathe in its aroma, what happens if you eat it? The short answer is that it benefits your memory. The aromatic compounds in rosemary are neuroprotective, playing a role in the prevention of neurodegenerative brain disorders. And its natural antioxidant, rosmarinic acid, helps destroy peroxynitrate, a harmful oxidant that contributes to Alzheimer's-related memory loss.

HOW TO USE

Add rosemary as an aromatic herb to your potatoes, bean dips, or casseroles to awaken your senses—and brain. Or, you can add the essential oil to one of your unscented candles and let it infuse throughout your home (or office!).

Oily Fish

Move over, Einstein. Oily fish—such as salmon, halibut, sardines, and scallops—are loaded in brain-boosting power guaranteed to keep your mind razor sharp. Not only do they help boost your mood, as we talked about in the previous chapter, but they also boost your memory.

Omega-3s help ensure that communication is sent and received between brain cells as quickly and efficiently as possible. They enable you to pull those memory files and information from your brain's data center (hippocampus) to make quick, informed decisions.

Omega-3s' powerful antioxidant and anti-inflammatory properties also help reduce damage to brain cells, slow down the buildup of amyloid plaque, and even mitigate the effect of toxins. Not willing to give up your sweet tooth? Omega-3s can actually help counteract the negative effect sugar has on your brain. (But that's no reason to run for the vending machine. When omega-3s are working hard to mitigate the effects of self-indulgent behavior, it means they can't help other areas of the brain that need work!)

In addition to their omega-3 benefits, fish such as salmon, scallops, and shrimp are rich in memory-boosting choline. Brilliant!

DID YOU KNOW?

Researchers have found that, compared with those who avoided fish, people who ate fish high in omega-3 fatty acids three times or more per week had a nearly 26 percent lower risk of having the silent brain lesions that can cause dementia and stroke.[35]

HOW TO USE

Incorporate fish into your weekly meal plan. Grill it on its own, add it to a pasta or quinoa dish, or wrap it up with sprouts, salsa, and guacamole ... fish tacos, anyone? Always choose wild fish over farmed. Smaller fish, such as sardines, have lower contamination of heavy metals. And if you don't like fish, try taking a daily fish oil supplement, or up your omega-3s by adding sacha inchi, hemp, and chia seeds to your diet.

Red Beets

Red beets are rich in anthocyanin, a phytochemical antioxidant that gives veggies, berries, and other fruits their rich shades of red, blue, and purple. But anthocyanin is more than just a pretty face. This antioxidant protects the brain from oxidative damage and age-related memory decline. Studies show that it actually reverses age-related memory loss, and helps boost cognitive function as well.

Beets are also an excellent source of folate, which is good for lots of things, like your brain. Low folate levels have been linked to cognitive decline and dementia in the elderly.

And one more place beets shine is in nitrates. Red beet juice has a lot of them, which act as vasodilators, thereby increasing blood flow to the brain. This is good, because the more oxygen-rich blood the brain gets, the better it is at processing information and fighting memory loss.

Sacha Inchi Seeds (aka Savi Seeds)

The brain, as I've mentioned, is mostly made up of fat. But before you take that as reason enough to go on a cupcake binge, know that the TYPE of fat is important. Omega-3 fatty acids improve the transmission of neurotransmitters so that information is sent and received efficiently and fluidly, which increases mental acuity and cognitive performance.

Savi Seeds contain the highest plant-based source of omega-3 fatty acids out there! So if you're looking to boost your brainpower, nosh on these. But don't inhale a huge bag of them (which can be really easy to do), since a little goes a long way. Just a single small, one-ounce serving a day packs a powerful punch, providing you with a healthy brain boost of omega-3s.

Savi Seeds are also super high in protein and fiber, which stabilizes blood-sugar levels and provides mental energy, focus, and improved concentration. This—coupled with the fact that they're rich in tryptophan, which converts to mood and memory-boosting serotonin—makes these the perfect snack!

Broccoli

Broccoli boasts a seemingly infinite list of health benefits, but its winning combination of vitamin K and choline is what gives it a brain-boosting A+! Choline helps you retrieve stored memories and thoughts from the brain, while vitamin K helps develop and strengthen cognitive function. And just because it can, broccoli also provides nearly a quarter of your daily folic acid requirement, which translates to unstoppable brain-boosting power.

Wild Blueberries

Remember red beets and their phytochemical antioxidant, anthocyanin? The power-house that reverses age-related memory loss? Well, wild blueberries are rich in antho-cyanin too, which helps reduce inflammation in the brain while boosting cognitive functioning and protecting the brain from short-term memory loss.

Interestingly, blueberries also have polyphenolic compounds that defend against age-related decreases in neuronal function. (Neuronal function declines in all of us as we age; it's what causes our memory, cognition, and motor skills to go.) Scientists aren't sure how the compounds work—they either lower oxidative stress and inflammation or they enhance neuronal signaling—but the good news is that blueberries make an effective weapon against the sort of mental decline most of us dread.

HOW TO USE

Wild blueberries are smaller and contain a higher dose of anthocyanins than regular blueberries (although regular blueberries are still AMAZING!). Eat them on their own, blend them into a smoothie, sprinkle them on salads, add them to baked goods, layer them into a fruit parfait, and mix them into blended frozen bananas for a guilt-free treat!

Walnuts

Don't be creeped out by the fact that these nuts actually look like brains. Instead, con-sider their appearance a friendly reminder to eat them daily for a high-functioning nog-gin. That's right—daily. Sprinkling these guys on your lunchtime salads may improve memory, cognition, and learning over time, thanks to their ability to enhance serotonin metabolism in the brain.

Walnuts are also rich in omega-3 fatty acids, antioxidants, and vitamin E. This translates to improved chemical messenger communication in the brain, protection from oxidative damage, and improved cognitive functioning. Go nuts for them!

Quinoa

To achieve optimal functioning, the brain needs glucose. And the best way to get glucose isn't through sodas and cookies but through complex carbohydrates. Enter quinoa.

Quinoa has slowly but surely earned a faithful following thanks to its many health benefits, one of which is its abundance of B vitamins. (B vitamins are essential for healthy brain function.) Since quinoa is a slow-releasing carb, and since it's also loaded with fiber and protein, it provides stable, energizing fuel for your brain.

PART 2

The Food–Weight Connection

Discover the top nutrients and foods to help
boost your metabolism and keep those muffin tops
and man boobs at bay!

You get up early for a run, watch *Friends* reruns on the elliptical, take the stairs instead of the elevator, eat clean, avoid sugars, and nix extra calories—but you still aren't dropping the pounds. Frustrated, yet unwilling to give up on those barely worn skinny jeans you've had in your closet for years now, you decide to pull yourself together and opt for a plain ol' salad with dressing on the side at your next meal. As you sit there gnawing on your lettuce, out comes this perky, skinny little thing who orders a burger without a flinch of guilt. What's up with that?

The difference between the two of you isn't necessarily the calories you consume, but *how your body responds to the calories you consume.*

In Chapter 8 we'll talk further about how your metabolism is affected by the food you eat. But here I want to shed some light on some sneaky things that could be sabotaging your weight-loss efforts.

Sneaky Seductions
Fat-Free Foods

Ever notice how many fat-free foods have been creeping up on our grocery shelves over the past several years? And that at the same time more and more people are becoming overweight or obese? North Americans are in fact the highest consumers of fat-free foods, but they also have the highest rate of obesity in the world. That's because there's a direct correlation between the increase in fat-free foods and societal weight gain.

When fats are removed from foods, they're typically replaced with excess sodium, refined sugars, artificial sweeteners, and chemical fillers to make the food taste good—all of which contributes to weight *gain.* These foods also tend to have the same number of calories as the fat-free versions, so your body will store any excess calories as fat anyway. And the thing is, our bodies actually need fat. Fat triggers our satiation levels, keeping us fuller longer with smaller amounts of food. And since fat-free varieties don't provide the same level of satiation, we eat approximately 28 percent more calories per day. So it's not the fat content that's the problem—it's all the excess sugar!

Sugar

Sugars are stored in your body as stubborn *fat!* No more than 10 percent of your daily caloric intake should come from sugars. For the average person, this can translate to around 40 to 50 grams. To put things into context, some fat-free, fruit-flavored yogurts can have up to 21 grams of sugar. One cup of 100 percent fruit juice has 25 grams of sugar—half of our recommended daily intake!

As sugars are absorbed into your bloodstream, your blood-sugar level rises. In response the pancreas releases a hormone called insulin, which moves sugar from the blood into your cells, where it can be used as a source of energy. The more refined the sugar, the greater stress on your pancreas, which can eventually lead to weight gain and illnesses like diabetes.

Your body also needs sugar for brain function and for muscle and liver glycogen. However, excess sugar is stored in your cells as fat. Now, glucagon is a hormone that takes the fat out of storage and releases it so that your body can burn it off. But when your body is producing insulin to bring your sugar high down, it can't produce glucagon. The result: not only are you storing extra fat, but your body can't burn the fat that's already stored—double fat whammy!

What's worse is that most fat-free foods contain poor-quality, highly refined sugars like high-fructose corn syrup. Even extremely small dosages have a tremendously negative impact on blood-sugar levels—and make you crave even *more* sugar.

Many high-sugar, fat-storing foods masquerade as "health foods" and should be avoided. These include fruit juice, non-fat fruit-flavored yogurts, breakfast cereals, high/refined-sugar granolas, and sauces like BBQ sauce, ketchup, and teriyaki.

Here's a look at the amount of sugar in some everyday foods. I'll bet some of these will surprise you!

Food Item	Grams of Sugar
Ben & Jerry's vanilla ice cream	16
Starbucks grande latte	17
Subway 6-inch sweet onion teriyaki chicken sandwich	17
Pizza Hut meatball sandwich	20
Organic non-fat yogurt	21
Tropicana 100% orange juice (8 oz.)	25

Food Item	Grams of Sugar
Vitamin water (20 oz. bottle)	33
Oscar Mayer Lunchables (crackers, turkey, cheese)	36
Pizza Hut crispy chicken salad (without dressing!)	37
Coke (1 can)	39

Zero-Calorie Sweeteners

In our effort to avoid sugar, we may reach for artificially sweetened foods and drinks, thinking they'll help shrink our waistline. Not so much. As with fat-free foods, studies show they can actually *expand* our waistline.

Studies have shown that those who drink one can of diet soda a day have a 34 percent higher risk of developing metabolic syndrome and a 41 percent higher risk of becoming overweight and/or obese.[36] In fact, those who drink diet soda have an even greater risk of becoming overweight or obese than the regular, full-sugar soda drinkers! How is this so?

The theory is that artificial sweeteners interfere with the body's hormonal response to foods. The sweet taste tricks our body into thinking we've eaten something sweet, but when the calories aren't there to match up, it starts to crave them—causing us to eat more sweet foods and calories to satisfy the deficit. In a study conducted by Purdue University, rats that ate yogurt sweetened with zero-calorie sweeteners gained more weight and body fat.[37] Artificial sweeteners confuse our hypothalamus. Our innate ability to detect that we've eaten enough becomes inefficient, and so we just keep eating and eating and eating.

In addition, artificial sweeteners like aspartame block the brain's production of serotonin, the feel-good neurotransmitter that also controls appetite. Low serotonin levels trigger the craving for sugar and carbs, foods that increase serotonin levels. Therefore, eating artificial sweeteners will cause us to keep craving—and eating— more sugar and carbs.

What to Do

Choose naturally fat-free foods, such as fruits and veggies, that aren't laced with chemical fillers, refined sugars, and artificial sweeteners. Opt for small amounts of healthy fats like nuts, seeds, extra virgin olive oil, and avocado. These will keep you fuller longer, causing you to eat less and delivering a much higher nutritional punch than artificially created fat-free foods.

Now that you're ditching artificial sweeteners, you may still want a little sweetness from time to time. White or brown sugar may seem like the only options left but don't be fooled; just because they're not synthetically produced, it doesn't mean they're good for you. Although white sugar is derived from the cane or beet plant, all the nutrients and minerals have been stripped away, leaving nothing but a sweet, nutritionally void substance. White sugar is extremely high glycemic, which causes blood sugar imbalances, and is a leading cause of weight gain, obesity and diabetes.

Not only that, but sugar also suppresses the immune system and feeds diseases, viruses, bacteria, and yeasts including candida. And brown sugar's no better; it's just white sugar with added molasses! Although it can be hard to cut out sugar completely, here are some better alternatives to the highly refined white stuff.

Stevia

Stevia is a natural sweetener derived from stevia leaf, an herb native to South America. It is virtually calorie-free and has no impact on blood-sugar levels, making it a great alternative for diabetics, those on sugar-reduced diets, or those watching their weight. It is much sweeter than sugar—about 100 to 400 times—and can have a bitter or pungent aftertaste, so a little goes a long way.

Coconut Palm Sugar (Coconut Palm Nectar)

Coconut sugar is a natural sugar derived directly from the sap of the coconut tree's flower blossoms. The sap is collected, boiled, and crystallized into sugar crystals. It's low on the glycemic index and puts less stress on the liver than agave nectar. It's rich in minerals—magnesium, potassium and zinc—and vitamins B and C. And it tastes delicious! Kind of like caramel or the top of crème brûlée!

Raw Honey

Although honey is higher on the glycemic index, raw honey (not to be confused with the processed honey found in most cupboards) is loaded with nutrients. Raw honey is a thick, cloudy color with a waxlike consistency. Raw honey has anti-microbrial properties and is rich in antioxidants, phytonutrients, and enzymes.

Yacon Syrup

Yacon syrup is a natural, low-calorie sweetener that actually helps to balance blood sugar. It's made primarily of fructooligosaccharide (FOS), which acts as a prebiotic and stimulates colon health, helps increase the absorption of vitamins, and improves healthy intestinal flora. FOS also helps with the absorption of calcium. It can be used as sugar or a molasses substitute in recipes; however, you want to use less than half the amount of yacon, as it has a stronger taste.

7. Estrogen Dominance: Thuttocks and Man Boobs

That big zit you discover before a hot date. The muffin top that even your magic yoga pants can't contain. The mood swing that just sent your assistant running. All these things represent your endocrine system in action. That system is made up of your adrenal, thyroid, and pituitary glands, and is responsible for the manufacturing and distribution of hormones throughout your body. And hormones in turn are largely responsible for your mood, stress response, growth and development, sexual function, tissue function, hunger, fat burning, fat storage, and metabolism. Even the smallest imbalance in your endocrine system can throw your body, energy, emotions, and thoughts into a wicked frenzy.

What Is Estrogen Dominance?

For many, too much estrogen is a surprising cause of weight gain. Estrogens are a group of steroids that act primarily as the female sex hormone—a hormone that supports reproduction and menstruation as well as bone, cardiovascular, and cognitive health. But not all estrogens are created equal. There's the stronger (bad) estrogen and the weaker (good) estrogen.

Our bodies make three kinds of estrogen:

1. Estradiol (E2). The strongest and most prominent estrogen. It's produced in the ovaries and plays a key role in the menstrual cycle. It also stimulates sexual desire and vaginal lubrication, increases bone health, regulates blood sugar, and supports heart health, including cholesterol levels, and mental health. Although it's essential, too much estradiol leads to bad PMS, bloating, water retention, mood swings, and weight gain (so, pretty much hell). An excess of this hormone is also linked to an increased risk of breast cancer.

2. Estrone (E1). A weaker estrogen, yet the least fave. Estrone is produced by the ovaries and adrenal glands, and is also produced and stored in our fat cells, especially during menopause. Estrone is most prevalent in postmenopausal women. The more fat cells we have, the more estrone is produced. It can also increase the risk of breast cancer.

3. Estriol (E3). The weakest and the most fave estrogen. Estriol can block breast and uterine cells from the harmful effects of the "bad" estrogens. Estriol is dominant during pregnancy and is produced in the ovaries, in the placenta during pregnancy, and in the liver through the conversion of estrone and estradiol.

Estrogen isn't just a problem for women. Our bodies, both male and female, are portals of estrogen receptors, into which any type of estrogen can plug itself. The stronger the estrogen that plugs into the receptor site, the more "estrogenic," or estrogen dominant, we become. This isn't a good thing. Estrogen dominance not only contributes to weight gain, but also significantly increases the incidence of uterine, endometrial, and breast cancer. In fact, the National Institute of Environmental Health Sciences has listed estrogen as a known cancer-causing agent.

What Excess Estrogen Does

Excess estrogen can promote increased fat tissue in the waist, belly, and other estrogen-sensitive fat tissues: for men, typically in the belly and chest (man boobs), for women, in the belly, lower butt, and upper thighs (thuttocks), and sometimes in the back of the arms. These fats are called "stubborn fat" due to their high resistance to fat burning.

The birth control pill, aging, hormone replacement therapy, steroids, and excess body weight all contribute to excess estrogen. The more fat tissue a person has, the more estrogen is produced within his or her cells, which promotes more fat gain, which produces more estrogen, which promotes even more fat gain. No wonder we have a hard time losing weight!

As well, certain foods and environmental factors, known as endocrine-disrupting chemicals (EDCs), can actually disrupt the function of the endocrine system and the way the body uses and stores fat. All of us are exposed to estrogenic chemicals on a daily basis, many of which are capable of mimicking estrogen activity in the body.

Outside our bodies lie estrogen-mimicking chemicals: phytoestrogens, which are found in some plant-based foods, and enoestrogens, which are found in our environment.

Estrogen in Food: Phytoestrogens
Soy, What's the Deal?

The controversy surrounding soy can stir up more drama than an episode of *Jersey Shore*. While soy does have acclaimed healthy benefits, excessive amounts of highly processed soy may have the reverse effect. Here are the facts.

Soy contains estrogen-like substances called isoflavones that mimic estrogen in the body. They can increase the amount of estrogen that can bind onto estrogen receptors. How is this a good thing? Research suggests that since soy isoflavones are a "weaker" version of the body's regular estrogen, they may cause less harm binding onto estrogen receptors than the stronger "bad" estrogens kicking around in your body. So some phytoestrogens, like pomegranates and flax, can be highly beneficial in moderate quantities. But excess quantities and concentrations can lead to issues. And why settle for "not as bad" when you can kick it to the curb altogether?

Here's where it gets dirty. Highly processed soy products like soy milk and soy cheese contain concentrated amounts of soy isoflavones, which significantly increases their concentration of estrogenic compounds. For an adult woman, two glasses of soy milk per day is enough to throw off her menstrual patterns. And really, who needs that? In addition, soy contains a compound called goitrogen, which is a thyroid-disrupting chemical. Goitrogen inhibits your thyroid from absorbing iodine from the blood to manufacture and distribute hormones throughout your body, causing your metabolism to slow down. And this, as we know, puts the brakes on fat loss.

SOY, WHAT TO DO?

Since soy is found in over 60 percent of packaged foods, try to limit your consumption of highly processed soy products that have concentrated amounts of soy isoflavones. Instead, try fermented soy products like miso, tempeh, and tamari, which are healthier and easier to digest and assimilate. And try to increase your iodine levels when eating soy or other foods that contain goitrogens. Iodine is found in sea veggies (kelp), shellfish, and sea salt.

Pesticides

About 90 percent of commonly used pesticides found in food and beverages are harmful EDCs. Pesticides can alter your metabolic patterns and promote fat storage, wreaking havoc on your weight-loss goals. Studies show that eating an organic diet for just five days can reduce circulating pesticide EDCs to non-detectable levels.

Here are some of the worst pesticide-laden foods, which means you should choose the organic versions of these foods whenever possible: celery, peaches, strawberries, apples, blueberries, nectarines, sweet bell peppers, spinach, kale/collard greens, cherries, potatoes, and imported grapes.

The following foods aren't highly contaminated with pesticides, so you don't need to buy organic: onions, avocado, sweet corn, pineapples, mango, sweet peas, asparagus, kiwi fruit, cabbage, eggplant, cantaloupe, watermelon, grapefruit, sweet potatoes, and honeydew melon.

Estrogen in the Environment: BPAs and PVCs

We've heard about the dangers of plastics. Bisphenol-A (BPA) and phthalates (PVC), both commonly found in plastics, are compounds that mimic estrogen. Although we don't eat plastic, it's a common container for many of our foods and beverages—and 93 percent of North Americans have detectable levels of BPA in their bodies![39]

How to Kick the Estrogen Habit

So you've been indulging in too many soy lattes and heating your lunch in the same BPA-rich plastic container for the past month, but now you know better! What's a guy or gal to do? Here are some ways to remove excess estrogen from your body.

Indole-3-Carbinol/Diindolylmethane

Indole-3-carbinol (I3C for non-nerds) is a chemical compound created through the cooking and chewing of cruciferous vegetables, which include broccoli, cauliflower, Brussels sprouts, cabbage, turnips, mustard greens, and kale. This compound is then broken down into diindolylmethane (DIM) in the intestinal tract, changing the metabolism of estrogen to a weaker, more beneficial version, making us less estrogenic.

Calcium D-Glucarate

Calcium D-glucarate is a nutrient found in fruits and vegetables, especially apples, oranges, grapefruit, broccoli, cabbage, Brussels sprouts, and alfalfa. It helps to eliminate excess toxins and hormones from your body, preventing them from recirculating into the bloodstream.

Love Your Liver: Milk Thistle and Lemon Water

It's important that estrogen be broken down and excreted or otherwise detoxed from the body to prevent reabsorption. The breakdown of estrogen is metabolized in the liver and passed on to bile or urine. A backed-up liver due to toxins, crap food, or partying like a rock star can put a damper on this process. Simple things like adding a few drops of milk thistle extract to your water once a day can improve its function and help eliminate toxins. Starting your day by drinking a glass of water with half a squeezed lemon can also make a big difference. Take time daily to love your liver, so it can love you back!

Fiber

Fiber not only helps you feel fuller longer but also absorbs and binds onto excess toxins and hormones to help eliminate them from your body. Fiber is found only in plant-based foods, so start noshing on whole grains, veggies, and fruits.

Exercise

Get moving! While exercise burns extra calories and knocks off a few pounds, it also decreases blood estrogen levels and reduces the risk of breast cancer. One study from the National Cancer Institute in the U.S. showed that exercisers who lost more than 2 percent body fat had a 14 percent reduction in estradiol levels, whereas those who lost 2 percent body fat *without* exercise had no reduction in estradiol levels.[40]

Foods That Counteract Estrogen Dominance
Broccoli

Broccoli is an amazing superfood that is good for just about everything. It has tremendous anti-aging benefits and is rich in antioxidants like vitamin C, carotenoids, and lutein, which protects your eyes. It's high in B vitamins, helping to boost mood and lift depression. It's also jacked in fiber, helps protect against cardiovascular disease, and has powerful antiviral, antibacterial, and anti-cancer properties. Numerous studies indicate that it protects against breast cancer and prostate cancer in particular.

Broccoli's power is drawn from DIM, which gives this cruciferous veg its killer anti-cancer and immune-boosting properties. DIM is also what changes the metabolism of estrogen to a weaker, more beneficial form, helping to reduce the severity of the bad estrogens kicking around in our body. Be sure to chew your broccoli well, as it's through mastication that DIM becomes active.

In addition, this low-cal, high-fiber rock star should be your weight-loss BFF, since the fiber will keep you full without adding any extra calories. Broccoli is also rich in calcium (more absorbable calcium than milk!), which is an essential mineral for weight loss. Its high fiber content coupled with its powerful detoxification properties ensures that the bad, excess estrogen is broken down and eliminated from your body.

Green Tea

Green tea is much more than a great sushi companion. Its health benefits stem from its high levels of epigallocatechin gallate (EGCG). EGCG is a polyphenol, a class of phytochemicals found in high concentrations in green tea. These polyphenols are called catechins, and they give green tea its slightly bitter taste. EGCG, the dominant and most important catechin in green tea, is an extremely potent antioxidant. In fact, EGCG appears to be the most powerful of all catechins, with an antioxidant strength estimated to be from 25 to 100 times more potent than both vitamins C and E—which also contributes to its powerful anti-aging and skin-glowing benefits!

EGCG has a long list of amazing health benefits. It can help lower cholesterol levels and increase antioxidants in the blood. Studies have shown that EGCG helps protect against several types of cancer by blocking the action of carcinogens. EGCG in green tea is also very effective in increasing levels of friendly bacteria in the gut and helping regulate and promote bowel health. Green tea also blocks the attachment of the bacteria associated with dental cavities, making it a great post-nosh drink!

The EGCG found in green tea can promote healthy and natural weight loss. The effects aren't immediate, but they can be significant. Green tea can help you lose weight by increasing your metabolic rate and helping to burn fat in the body while reducing the storage of fat. Green tea's calorie-burning properties lie in EGCG's ability to increase heat production (or thermogenesis) by affecting enzymes in the metabolic process and increasing the amount of calories burned throughout the day. *Now that's hot!* And although green tea doesn't produce immediate weight loss, green tea extract has been shown to stimulate fat oxidation and boost the metabolic rate without increasing the heart rate. And a faster metabolism means a slimmer you!

A randomized, controlled trial conducted at Oklahoma State University, in which 35 subjects with obesity consumed either four cups of green tea or two capsules of green tea extract a day over an eight-week period, found that green tea consumption significantly decreased both body weight and BMI (body mass index) compared with the control group.[42]

HOW TO USE

Adding green tea to your daily regimen is a great idea both for weight loss and for all its fantastic health benefits. But since green tea contains caffeine, consuming it regularly in large amounts—or right before bed—isn't necessarily recommended. The polyphenols in green tea are also active in the body, and may interfere with medications you may be taking, so you should consult a physician before prescribing yourself a strict diet of green tea. However, go ahead and drink up in moderation, and enjoy reaping the wide range of health benefits EGCG has to offer.

Maca

Our favorite aphrodisiac from the chapter on sex can also help out in the hormone and weight-loss department. Maca is an adaptogen that helps to balance hormones naturally. It does this by nourishing, strengthening, and balancing the endocrine system including your thyroid, pancreas, and adrenal glands. Each plays an important role in weight loss and while maca doesn't actually affect hormone levels, it helps to improve the communication between receptor cells. In order for the body to function optimally, hormonal communication must be kickin' seamlessly. A balanced thyroid keeps your metabolism burning, and balanced adrenals keep cortisol levels in check. As you'll learn in Chapter 8, excess cortisol and insulin resistance are the main causes of excess belly fat. Plus, maca contains Indol-3-carbinol (I-3-C), which helps reduce the amount of bad, fat-storing estrogen that tends to sabotage weight-loss efforts. Wicked.

8. Metabolism

I try and try but the scale doesn't budge! Sound all too familiar? Your thyroid is directly responsible for your metabolism. Period. It produces two hormones (T3 and T4) that control your body temperature and the rate at which your body uses and expends energy (from carbs, fats, and proteins). The thyroid also regulates your hormones and hormonal communication.

How Your Thyroid Makes You Fat (or Skinny)

It's really quite simple: your thyroid drives your metabolism. When everything's in balance, it cruises along at a consistent speed. But when it gets out of whack—from things like poor nutrition or stress—your metabolism comes to a grinding halt that's worse than Friday afternoon traffic before a long weekend.

Here's a quick run-through of how it all works:

- Your pituitary gland is an endocrine gland, about the size of a pea, that sits in the base of the brain. The pituitary gland helps control many body processes, one being thyroid gland function.
- Your hypothalamus is an area at the base of your brain that acts as a thermostat for your whole system. The hypothalamus signals your pituitary gland to make a hormone called thyroid-stimulating hormone (TSH).

- Your pituitary gland then releases TSH—the amount depends on how much T4 (thyroxine) and T3 (triiodothyronine) are in your blood.
- Your thyroid gland regulates its production of hormones based on the amount of TSH it receives.
- Although this process usually works well, the thyroid sometimes fails to produce enough hormones.

To keep your thyroid performing at its peak, some nutrients are must-haves and others are must-avoids.

Iodine

Even the slightest dip in thyroid levels can send your metabolism to a crashing halt. For your thyroid to function optimally it needs to absorb iodine from your blood, which enables it to manufacture and distribute hormones throughout your body. If adequate amounts of iodine aren't absorbed, your thyroid and metabolism become sluggish, and you can kiss precious fat-burning goodbye.

Goitrogens

Goitrogens are naturally occurring substances that can interfere with the function of the thyroid gland. If you suffer from a sluggish thyroid, it's best to avoid raw foods containing goitrogens. But many of these foods are necessary staples in the food connection to vibrant health, so don't cut them out altogether! Instead, I would suggest eating them cooked instead of raw, as cooking will destroy goitrogens (and remember, this is only necessary if you have a sluggish thyroid).

Foods containing goitrogens:
- All soy products
- All raw cruciferous vegetables: broccoli, Brussels sprouts, cabbage, cauliflower, kale, kohlrabi, mustard, rutabaga, and turnips
- Millet
- Peanuts
- Radishes
- Spinach
- Strawberries
- Peaches

Foods That Help Support Thyroid Function
Kelp

Kelp is a sea veggie that gives you the best of both worlds: it satisfies your salt cravings while being low in sodium and packing a huge nutritional punch! It contains over 70 proteins, growth hormones, vitamins, enzymes, trace elements, and minerals, including potassium, magnesium, calcium, and iron. Kelp is also a rich source of iodine, which is critical for healthy thyroid function. So kelp can not only help you overcome iodine deficiencies, it also boosts metabolism, helping you shed some unwanted pounds. In addition, kelp is extremely alkaline, which supports the body's pH balance and improves overall health.

There's more: kelp helps boost energy levels and aids in digestion. The latter is key because undigested food particles become toxic, and fat binds onto toxins, making them harder to get rid of. And, of course, proper digestion helps your body assimilate nutrients, keeping you satisfied (and away from that bag of chips).

HOW TO USE
The saltiness of kelp granules makes them a great salt substitute—especially if you have high blood pressure or are trying to reduce your sodium intake. You can use them in soups, sauces, dressings, salads, and pastas, or to season any dish that requires salt. Kelp can also be taken as a supplement in tablet, capsule, liquid, or powder form. And you can purchase kelp noodles: at only 12 calories per cup, these make for a stellar skinny substitution!

Other foods rich in iodine:
- Sea vegetables
- Sea salt
- Fish
- Shellfish
- Eggs

Cayenne Pepper

This hot little number does a whole lot more than just spice up your meals—cayenne is increasingly seen as a miracle herb. Cayenne pepper, or *Capsicum annum*, is part of the nightshade family; its cousins include bell peppers and jalapenos. Its main ingredient is called capsaicin, which offers a plethora of important health benefits.

One of the most widely acclaimed of these benefits is its role in weight loss. Yes, that's right! The capsaicin in these peppers can burn extra calories in a way similar to

exercise. When taken regularly, cayenne pepper helps facilitate weight loss by incre
ing the body's metabolism. Cayenne is an active stimulant that increases blood flow,
which results in increased energy in the body. Increased energy comes from the almost
immediate strength the heart receives from the cayenne, which means it has to pump
less and leaves your body feeling energized.

DID YOU KNOW?

In a double-blind, placebo-controlled trial at the University of Maryland School of
Medicine, researchers studied the effects of capsaicin on metabolism and weight loss
in 40 men and 40 women over a period of 12 weeks. The capsinoid group showed a
decrease of abdominal fat that was not seen in the placebo group. Results showed that
capsinoid ingestion was also associated with a significant increase in fat oxidation.[43]

It's necessary to emphasize, though, that cayenne won't magically cause weight
loss; rather, it acts as a catalyst for weight loss to occur. Alongside a healthy balanced
diet and an active lifestyle, regular use of cayenne pepper can be a fantastic tool to help
increase metabolism and facilitate weight loss.

Cayenne pepper also has amazing benefits for the circulatory system, feeding the
veins and arteries, reducing blood pressure, cleansing the arteries, and helping rid
the body of "bad" LDL cholesterol. Capsaicin acts as a counter-irritant, bringing up
and carrying away blood toxins as well as reducing pain and inflammation. In fact,
the heat from capsaicin increases our feel-good endorphins—the same ones that are
released after an orgasm and that give us "runner's high" after a great workout. When
endorphins are released, they numb our pain receptors, reducing physical aches and
pains.

Cayenne supports digestive function, stimulating peristalsis movement in the
stomach and intestines and helping our bodies to properly assimilate nutrients and
eliminate efficiently. Believe it or not, cayenne is also thought to heal tissues of the
stomach when an ulcer is present, and its heat can do wonders to warm and soothe
the body internally.

Cayenne water has been proven to actually stop a heart attack or hemorrhaging
within 10 seconds of ingestion. Although the mechanism isn't completely understood,
its importance for heart health can't be overstated. In fact, a cayenne pepper drink
taken regularly is believed to significantly improve heart health and blood flow.

Yerba Maté

Yerba maté is a South American herb and a member of the holly family. It's rich in nutrients, including B vitamins; vitamins A, C, and E; the minerals calcium, magnesium, iron, potassium, and selenium; and powerful antioxidants. Yerba maté could also be beneficial as a weight-loss aid: researchers found a thermogenic effect in healthy individuals who took this herb, indicating a rise in the proportion of fat burned as energy.[44]

9. Insulin Resistance: Muffin Tops

Sick of using wide belts and tunics to hide that extra midsection bulge hanging over the top of your jeans? Or, even worse, the horror of your hottie putting his arm around your "love handle" only to find more than he bargained for? Fear no more, my friend. Off with the muffin top!

The two main contributors to belly fat are excess cortisol and insulin resistance. We're going to look at insulin resistance here; for more information on excess cortisol and tips on how to correct it, refer to Chapter 2 on stress—it's the same deal.

What Is Insulin Resistance?

Insulin is a hormone responsible for moving sugar (glucose) from the bloodstream and storing it as glycogen within the muscles and liver so that it can be used as a source of energy. As sugars are absorbed into the bloodstream through diet and the digestion of carbohydrates, blood-sugar levels rise. To lower these levels the pancreas releases insulin, which moves sugar from the blood into the cells. The more refined the sugar, the greater the stress on the pancreas.

How Excess Insulin Makes Us Fat

It's no secret that sugar causes weight problems and is linked to obesity, illness, diabetes, cardiovascular disease, and mental health disorders. Although we need some sugar to function, too much can lead to big trouble. Once insulin is released, sugar is first used for immediate energy, particularly within your brain. Then it's stored in your muscles, and then in your liver. Whatever is left over is stored in your fat cells as, well, fat—especially in the tummy, causing the dreaded muffin top. If that's not bad enough, insulin also shuts off our precious fat-burning hormones, such as glucagon and human growth hormone (HGH).

Glucagon takes the fat out of storage and releases it so that our bodies can burn it for energy. HGH is responsible for growth, cell production, and cell regeneration. It helps to build lean muscle and burn fat, and has superior anti-aging benefits. We love HGH! But when your pancreas is pumping out insulin in response to too much sugar, your body blocks the release of HGH and can't produce glucagon—two of the things that help us fight fat the most. So you end up storing extra fat while thwarting your body's attempts to burn it off at the same time.

The Lowdown on Sugar

If you need more reasons to kick your sugar and refined-carb habits, get a load of these:

- Sugar feeds bacteria, yeast, and candida, and contributes to both low blood sugar and high blood sugar. It also weakens the immune system and feeds diseases like cancer.
- Overconsumption of sugar may also lead to constant fatigue (physical and mental), headaches, fast heartbeats, aches, muscular pains, shakes, loss of consciousness, paralysis, troubled vision, and alcoholism.
- Hypoglycemia—low blood sugar brought on by too much insulin production—causes irritability, nervousness, moodiness, anxiety, fears and phobias, perception troubles, memory losses, and concentration problems.

How Insulin Resistance Happens

Remember, insulin isn't the enemy; it's required to move sugar from the blood into muscle and liver cells. But when your body is constantly circulating *excess* insulin, over time the cells get so used to it they start to ignore the fact that it's there. As the cells become less sensitive, their uptake of glucose from the blood declines.

Think of it as online dating. The first time you try it you think, "Wow! This is great!" Potential suitors are knocking on your inbox one after the other, and with each profile seeming to be the perfect catch, you eagerly open each message as soon as it gets delivered. But after months of going on random dates, either you find that special person who rocks your world (congrats to you) or, more likely, you want to throw your iPad out the freakin' window every time that annoying ping reminds you of a new match arriving in your inbox. The appeal has obviously worn off. You ignore them, and now unread messages are flooding your inbox. Joy.

Insulin works the same way. Cells become less "eager and excited" by insulin's constant presence. Blood glucose levels remain high, since the cells can't be bothered to take in some of the insulin knocking at the door. In an attempt to manage the blood glucose levels, the pancreas creates even more insulin and starts to get flooded, like your inbox of unread messages. Your cells resist the insulin completely, hence the term *insulin resistance*. Once this happens, losing weight becomes a nightmare.

Foods That Chop the Muffin Top
Yacon Syrup

Who would think a sweetener could help you lose weight? But it can! In fact, this sweetener can actually lower your body mass index, reduce blood-sugar levels, and shrink your waist circumference. It's also rich in potassium and antioxidant vitamins A, C, and E.

Yacon syrup is extracted from the tuberous root of the yacon plant, native to Peru. Yacon root resembles a sweet potato, but has a much more fruity taste, although it's low in sugar and calories. And its blood sugar–lowering properties make it not only safe but also beneficial for diabetics.

DID YOU KNOW?

A 2009 study published in the *European Journal of Clinical Nutrition* indicated that yacon syrup demonstrated positive effects on obese, premenopausal women with insulin resistance. Over a 120-day, double-blind, placebo-controlled trial, obese and slightly dyslipidemic (containing an abnormal amount of fat and/or cholesterol in the blood) premenopausal women who were given yacon syrup every day had a significant decrease in body weight, waist circumference, body mass index, and serum insulin levels. In addition, it helped increase satiety, helping them to feel fuller longer.[47]

The rock star properties mainly come from yacon syrup's high concentration of fructooligosaccharide (FOS), which acts as a prebiotic fiber and stimulates colon health by improving intestinal flora. Because it's not digested, fiber is our fat-loss BFF, as it gives us the full feeling without any calories. And since 30 to 50 percent of this sweetener is FOS, up to half of it can't be absorbed into the body, making it naturally low-cal and low-glycemic. FOS also helps with the absorption of calcium, another great weight-loss aid.

HOW TO USE

Yacon syrup has a thick, fruity, molasses-y taste and makes an awesome substitute for sugar or molasses in recipes, teas, cereals, oatmeal ... or anywhere you can use a little sweetness in your life. However, because it has a pretty strong taste (and is slightly on the pricey side), you'll want to use less than you normally would with regular sugar or sweeteners.

Cinnamon

Cinnamon is a great way to add a little sweetness to your life, helping to nix the muffin top sans the calories. This naturally sweet spice is found in the inner bark of the cinnamon tree. It has exquisite antimicrobial and antibacterial properties, and is also a great source of calcium, fiber, manganese, iron, and antioxidants.

Cinnamon's innate sweetness can not only replace sugar in your meals but also lower the glycemic index of your food by stimulating your cells' insulin receptors, increasing their ability to absorb glucose and effectively lowering blood glucose levels. A study led by Pakistani researchers indicated that half a teaspoon (or one gram) of cinnamon a day can lower blood-sugar levels in type 2 diabetics by 20 percent. After the 40-day study period, not only were fasting glucose levels lowered, but so were triglycerides, "bad" LDL cholesterol, and total cholesterol levels.[48] In cooperation with the Beltsville Human Nutrition Research Center at the USDA, Richard Anderson, who was part of that study, went on to research the effects of cinnamon in 22 obese subjects who were classified as pre-diabetic. He concluded that water-soluble antioxidants found in cinnamon improved antioxidant levels by 13 to 23 percent, which correlates to a reduction in fasting glucose levels and aids in weight loss.[49] As well, cinnamon is known to increase the body's thermogenic properties, temporarily boosting metabolism. The water-soluble antioxidant also has anti-inflammatory properties.

Want to know what else? Cinnamon sticks are the perfect thing for getting rid of bad breath! They're antibacterial, and the most effective way to eliminate bad breath is to kill the sulfur-producing bacteria that's causing the odor. Besides the fresh taste cinnamon leaves in your mouth, it's naturally calorie- and sugar-free. A cinnamon stick is easy to stash in your purse for when you want to freshen up: keep some pieces in a mint container and just pop one in your mouth! Plus, the sucking and chewing will stimulate saliva flow, which helps to wash out the odor-causing bacteria.

HOW TO USE
Sprinkle ground cinnamon on your favorite dishes, use it as a natural sweetener in your coffee or tea, or add it to breakfast cereals or a baked sweet potato or squash. Try baking some apple slices sprinkled with cinnamon for a guilt-free treat.

Chia Seeds

Cha-cha-cha chia! Yep, I'm talking about the same seeds that grow on that odd-looking eighties-retro Chia Pet plant. But lo and behold, it doesn't only grow on your countertop. Chia (*Salvia hispanica*) is a plant native to Mexico and Central America. Its seeds are one of the world's highest plant-based sources of fiber (with four times more fiber than flax!), making it an amazing weight-loss aid and blood-sugar stabilizer.

Chia seeds are a good source of omega-3 fatty acids (which also aid in weight loss) as well as a plethora of antioxidants and other nutrients, such as calcium and iron. Its high concentration of insoluble fiber soaks up fluids like a sponge, increasing satiety levels and keeping you fuller longer. Fiber slows down the absorption of carbohydrates and improves the intake of sugar by cells and tissues. This helps balance blood-sugar levels and wards off cravings. Fiber also lowers cholesterol levels, boosts heart health, pulls toxins from your body, and improves digestive health. And as the toxins are eliminated, they take fat with them!

Chia seeds are also rich in protein, which delays hunger and has thermogenic properties, requiring more energy to be burned. Remember, your body craves nutrients, NOT calories! And because chia seeds are so nutritionally dense, your body won't be left craving more.

Bilberries

Bilberry is the euro-chic relative of the Westernized blueberry. Closely resembling wild blueberries, bilberries are smaller in size but have a darker interior flesh due to their high-antioxidant anthocyanin pigments. In addition to their antioxidant, anti-inflammatory, skin-loving, belly-bloat-busting properties, bilberries have been used traditionally to balance blood-sugar levels and even treat diabetes.

Bilberry is an extremely rich source of chromium, a mineral that helps maintain normal blood-sugar and insulin levels and reduce carb cravings. Studies have shown that those who supplemented with chromium had the largest reduction in carb cravings. Bilberry leaves are particularly rich in tannins and myrtillin, a compound that also controls blood-sugar levels.

Romaine Lettuce

Romaine lettuce not only makes a great salad staple, but can actually help shrink your muffin top! Its secret ingredient? Chromium. This mineral is key in carbohydrate and fat metabolism. Not only that, but it helps reduce sugar cravings!

Chromium plays a lead role in controlling blood-sugar levels and is the active component in the body's glucose tolerance factor (GTF), which essentially helps fulfill insulin's mission in life—bringing glucose to cells to be used up for energy. Chromium lights a fire under your insulin receptors' ass, so instead of resisting insulin, they actually increase their uptake, helping stabilize and lower blood-sugar levels. This is especially key in the prevention and treatment of type 2 diabetes. Plus, it curbs weight gain and visceral fat (the harmful fat that hugs your organs).

> **TIP**
> For those who are insulin resistant, 200 to 400 milligrams of chromium is recommended per day, which may be best to take in supplement form.

And if you're the type that has a secret love affair with carbs and fats—especially during those "emotional eating" times—chromium can kick those crazy cravings to the curb too! A study published in the *Journal of Psychiatric Practice* indicated that when those who suffered from event-driven mood swings (i.e., atypical depression) supplemented with chromium, they experienced a decrease in appetite and overeating, reduced carbohydrate cravings, and fewer mood swings.[51] So you can kiss that tub of ice cream goodbye.

These crispy leafy greens are a great source of dietary fiber. Three cups of romaine contain 12 percent of your daily recommended intake, helping to slow down and stabilize blood-sugar levels and supporting proper digestion, elimination, and weight control. Romaine lettuce is also high in vitamins A, C, K, and folate, which are all essential vitamins and minerals for the body.

Manganese is an important trace mineral found abundantly in romaine lettuce. Like chromium, it plays a role in maintaining healthy blood-sugar levels in the body, and acts to prevent or treat type 2 diabetes.

Other foods rich in manganese:

- Kale
- Collard greens
- Chard
- Spinach
- Mustard greens
- Raspberries
- Pineapples

Although romaine lettuce is one of the richest sources of plant-based chromium, four cups accounts for only 26 percent of your required daily intake. So combine it with other sources of chromium, which include onions and ripe tomatoes as well as whole grains, oysters, and potatoes.

Other foods high in chromium:

- Onions
- Brewer's yeast
- Sweet potato
- Garlic
- Broccoli
- Green beans
- Potatoes
- Basil

HOW TO USE

Not only does romaine make for a great Caesar salad, but the crisp romaine leaves are a fun and super slimming substitution for taco shells, sandwich wrappers, and dippers for hummus, guacamole, salsa, and canapés. Try filling a romaine leaf with hummus, salsa, Kalamata olives, and sprouts for a satiating, fiber-rich snack.

PART 3

The Food–Beauty Connection

The secret to the fountain of youth is found right in your fridge. Let the Kitchen Beautician in you shine through and discover all the tips and tricks for a clear, glowing complexion; smooth, supple skin; and shiny, lustrous locks!

Do you want to glow? Here's the first thing you can do for a radiant, flawless complexion. Walk into your bathroom. Grab your most expensive synthetic, over-the-counter anti-wrinkle cream and throw it out. Yes, I said throw it out. Some of these toxic anti-aging creams may contain a few "effective" compounds, but they're also laced with chemical solvents that do more damage than good. And do you know what kind of damage? Wrinkle-causing ones! Yes, anti-wrinkle creams can actually *cause* wrinkles! The chemical ingredients that make up these expensive products can stress the skin. An allergic or anti-inflammatory response can occur, causing free-radical damage. The result: premature aging.

But that's not all. These toxic, perfumed skin (and hair) care products can also disrupt the endocrine system, wreak havoc on hormones, cause diseases such as cancer, and lead to weight gain. It's not just that extra scoop of ice cream you need to worry about; your shampoo could also be making you fat.

The following two pages list a sample of a few toxic chemicals to avoid and the effects they have on your health. For more specifics, the Environmental Working Group (www.ewg.org/skindeep) ranks the safety of over 78,000 beauty products. Give yours a go to see how they stack up.

Chemical	Why It's Used	Products Found In	Health Impact
Parabens methylparaben, propylparaben, and butylparaben; any ingredient ending in "paraben"	Used as preservatives	Cosmetics Shampoos/ conditioners Moisturizers Shaving foam Toothpaste Sunscreen lotion	Estrogen-mimicking chemicals disrupt the endocrine system/hormones; may cause things like • Breast cancer (found in breast cancer tumors) • Uterine cancer • Prostate cancer • Estrogen-dominant weight gain
Sodium lauryl sulfate (SLS) Sodium laureth sulfate (SLES)	A foaming agent used in cleaning products; it makes products foam, lather, and bubble	Shampoos Soaps Face cleansers Toothpaste Bubble bath	• Damages the skin and causes rashes, irritation, and inflammation • Can cause eye irritations • Inhalation of SLS can irritate the respiratory tract and induce coughing
Petrochemicals, mineral oil, petroleum, petrolatum, paraffin	An inexpensive oil used in skin products	Cosmetics Creams Ointments Baby lotion Vaseline	• Clogs pores and inhibits skin from perspiring • Mineral oil, a byproduct of making crude oil into gasoline, could contain carcinogens

(Continued)

Chemical	Why It's Used	Products Found In	Health Impact
Phthalates All chemicals with the suffix "phthalate," including dibutylphthalate (DBP), dimethylphthalate (DMP), and diethylphthalate (DEP)	Act as solvents and make products more flexible	Nail polish Hair spray Cosmetics Perfume Skin creams	Endocrine disruptor can be linked to • Low sperm count • Low testosterone production • Breast cancer • Liver damage • Decreased kidney function • Respiratory distress
Synthetic fragrances	Used to add scent to products; any synthetic fragrance contains phthalates	Shampoos/ conditioners Cosmetics Creams Cleansers Moisturizers	• Some synthetic fragrances can contain phthalates (look for products containing natural fragrance or essential oils) • Common allergen
PEG polyethylene, polyethylene glycol, polyoxyethylene	Petroleum-based chemicals serve as emulsifiers, thickeners, solvents, cream bases, and skin conditioners; used in cleansers to dissolve oil and grease	Shampoos/ conditioners Skin cream Lubricants Toothpaste	• Reduces skin's natural moisture and increases appearance of aging • May contain the carcinogenics ethylene oxide and 1,4-dioxane • Can irritate damaged skin
Triclosan/ Triclocarban	Adds antimicrobial properties to soap	Liquid/bar soaps Toothpaste Shaving cream	• Disrupts endocrine system, thyroid function, and hormones

This doesn't mean you need to throw hygiene out the window (please, don't). Manufacturers are smartening up: some amazing beauty products are on the market these days that are full of natural beauty-boosting goodness and free of all the toxic crap. Choose those! Check out some of my faves in the Resources section at the back of the book. And for a self-indulgent treat, I've equipped you with tons of DIY beauty products with ingredients found in your kitchen. See, I've got your back.

Beauty really does come from within. I'm not just talking about the nutrients (or lack thereof) you put inside your body, but also what goes on in your thoughts—your mental state, your attitude toward yourself, your body image. Nothing radiates more beauty than pure happiness, being filled with love, and most important, the love of self. And, as we've seen in the previous chapters, food *does* affect all this. So to look glam on the outside, you need to start by feeling glam on the inside. Sure, you can use a good bronzer, but what happens when you're watching a rom-com with your sweetie and tears begin to trickle down your face, washing away that sun-kissed glow? You turn into a hot mess. Not feeling so fab then, are ya?

Nourish your body inside and out and watch those worry lines soften, skin glow, eyes brighten, and your natural beauty shine through!

10. Beauty and Anti-Aging

What you see on the outside directly reflects what goes on inside you. Our body is made up of trillions of cells, and over time these cells accumulate free-radical damage. This damage results from many factors, including metabolism, poor diet, environment, pollution, UV rays, stress, allergies, pesticides, radiation, and overexertion. All of these things can cause the atoms or molecules that make up a cell to become unstable, which leads to premature aging and diseases such as cancer and heart disease.

Free Radicals vs. Antioxidants

Free-Radical Damage

Here's how free-radical damage works: when a cell oxidizes—that is, when it comes into contact with another substance, typically (but not always) oxygen—it loses an electron, leaving it with an unpaired electron and thereby making it unstable. Because it's missing an electron, the molecule will scavenge your body, trying to either steal an electron to complete its pair or dump an extra electron it has no room for. Once a molecule either loses or gains an electron, the chemical structure changes and damage occurs. If free radicals go unchecked, they damage cells and can even alter DNA— mutating or deforming your genetic blueprint.

To illustrate, let's say you're almost finished a jigsaw puzzle when you realize that one of the pieces is missing. Annoyed that this beautiful picture has a gaping hole right in the middle, and blanketed by a feeling of defeat, you decide to take a jigsaw piece from a totally different puzzle sitting in your closet. You squeeze it right in there. Of course it doesn't fit properly, and totally distorts the image of your puzzle, but at least it's complete. So you feel a tiny dose of accomplishment.

But now the other puzzle is incomplete. So when it comes time to start (and finish) that puzzle, the same sequence of events occurs. One puzzle will always have a missing piece, and each puzzle's image will get distorted.

This is what happens to your cells. If an atom or molecule loses an electron, it becomes unstable. During this process, oxidative damage occurs and the cell begins to break down. So it becomes highly reactive, and begins the process of hunting down an electron from other cells in your body. A vicious chain reaction occurs, causing widespread cellular disruption, oxidation, breakdown, and damage.

Antioxidant Prevention

Antioxidants prevent oxidation by neutralizing free radicals. They do this by taking up the space of the missing electron, making it complete (like the missing puzzle piece that magically appears without having to ruin the other puzzles). However, once these antioxidants give up one of their own electrons, they become inactive, which is why we need to consistently add them to our diet. They help by donating themselves to the cells within our body (such as skin, muscles, heart, liver), keeping them intact. How sweet!

These chain-breaking antioxidants include vitamin A (beta carotene), vitamin C (ascorbic acid), vitamin E, phytochemicals found in plant-based foods, ubiquinone, uric acid, and preventative-type enzymes like superoxide dismutase, catalase, and glutathione peroxidase. These work by destroying free radicals and making them "passive" so that they don't react.

Key Nutrients for Looking Your Best
Vitamin C (Ascorbic Acid)

Vitamin C firms and tones up the skin. It prevents free-radical damage, protects your skin cells, and slows down the appearance of aging by preventing wrinkles. It's required for collagen production, as well as for the protection of collagen fibers that keep skin firm. Collagen is a protein molecule that makes up the dermis. It acts as the skin's foundation and determines its firmness: the stronger the network of collagen fibers, the firmer the skin.

Foods rich in vitamin C:

- Kakadu plums
- Camu camu
- Rosehips
- Sea-buckthorn
- Guava
- Black currants
- Red peppers
- Parsley
- Kiwis
- Broccoli

Vitamin E

Vitamin E keeps moisture in the skin and protects the oils in the skin's moisture barrier from free-radical damage. It soothes dry skin and can minimize the appearance of wrinkles when applied topically. Vitamin E also reduces the effects of sun exposure on the skin and can help prevent skin cancer.

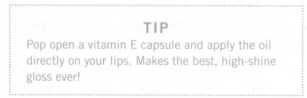

TIP

Pop open a vitamin E capsule and apply the oil directly on your lips. Makes the best, high-shine gloss ever!

Foods high in vitamin E:

- Sunflower seeds
- Almonds
- Walnuts
- Mustard greens
- Swiss chard
- Spinach
- Collard greens
- Tomatoes
- Turnip greens
- Avocados
- Mangoes
- Pine nuts

Vitamin A

Vitamin A helps normalize oil production in the skin and fights acne and inflammation. It also revitalizes the skin by increasing cell turnover and encouraging new skin cell growth. Eating real-food sources of vitamin A or beta carotene (a precursor to vitamin A) is the best way to ingest this nutrient. Too much vitamin A (in supplement form) can have negative health implications and increase your risk of hip fractures.

Foods high in vitamin A:

- Sweet potatoes
- Pumpkins
- Carrots
- Red peppers
- Spinach
- Kale
- Collards
- Watercress
- Turnip greens

Carotenoids

Carotenoids are strong antioxidants that protect against free-radical damage, provide anti-aging benefits, and enhance the immune system. There are roughly 50 different carotenoids. Here are a few:

Lycopene, the bright red carotenoid, acts as a natural sunscreen to protect the skin from UV damage, which causes free radicals and results in wrinkles, dry skin, and sun spots. Lycopene also helps build our skin-firming collagen.

> **TIP**
> For best absorption, combine foods high in lycopene, like tomatoes, watermelon, and papaya, with foods containing healthy fats, like extra virgin olive oil, nuts, and avocado.

Beta carotene, the most popular carotenoid, converts in the body to retinol, which is an active form of vitamin A. It has strong anti-aging benefits and protects against oxidative stress and UV damage. Beta carotene also enhances immune function and is known to help with male reproductive health. It provides the yellow-to-red pigments found in foods.

Lutein, another carotenoid, is excellent for eye health. Foods rich in lutein include spinach, chlorella, and kale, so load up on those greens if you want to keep your eyes shining bright.

Polyphenolic Antioxidants

Anthocyanins are powerful antioxidants that provide the deep red, purple, and blue pigments found in plant-based foods; they're also what give berries their claim to fame. They slow down the aging process—not only physically, but also mentally by keeping the brain sharp and preventing neurological decline. Plus, they boast amazing anti-cancer properties and protect against diabetes.

Foods high in anthocyanins:

- Purple corn
- Chokeberries
- Black raspberries
- Wild blueberries
- Red grapes
- Cherries
- Black currants
- Raspberries

Resveratrol has anti-aging, anti-cancer, and anti-inflammatory benefits, and can help control blood-sugar levels. It's found in the skin of red grapes, and becomes most active during fermentation, making red wine the highest source. Wahoo!

Polyphenols are antioxidants with amazing health benefits. Red grapes, black currants, green tea, and red wine are all great sources.

Selenium

Selenium aids in the production of the antioxidant enzyme glutathione, which repairs cell damage and slows down the skin's aging process. Selenium also supports the elasticity of our tissues and protects against sunburn and skin cancer.

Foods rich in selenium:

- Brazil nuts
- Tuna
- Oysters
- Crimini mushrooms
- Mustard seeds
- Barley
- Oats

Zinc

Remember zinc, our super sex-drive-boosting nutrient? Zinc helps you not only feel good, but look good too! It's essential in the creation of new skin cells and aids in protein synthesis and collagen formation. It controls the production of oil in the skin and adds color and brightness to the complexion. Got an acne problem? Acne is often a sign of zinc deficiency. So if you want clear, bright skin, get more zinc in your diet. It'll have you looking 10 types of adorable.

Zinc-rich foods:

- Oysters
- Clams
- Wheat germ
- Sesame seeds

- Pumpkin seeds
- Crimini mushrooms
- Spinach
- Summer squash

- Cocoa powder
- Miso
- Maple syrup

Copper

Copper is one of the most abundant minerals in our body, and along with zinc and manganese, it's essential in the production of superoxide dismutase—the enzyme found in the skin that repairs all damage caused by free radicals and produces skin-building cells. It also aids in the production of collagen and is what gives color to hair, skin, and eyes. A copper deficiency could cause premature graying, so you might want to swap your hair dye for some copper-rich foods.

Foods rich in copper:

- Crimini mushrooms
- Sesame seeds
- Cashews
- Quinoa
- Miso

- Chickpeas
- Turnip greens
- Swiss chard
- Spinach
- Mustard greens

- Asparagus
- Walnuts
- Olives

DID YOU KNOW?

Adding more copper-rich foods to your diet may help prevent and treat graying hair!

Silica

Silica is a trace mineral essential for healthy skin. It strengthens connective tissues, tendons, cartilage, muscles, hair, and nails. Silica improves your skin's elasticity and helps repair wounds. The best sources of silica are extracts derived from bamboo or horsetail. If horsetail's not your thing, try these other suggestions!

Foods rich in silica:

- Leeks
- Cucumber skin
- Green beans
- Chickpeas
- Strawberries

Omega-3 Fatty Acids

We covered omega-3s in detail in Chapter 5, so you know how good they can be for boosting your mood. But omega-3s also help slow down the aging process and restore moisture to dry skin.

Foods rich in omega-3s:

- Wild salmon
- Anchovies
- Algae
- Sacha inchi seeds
- Flax
- Chia seeds
- Walnuts

Foods That'll Make You Look Smokin' Hot
Goji Berries

Goji berries (also known as wolfberries) are one of the most beautifying fruits around. They're like a makeover for your whole body—inside and out! Start adding this super-food to your diet and watch the transformation begin.

Goji berries are among the highest antioxidant-containing foods. They're thought to help fight heart disease, defend against cancer and diabetes, strengthen the immune system, improve vision, and enhance the complexion. Their claim to fame is their high concentration of carotenoids, in particular beta carotene and zeaxanthin, both of which are essential for eye health and night vision (as well, beta carotene converts into antioxidant vitamin A, which helps treat acne). Goji berries are also rich in polysaccharides. These polysaccharides, in combination with the goji berry's exceptionally high source of antioxidant vitamin C, help strengthen the immune system and prevent age-induced free-radical damage. One of the polysaccharides in particular appears to stimulate the pituitary gland's secretion of HGH (human growth hormone), which not only helps keep your skin young and firm, but also increases lean muscle mass and aids in fat loss.

Goji berries' therapeutic applications include relieving fatigue, promoting visual health, protecting against diabetes, enhancing male sexual function, and supporting a healthy life span. They contain 18 amino acids—including all the essential ones. And as a rich protein source, goji berries are great for healthy-looking hair. They also contain 21 trace minerals and are rich in B vitamins and vitamin E. Goji berries have been traditionally regarded as a longevity- and strength-building food—and no wonder!

HOW TO USE

Goji berries are a tiny dried fruit with a tart taste. Toss them into oatmeal, cereals, or muffin and cookie recipes. They can be rehydrated in water and blended into a purée to be drizzled on your favorite treat (try some over a sliced-up mango) or stirred into yogurt. They can also be added to boiling water and steeped into a tea.

Camu Camu Berries

The camu camu tree, grown in the rainforests of Peru, produces a powerful little fruit called the camu camu berry. Camu camu berries are one of the world's richest plant-based sources of antioxidant vitamin C, which helps with collagen formation. Collagen is the protein that gives your skin its structure, elasticity, and tautness—in other words, youthfulness. Camu camu is also rich in antioxidants and flavonoids, both of which help prevent the free-radical damage that causes premature aging and disease. In addition, the vitamin C in camu camu is great for boosting the immune system and keeping you healthy and radiant inside and out!

HOW TO USE

Camu camu can be found in powder or supplement (capsule) form. The powder can be blended into smoothies or even applied topically. Because vitamin C is best used topically for the synthesis of collagen production in the skin, you can blend camu camu powder with coconut oil or extra virgin olive oil. Gently massage the mixture into your skin then wipe off with a damp cloth.

Olives/Extra Virgin Olive Oil

Olives aren't just for martinis! Olives (and extra virgin olive oil) are one of the healthiest fruits around—and one of the best-kept beauty secrets. Their high-antioxidant, antiviral, antibacterial, anti-inflammatory, antifungal properties treat a large number of diseases and ailments, including heart disease, several cancers (breast, prostate, and colorectal), candida, fungal infections, the flu virus, and yeast infections. Olives can be used to lower cholesterol, protect the liver, guard against colitis, reduce inflammation, and improve the look of your hair and skin, giving you the glow!

Olives are a rich source of vitamins A and E, both of which protect the oils on the surface of your skin from free-radical damage. Olives also help strengthen connective tissues, improving skin tone and protecting against UV radiation. The rich phenol content protects skin against oxidization. By using extra virgin olive oil topically, you can prevent and treat aging skin. In addition, used topically, olive oil's antibacterial and antifungal properties can treat acne, eczema, and psoriasis. It helps repair cells, protects against damage, and soothes the skin, helping it renew and regenerate.

Extra virgin olive oil also helps with the absorption of calcium, contributing to bone health. The fats are made up primarily of monounsaturated fatty acids (heart-healthy because they raise good cholesterol) and cancer-fighting oleic acids, which moisturize and lubricate skin cells. Extra virgin olive oil is naturally rich in squalane, which is a key ingredient in many store-bought skincare products. Squalane absorbs easily into the skin, keeping skin moist as well as restoring lost moisture.

BUYING OLIVES

It's best to choose dark purple or black olives due to their higher antioxidant properties and richer nutrient profile. Kalamata olives are my personal fave. It's the Greek in me! These olives contain the antioxidant anthocyanin, which is anti-aging, antibacterial, and anti-inflammatory, and can prevent and slow down the effects of cancer. However, don't buy those black, processed olives found in cans. They've been chemically ripened and processed, and their nutrients destroyed.

Here are some things to keep in mind when you're buying extra virgin olive oil (EVOO):

- EVOO is the highest-quality olive oil. It's made through an extraction process that doesn't alter or treat the oil in any way. When purchasing EVOO, make sure it's in a dark glass bottle, as light, heat, and oxygen destroy its nutrients and antioxidant properties and accelerate the oxidization process. Olive oil starts to degrade the moment it's squeezed from the olive, which is why it's essential that the oil be stored in a dark bottle away from light.
- Use EVOO raw or cooked at extremely low temperatures. Drizzle it on food after the food has been prepared or use as a dressing. Heat destroys the phenols and antioxidant properties of the oil. EVOO has a low smoking point, around

250°F (120°C). Beyond that point the oil will smoke, oxidize, and become rancid, resulting in further free-radical damage—which will cause, not prevent, premature aging!

- Know how extra virgin differs from virgin. Virgin olive oil undergoes the same process as extra virgin olive oil but is made from olives harvested later in the year, giving it higher levels of acidity (between 0.8 and 2 percent, which distinguishes it from EVOO, which has an acidity of less than 0.8 percent). Virgin olive oil has a higher smoking point than EVOO (around 350°F, or 175°C), which makes it better for cooking, but still, keep it at a low temperature.
- If it's not extra virgin or virgin, don't buy it. The "olive oil" sold in clear glass bottles shouldn't be used at all—ever! These have been refined and chemically treated, and are hence devoid of nutrients and antioxidants. Oxygen attaches to the fats (oxidization) to produce hyperperoxides. Then the hyperperoxides break down and cause rancidity. Rancid oils cause free-radical damage in our body, which leads to disease and premature aging.

HOW TO USE

- Add olives to salads, tomato sauces (olives and tomato sauce make a great antioxidant combo, especially in protecting against and helping prevent UV damage), and other dishes to add a natural saltiness. When making a decadent chocolate dessert, blend in one black olive instead of the pinch of salt to bring out the richness and depth of the chocolate flavor. You won't even taste the olive, but it does an amazing job of accentuating the richness of the chocolate. Olives are also great blended in chocolate smoothies.
- Drizzle EVOO onto already cooked dishes and use in salad dressings.
- Use EVOO topically as a moisturizer. Your skin will absorb the oil and it won't leave you greasy.
- Smooth EVOO onto lips as a natural moisturizer and lip gloss.
- Use EVOO as a facial moisturizer before bed, especially around the eye area.
- Add the oil to a warm bath and soak in it for supple skin.
- Soak your fingernails in EVOO to soften cuticles and strengthen nails. Adding fresh, minced garlic increases the antifungal properties.
- Mix EVOO with sea salt and rub onto skin as an exfoliant to remove dead skin cells.

Coconut Oil

If you want the glow, you have to get fat—the healthy kind of fat found in foods like coconut oil, that is! Coconut oil is a great way to get those beauty-boosting essential fats without the extra calories that will lead to the *wrong* kind of fat. By weight, coconut oil has fewer calories than any other fat source. Although it's a saturated fat, the medium-chain fatty acids make it easily absorbable by the small intestine (not requiring the full digestive process). This means it provides increased energy faster than any other fat. Coconut oil has immune-boosting properties and is antiviral, antimicrobial, and antifungal. It's especially beneficial for those who suffer from candida or fungal infections, which can lead to acne and skin irritations. So by adding more of this to your diet, you may begin to see your face clear.

Due to its fatty-acid profile, coconut oil is also great for topical use as a moisturizer. It can smooth and clear skin and may help reduce the signs of stretch marks. Because it's a saturated fat, it can help firm up saggy skin. Saturated fats are required to strengthen cell walls, and plant-based sources are the healthiest. And, contrary to popular belief, research shows that coconut oil can help lower cholesterol levels. It's also great for diabetics, as it helps normalize blood-sugar levels. Whether it's eaten through food or used topically as a moisturizer, it does wonders for improving skin ... making it totally succulent!

Aloe

Aloe is a great plant to have around the house or in the garden—it's a medical power-house in a pot! The aloe plant is highly regarded for its anti-inflammatory and healing properties. It's especially beneficial in the treatment of skin conditions like psoriasis, eczema, rosacea, and herpes, and can be used to quickly heal wounds, burns, and frostbite if applied topically. Aloe can speed up the healing of bad burns by nearly nine days. The anti-inflammatory properties may be partly attributed to the plant's high concentration of methylsulfonylmethane (MSM), a natural sulfur compound that helps alleviate arthritic joint pain and inflammation and improve joint flexibility and strength. This also makes aloe gel great for muscle recovery after a workout. However, MSM is found only in outdoor plants fed by rainwater or sulfur-rich water. Ingesting aloe can also decrease the number and size of papillomas and reduce the incidence of tumors by more than 90 percent in the liver, spleen, and bone marrow.

Aloe is rich in polysaccharides, which also have anti-inflammatory properties and aid in the growth of new tissue. Polysaccharides have superior intestinal health bene-fits (such as improving digestion and reducing risk of colon cancer) and help your body absorb precious nutrients, helping to maintain your health and glowing complexion. Since aloe is more absorbable than vitamin E, it makes a phenomenal emollient that soothes and softens dry skin.

Green Tea

If ever there were a drink of the beauty gods, it would be green tea. Originating in China over 5,000 years ago, green tea is made from the leaves of the *Camellia sinensis*, which grows abundantly in the Himalayas, and is rich in antioxidant compounds, essential oils, and caffeine. The most important of its many antioxidants is EGCG (epigallocatechin gallate), which can be more active than vitamins C and E!

In a study conducted at Western Reserve University, researchers coated human skin with green tea and exposed it to direct sunlight; the tea was found to protect skin from the harmful UV rays that cause premature aging.[52]

Green tea isn't only an amazing anti-aging tonic; it keeps the skin acne-free as well. Plus it washes away dental plaque, keeping your pearly whites as brilliant as your complexion. It also boosts metabolism to help you shed pounds; it aids digestion; and it helps treat impaired immune function, rheumatoid arthritis, and cardiovascular diseases.

Cupuacu

Many of the foods featured in this chapter help diminish wrinkles and lines, and the cupuacu fruit deserves the spotlight. Hailed as a "super-fruit," cupuacu is related to cacao (hence the hint of chocolate in smell and taste) and loaded with antioxidants. It's like the fruit won the antioxidant lottery: its pulp contains more antioxidants than even the popular acai berries and blueberries.

Cupuacu's bioactive polyphenols are its magic ingredient. They provide protection against ultraviolet radiation, which helps prevent premature aging.

11. Pimples, Dots, and Age Spots

We all know that moment. The one when you have a huge day ahead of you, whether it's a date, a job interview, or a very important meeting. You wake up, walk to the bathroom, look in the mirror—and there it is: that big red nodule glowing right at you from the middle of your face. No!

Acne, while not life-threatening or rare, can totally detract from a person's inner and physical beauty in a most grotesquely unfair way. Plus, no matter how severe or mild, it can affect one's self-confidence. Whether you have one zit or ten, don't you feel as if that's what everyone is *really* looking at when they speak to you? Whether you're emerging from your teens and hoping to leave acne behind for good or heading into menopause and still battling the breakouts, acne can affect anyone anytime. And while commercials would have us believe that the solution lies in medications, serums, and antibiotics, the truth is that we need to start with what we put in our mouths. Here's how to feed a flawless complexion!

Blemish Breakdown

Acne is sort of like a busted sprinkler system. Think of your face as the lawn and your pores as the sprinkler heads. Now when dirt and bits of grass work their way into the sprinkler heads, the water is usually able to push it all out in the torrent that showers the lawn. But if too much dirt and clippings get lodged in a sprinkler head and enough pressure builds up, that sprinkler head is going to swell and blow up completely.

The same thing goes for your face. Its pores (or sprinkler heads) are actually hair follicles that connect to sebaceous glands, which produce an oily substance called sebum. When everything works as it should, the sebum drains to the surface of the skin, carrying with it the dead skin cells it's washed out of the follicles. Plus, the sebum provides some nice moisture to your skin. But if you produce too much sebum, or if dead skin cells, hair, and/or bacteria block the follicles and trap the sebum inside, watch out. Excess sebum is a breeding ground for bacteria, which infects the follicle and gives birth to those nasty zits.

All breakouts, however, are not created equal.

Whiteheads

The most innocuous are whiteheads, which occur when there isn't a broken follicle or inflammation, just bacteria and sebum below the surface of the skin.

Blackheads

A blackhead happens when the hair follicle opens at the skin's surface and exposes the blocked sebum to oxygen. The oxygen oxidizes the sebum and turns the head of the bacteria black, hence the name *blackhead*—such creative nomenclature. All the bacteria hide out just below the blackhead, which you can see when you do an extraction. Ever try one of those blackhead remover strips? I used to use them occasionally as a teenager, and after pulling the strip off my nose it was so cool seeing the tiny little blackheads standing erect with their soft white tips. Those tips were full of bacteria, oil, dead skin cells, and other debris. Lovely. I do recommend getting blackheads extracted professionally during facials or through exfoliant scrubs and masks (see recipes in Chapter 13). It gets rid of the bacteria and lets the sebum drain normally again.

Pimples

Throw a little inflammation into the mix and you end up with a puffy red pimple. Since bacteria live in our skin and LOVE excess oil, they essentially throw a party and multiply when there's an abundance of sebum. This irritates the follicle, which calls the cops (also known as white blood cells) to come break it up. The white blood cells rush to the scene and, as a result, inflame the whole area. At this point, you can actually feel it brewing. You place a finger on the area and feel a hardened lump just below the surface of your skin. You rush to a mirror, and there it is: a reddish little bump that portends all manner of superficial woe. Damn it!

You could try squeezing it, but nothing would come out—everything is still below the skin's surface at this stage. So leave it alone! Premature popping does way more damage than good, internally. Give the beast a few days, and the white blood cells will work their way up to the surface of the skin to become the revolting white pus of a full-fledged zit.

What's Behind the Breakouts

If too much sebum leads to zits, it stands to reason that you have only to remove the excess to get the complexion you've always dreamed of. Not necessarily true. Excess sebum is the symptom, not the problem. While many reasons are still undetermined, here are some documented triggers that cause acne:

Raging Hormones

There are two sides to every coin, and while raging hormones might've once meant hooking up during adolescence, it can also mean your complexion takes a nosedive into a rocky sea of breakouts. Hormones, it turns out, are rather sensitive, and it doesn't take much to upheave them.

Androgens are the group of male hormones that control sebum production, testosterone being the most prominent and well-known of these. Thanks to an enzyme called 5-alpha-reductase, the body can convert testosterone into a more active form called dihydrotestosterone (DHT), which opens the floodgates on sebum production. And this, as we've seen, leads to a river of pimply pain.

Excess Androgens = Increase in Sebum Production = Increase in Acne

But testosterone isn't always to blame either. A fluctuation among any hormones can throw things out of whack. What's important is that hormones are balanced in optimal ratios. So while it *may* be that your body is producing too many androgens, it could ALSO be the case that androgen levels are about normal but other hormone levels are relatively too low. Or it could be that a hormonal imbalance increased the production of 5-alpha-reductase, which then converted a more than normal amount of testosterone to DHT. So the goal isn't necessarily upping one hormone or reducing another. It's to achieve a happy, blemish-free balance between all hormones.

Other factors that throw hormones out of whack:

- Birth control pills
- Stress
- Xenoestrogens (estrogen-mimicking chemicals found in our environment; see Chapter 7)

Stress

Whether it's physical, mental, or emotional, stress ramps up cortisol production. This leads not only to chronic inflammation (which then manifests as acne) but also to an imbalance of hormones like insulin, testosterone, and estrogen. Stress suppresses the immune system and compromises the digestive system as well, which could trigger the harboring of more harmful bacteria.

TIP

Adding adaptogenic herbs like maca, holy basil, and ginseng to your diet can help your body manage stress and balance hormones.

Digestive Issues

Digestive issues can also encourage breakouts, since there's a direct correlation between poor digestive function and the onset of acne. This makes sense when you consider that the bulk of our immune system resides in the gut. If we don't have enough beneficial bacteria swimming around in there, inflammation occurs and bad, acne-forming bacteria mutiny to wreak havoc on your complexion.

DID YOU KNOW?

A study published in the *Journal of Dermatology* found that in a group of 13,000 adolescents, those with acne were more likely to experience symptoms of gastrointestinal distress like constipation and heartburn.[53]

But one of the biggest-known triggers is ... the food we eat. Here's what puts your complexion in a tizzy.

Sugar and Refined Grains

Let's just say that *real* chocolate does not give you zits. Honest-to-goodness dark chocolate is probably the biggest victim of character assassination in the food world, all because of those highly processed pseudo-chocolate bars on the shelves. You know, the ones packed with highly refined sugar, preservatives, and milk solids. And it's *those* ingredients that can lead to acne. Leaving real chocolate uneaten is such a shame.

What you should watch out for are things like sugar, refined grains, and processed, high-glycemic foods like cereals, baked goods, pasta, and fruit juice, all of which can cause acne. These foods cause a spike in blood sugar, which forces a spike in insulin—one of those hormones that hang in a precarious balance. Insulin affects the production of androgen, so a bump in insulin means a bump in androgen, which means a bump in the production of sebum. And that means more bumps on your face.

If your androgen production already runs on the high side, more insulin won't help things. Additionally, sugar feeds yeast and candida (a type of fungal yeast infection) in your body, resulting in an imbalance of gut flora and inflammation and creating a breeding ground for acne.

Dairy

Guess what? Dairy does the same thing.

That's right. Years of drinking wholesome milk, and all you have to show for it is a haywire hormonal system. Dairy, you see, contains loads of lactose, which is essentially sugar. But even worse than the insulin spike lactose causes are the naturally occurring hormones in milk. Think about it: cows make milk to feed their calves so they can grow into enormous cows. What do you think makes them grow? Hormones! Just as a mother's breast milk contains naturally occurring hormones, so does cow's milk. But their milk is intended for their calves, not us humans.

That's not the end of it. Those hormones increase testosterone and other androgens while also triggering inflammation. Even worse, cow's milk comes intact with the enzyme that converts testosterone into DHT, the most active form of the androgen.

Hormones found in any food product run counter to balancing your own, but dairy is a major threat to clear skin. In a study conducted by Harvard University and published in the *Journal of the American Academy of Dermatology*, a direct correlation was established between high school dairy intake and acne, where the more milk was consumed, the higher the incidence of acne was. And unlike most teenage horrors, acne didn't stop after the diploma was handed out. Those who consumed more milk during high school also experienced more acne later in life, ESPECIALLY if they drank skim milk![54] This actually makes sense, though, when you consider that skim milk includes a higher concentration of sugar to compensate for the loss of flavor caused by taking out the fat. And where there's more sugar, there's more insulin, and ultimately more acne.

Food Toxins

The word toxins can be a little misleading, I grant you. It's not as if there's a "Caution: Poison" sign on the foods you eat. But foods that contain chemicals, pesticides, artificial additives, and highly processed oils do act as toxins in your body. They stress the body as it tries to process them, and any food that stresses your body can cause acne.

So how do toxins stored deep within your fat cells lead to acne? Your skin is your largest eliminative organ, and it's through it that many toxins are released. But your skin can only handle so much. And when it's constantly bombarded by unhealthy fats and chemicals, acne is its way of revolting.

Detoxes are a great illustration of this. Have you ever gone on a cleanse expecting to feel and look great as a reward for consuming nothing but green juice for seven days, only to be plagued by acne? That's because a cleanse can mobilize the toxins that have burrowed deep within your cells, and as your body purges them, they make their pimply exit through your skin.

Some toxins promote inflammation as well, like highly refined vegetable oils (and the foods fried in them), trans fat, animal-based saturated fats, and even omega-6 fatty acids.

Food sensitivities—usually to things like dairy, wheat, gluten, soy, eggs, shellfish, and peanuts—also result in inflammation. And inflammation just encourages bacteria to grow in the blocked pores, giving rise to a nasty case of breakouts.

Blemish Busters

It seems as though everywhere you look someone is trying to get you to sign up for a "revolutionary" diet. But as with money, romance, and shoes, your dietary needs are intensely personal.

So if your primary objective is to clear up your skin, you need to start with a clean, natural diet that features drinking plenty of water and lots of plant-based, nutrient-dense, antioxidant-rich, high-water-content foods. Not only will these clear up your complexion, they'll also make you feel as good as you look!

Here are some anti-acne nutritional warriors.

Probiotics (Beneficial Bacteria)

Gut + Probiotics = Love

That's right, probiotics are the heartthrob of your intestinal tract, and for good reason. They're essentially "good" bacteria: they ensure that nutrients are delivered to your cells, they keep bad bacteria in check, and they reduce inflammation in your intestines. Studies suggest that taking a probiotic supplement or eating probiotic-rich foods like miso or kimchi actually promotes clear, healthy skin. That calls into question the practice of taking antibiotics to curb acne. Not only do antibiotics eliminate ALL bacteria in your system (good, bad, and otherwise), they don't correct the underlying problem—just the symptom.

FERMENTED FOODS

Fermented foods like miso, kimchi, and raw sauerkraut are rich in naturally occurring probiotic cultures and have the same benefits as probiotic supplements.

While I personally LOVE fermented foods, if acne is a result of yeast overgrowth (candida), some fermented foods, such as vinegar and pickles, may aggravate it. Plus, these foods are typically pasteurized, which reduces the probiotic benefits, and are loaded in salt—not always good for your face. Raw, unpasteurized versions are the best, like unpasteurized miso, which is also high in zinc.

Zinc

Your gut may love probiotics, but the mineral that really gets your skin pumped up is none other than zinc. In addition to soothing inflamed skin, regenerating skin cells, and speeding up the healing process, zinc inhibits 5-alpha-reductase activity. (Remember that enzyme that converts testosterone into its more active, pimple-promoting form?[55] Yeah. Zinc puts the kibosh on all that.) In fact, acne is often associated with a zinc deficiency. Consuming just 30 milligrams per day helps fight acne, and a quarter cup of raw pumpkin seeds provides just over half that recommended amount.

Vitamin A

Vitamin A helps normalize oil production in the skin and fights inflammation, making it an anti-acne superhero. Vitamin A also encourages the turnover of skin cells, which helps keep follicles free and clear, a crucial step in preventing acne.

The absolute best (and healthiest) way to get vitamin A is through food. Try sweet potatoes, pumpkin, carrots, red peppers, kale, collards, watercress, and turnip greens for a vitamin A boost.

Vitamin E

Vitamin E is a clear-skin must-have. This powerful antioxidant helps repair and heal tissues while also fighting free-radical damage. Great sources include sunflower seeds, almonds, walnuts, mustard greens, and Swiss chard.

Omega-3 Fatty Acids

Omega-3 fatty acids are king among anti-inflammatories, and their benefits are more than skin-deep. Omega-3s help heal and reduce inflammation underneath the skin's surface, which speeds up healing and reduces the severity of acne.

Other Dietary Changes for Zit-Free Skin

- Cut out dairy, sugar, refined grains, and other foods with a high glycemic index. (These cause significant insulin spikes that result in a hormonal imbalance.)
- Start stress-busting! Freaking out or overly taxing your body is bad for lots of things, including your skin. B vitamins help your body manage stress (see Chapter 2 for more ideas).
- Just say no to food-based toxins like hormone disrupters (xenoestrogens), pesticides, and packaged/highly processed foods. Your liver, no longer bogged down with toxins, will thank you with clearer skin.

Clear-Skin Cravings

So how do you turn this week's menu into a blemish-blasting strategy? Start with these foods, which do the hard work for you.

Raw Honey

Need a little sweetness in your life? Try some raw honey to satisfy those sugar cravings while helping your body look and feel amazing! Raw honey is one of nature's most wondrous promoters of general health. This pure source offers so many health benefits that it's truly one of the world's food treasures. Raw honey is the only absolutely unprocessed honey: it's unheated, unpasteurized, and 100 percent pure. Its health benefits come mainly from its abundance of naturally occurring nutrients. Raw honey is nutritionally superior to all other forms of honey, as it contains loads of vitamins, minerals, and amino acids, and over 5,000 live enzymes. So it's not surprising that honey in its raw form acts as a powerful immune booster in the body. It is these powers that help your body fight off illness and disease and that can give your digestive system a real kick-start.

Unlike most of the honey found in supermarkets, which has been pasteurized (heated) and filtered to look more appealing to the consumer (not to mention easier to spread), raw honey is in its pure form. The heating undergone by most commercial honey causes a destruction of many of the enzymes and yeasts that benefit the body. The bottom line: raw honey is much more nutritious than your average grocery-store version that has undergone any of these treatments.

Raw honey has antiseptic, antibiotic, and antibacterial properties, and for these reasons it's been used for centuries to heal wounds, cuts, and burns. These properties allow honey to inhibit bacterial growth and infection and minimize pain and inflammation while promoting the body's natural healing processes.

Research published in the *Journal of the Federation of American Societies for Experimental Biology* shows for the first time how honey kills bacteria: bees make a protein added to the honey, which can be used to treat burns and skin infections—and which could one day help combat antibiotic-resistant infections.[57] Now, that's what you call superfood power!

Sweet Potatoes

They're dense, slightly sweet, and full of mood-boosting orange color. But sweet potatoes are more than just a pretty face—they help yours look a lot better, too.

Sweet potatoes are rich in vitamin A, which is an anti-inflammatory AND helps fight off acne-causing bacteria. Vitamin A and another of sweet potatoes' abundant nutrients, vitamin C, work hard both to prevent acne and to heal it should it strike.[58]

But sweet potatoes fight acne on another level, too. In addition to their vitamins and antioxidants, they have a relatively low glycemic index, which helps maintain a steady insulin level and avoid the pimply dangers associated with hormonal imbalance.

Walnuts

Walnuts may be good for the brain, but they have a superficial side, too. Known as the nut of the gods, their nutritional properties provide regal beauty benefits.

Walnuts are used in the makeup and beauty industry now more than ever. Their rich stores of omega-3 fatty acids not only keep your skin healthy and glowing, but also reduce inflammation. And, since inflammation leads to breakouts, walnuts make a nutty, tasty anti-acne treatment.

Along with omega-3s, walnuts are rich in vitamin E and other powerful antioxidant and anti-inflammatory compounds, reducing inflammation and the incidence of breakouts. Plus they provide moisture to the skin and prevent sun damage.

Coconut Oil

As we talked about in the preceding chapter (page 126), coconut oil has amazing acne-zapping and preventative benefits due to its antiviral, antimicrobial, antifungal properties. It's especially beneficial for those who suffer from candida or fungal infections, which can lead to acne and skin irritations.

Kimchi

Kimchi, a spicy, fermented Korean staple, adds a nice kick as well as a healthy dose of probiotics to your meals. It's a fermented cabbage (and often radish) slaw that provides the same benefits as many probiotic supplements.

When it comes to acne, a clear complexion begins in your gut. Adding fermented foods like kimchi to your diet replenishes your GI tract with beneficial bacteria. This is especially advantageous for those who've been heavily dosed with acne meds that kill ALL bacteria, which can often make your complexion even worse.

HOW TO USE

Add kimchi to your favorite sandwiches, on top of your pizza, or to stews or stir fries for an extra kick.

TIP

Anti-inflammatory foods such as turmeric and ginger also do wonders in promoting a clean, clear complexion.

Lavender

Okay, so it's not exactly a food for eating, but lavender has antibacterial, anti-inflammatory, painkilling properties that make it a killer weapon against acne. It's also great for normalizing the skin, whether yours tends toward oily or dry and sensitive. (Lavender has something for everyone!) Pair it with lemongrass or raw honey for an even more fragrant way to clear up your skin.

HOW TO USE

Apply a few drops of lavender essential oil directly onto blemishes with a cotton swab to eliminate them.

Licorice Oil

Once used to inspire passion, licorice nowadays can still get you excited about at least one thing: spot-free skin! Licorice oil can lighten dark spots on skin, including age spots. And since it's also antibacterial, anti-inflammatory, antiviral, and even antispasmodic, it can help clear up your complexion too, treating and preventing acne. In fact, it also works great for rosacea!

Lemon

No one can accuse lemon of slouching about. In addition to working well as a toner or an uplifting scent in moisturizers and scrubs, lemon juice can help lighten dark patches and age spots on the skin.

DIY TOPICAL ZIT-ZAPPING REMEDIES

Dollop the following directly on your zit, using a cotton swab to zap it.

For sensitive skin or when applied to a larger surface area, it's best to dilute essential oils with a carrier oil, such as extra virgin olive oil.

RAW HONEY	Antiseptic, antibiotic, and antibacterial properties Speeds up healing and reduces inflammation
LAVENDER OIL	Antibacterial, anti-inflammatory, and painkilling properties Reduces redness and swelling
LICORICE OIL	Reduces inflammation and redness (also good for rosacea)
TEA TREE OIL	Antibacterial, anti-inflammatory Gets rid of redness and scars
APPLE CIDER VINEGAR	Antiseptic, antibacterial, balances pH Dilute with water!

DIY Blemish-Busting Face Mask

Here's a weekly face mask that can help keep your skin and acne in check:

2 Tbsp (30 mL) raw honey

3 drops lavender essential oil

1 Tbsp (15 mL) matcha green tea powder

1 Tbsp (15 mL) lemon juice

¼ cup (60 mL) lukewarm water

Mix all ingredients in a bowl to create a paste and massage onto skin. Let sit for 15 minutes, then wash off.

12. Kitchen Beautician: Body

Remember when playing with your food was absolutely, positively not allowed? When you were denied dessert if you so much as stirred your mashed potatoes or pretended croutons were ships at sea in your soup? Oh, how things have changed! Not only are today's parents a lot more lenient, but playing with your food can actually make you look better!

That's right—just as eating certain foods can improve your health, WEARING certain foods can improve your looks. You've seen women with cucumber slices on their eyes, and you've probably tried a green tea scrub or pomegranate facial at the spa at some point. But what I'm talking about is harnessing the power of a wide variety of foods to make you look better ... and doing it from your own kitchen! Just to prove I'm perfectly serious, let's start with everyone's favorite beauty problem: cellulite.

Surrender Your Cellulite

I'll be honest with you: there's no magic food, lotion, cream, or chemical that will banish cellulite forever, no matter what a cosmetics clerk says or a firming cream promises. Cellulite is a buildup of fat, water, and toxins that pushes up against connective tissues just underneath the skin, usually in places like the butt, thighs, and belly where circulation is low. Exercise and a healthy diet can help reduce the appearance, but even the fittest and skinniest of chicks usually have some to hide. Factors like stress, poor diets high in sugars and refined carbs, hormonal imbalance, cigarette smoke, contraceptives, and, to put it bluntly, couch-potato syndrome just exacerbate the problem. Really, it's almost enough to make you want to give up and eat another candy bar.

But don't do it! There ARE temporary fixes that can help reduce the cottage-cheese effect under your butt. (Or wherever it may be.) Here's what works.

Dry Skin Brushing

Dry skin brushing is ah-may-zing! Find yourself a natural bristle brush and, when your skin is dry, brush your body with strokes in the direction of your heart. (For example, if you're dry-brushing the backs of your legs, you should be brushing upward.) It's best to do this for a good 10 minutes before jumping into the shower. Not only will it get rid of dead skin cells and exfoliate your entire body, it will also increase circulation and stimulate your lymphatic system to wake up and eliminate toxins from your body.

Infrared Sauna

Sweating is one of the best ways to expel toxins from your system, and the infrared sauna is a fantastic way to do it. It's not as hot as a typical dry sauna where you feel the heat as soon as you step inside. In an infrared sauna, you'll probably wonder what's going on and start to fiddle with the temperature panel to make it hotter. But if you just give it 5 or 10 minutes, you'll be sweating buckets! Creating more of an inside-out heat, these saunas stimulate the cells deep within your body to create heat and mobilize toxins. Bonus: infrared saunas stimulate your metabolism as well, so you burn tons of calories!

Caffeine

There's a reason why caffeine is found in nearly every over-the-counter cellulite cream: wearing your coffee is a great way to reduce the appearance of lumps and bumps. Caffeine is a natural anti-inflammatory that temporarily reduces the appearance of dimples by smoothing out the area. It also helps tighten skin and blood vessels, break down fatty deposits, and reduce water retention by sucking excess fluid out of cells.

Water

As in, drink some! Yes, it's that simple. Water helps flush out toxins and excess fluids from your body, minimizing the puffiness of the protruding fat deposits. Drink half your body weight in ounces each day. Your dimpled bottom will thank you.

Bentonite Clay

This potent, high-mineral clay is made up of volcanic ash deposits and comes straight from the sea. Toxin buildups, whether in the skin or in fat cells, are no match for bentonite clay, which helps to pull toxins stored deep within your skin. You may notice a little breakout at first use, but this is totally normal. It means that it's working—that toxins (along with lumps and bumps) are on their way out the door. Mix bentonite clay with water in a one-to-one ratio and lather up.

Berries and Greens

Eat them or wear them, berries and leafy greens are going to do you a world of good. Blueberries, raspberries, blackberries, and the like are rich sources of antioxidants that keep cells healthy and fresh. They also contain anti-inflammatory properties, which reduce puffiness. Leafy greens, like kale and Swiss chard, are loaded with phytonutrient goodness. They help cleanse the body of toxins and waste (something your liver also benefits from!). Both berries and greens are high in fiber, which helps pull toxins from your body—and fewer toxins in your body means fewer dimples on your thuttocks.

Whip It, Whip It Good: Scrubs for Smoothing

Knowing how effective ingredients work is half the battle. But before you plastic-wrap yourself with leafy greens or pour coffee into your bath, have a go at any (or all!) of these three scrubs. I've formulated them for optimal results, and they all increase circulation, eliminate fluid retention, and make skin appear smoother. Best yet, these are recipes you can whip up in your kitchen to whip your cellulite into shape.

The Rise and Shine Scrub	¾ cup (175 mL) coffee granules

The Rise and Shine Scrub
(I also love using this on my face!)

¾ cup (175 mL) coffee granules
½ cup (125 mL) carrier oil (Try coconut oil, extra virgin olive oil, almond oil, or sea-buckthorn seed oil. The oil hydrates, moisturizes, and soothes skin.)

Use circular motions to massage well onto damp skin in the direction of your heart. (The massage yields the greatest benefit!) Let sit for 15 to 20 minutes and then wash off.

The Detox

½ cup (125 mL) bentonite clay powder
½ cup (125 mL) water
2 Tbsp (30 mL) apple cider vinegar

After bathing and while skin is still moist, use circular motions to rub the mixture in the direction of your heart. You can either let it sit on your body for 15 to 20 minutes or wrap it in warm damp towels. After 20 minutes, rinse off completely.

The Tropical Breeze

½ cup (125 mL) pineapple, peeled and cubed
½ cup (125 mL) papaya, peeled and cubed
½ cup (125 mL) matcha green tea powder

Add all ingredients to blender and blend. Massage the mixture onto cellulite-prone areas in circular motions in the direction of your heart and then wash off.

Pineapple and papaya contain the papain enzyme, which helps to smooth skin, and vitamin C, which strengthens the connective tissues. Those tissues are the only thing standing between the fat and your skin, so give them a workout!

Oil Change

If you're like me, your skin can never be too soft. Most of us spend a lot of time reading magazines, trolling department stores, and investing in the latest and greatest body crème to hit the shelves. If it promises us smoother, softer skin, we're in. The reason, of course, is that it feels like a Sisyphean task to stay moisturized. We slather on the lotion morning, noon, and night, and yet still we can't seem to banish the telltale white layer of flaky dryness on our arms and legs. It seems as if we'll never get the dewy skin we crave!

The fact is, however, it doesn't take expensive creams or moisturizing misters to restore your skin to a silky smooth state. The best thing for it is simple fats saturated in antioxidants and vitamin E. And since about 60 to 70 percent of what you put on your skin is absorbed, whatever you're slathering on your bod should be pronounce-able and directly useful.

That brings us to oils. Apricot, almond, coconut—the stuff that works on the inside just happens to work on the outside, too! Plus, it smells divine. The best time to apply your oil of choice is right after you shower. Like, immediately. Like, don't even step out the door! Just grab a towel, pat yourself down, and slather on the oil. This is the most effective way to absorb all that natural, hydrating goodness. Then just dab off any excess oil with your towel, and step out to admire your glow.

But which oil is for you? Here's the scoop on a few of my favorites.

Apricot Oil

Loaded with antioxidant vitamins A and C, apricot oil is easily absorbed and has a mild scent (as opposed to its more odorous cousin, extra virgin olive oil). But the best part about it is that it aids collagen production. You know that stuff that makes your skin resilient and young-looking? Yep, this is where you get it. And, since it's comparatively inexpensive, using apricot oil will save you money now (when using it as a moisturizer) and later (in delaying trips to the cosmetic surgeon).

> ### TIP
> The best way to use these oils is to keep them in your shower, and as soon as you're done bathing, saturate your body with them. When your skin is moist, it yields the greatest absorption. You may also add your own natural fragrance using essential oils like lavender, lemon balm, angelica, cinnamon, citrus, or whatever your heart, and nose, fancies. Grapefruit will uplift and refresh you, while lavender can help relax you after a long day.

Almond Oil

Who doesn't love the smell of almond oil? At once mild and exotic, it brings to mind the best parts about a far-flung vacation. Your skin, meanwhile, loves that it's a great source of vitamin E, which protects skin from UV damage while rejuvenating and deeply moisturizing it. Almond oil's emollient properties soften and smooth skin, and this little beauty also evens out skin tone to improve your complexion. So what if you're using it on your thighs? They want to be pretty, too!

Extra Virgin Olive Oil (EVOO)

Got acne, eczema or psoriasis? EVOO's antibacterial, antiviral, anti-inflammatory, anti-fungal properties make it an effective treatment for these and other conditions. And, since it's also rich in vitamins A and E, EVOO helps repair cells and protect against free-radical and UV damage while simultaneously promoting skin-cell renewal and regeneration. Oh! And did I mention it's incredibly soothing, too?

Even if you're not battling a skin condition, EVOO is a hydrating beast—if a little pungent in the olfactory sense—and loaded with antioxidants. It's also rich in squalane, a key ingredient in many a store-bought skincare product that's easily absorbable and really good at getting skin to recapture and hang on to moisture.

Coconut Oil

Yes, coconut oil is one of my favorite oils to cook with, because it is SO good for your body. (And much better than other oils that don't do well with high temperatures.) But coconut oil knows how to treat you right all over, not just in the kitchen. For starters, it can help firm up saggy skin. That's because it's a saturated fat, which is necessary for strengthening cell walls. (And plant-based saturated fats do this better than the other kind.) While it doesn't absorb quite so readily as other oils, its good qualities—smoothing and clearing your complexion and possibly even reducing the signs of stretch marks—help make it a net gain.

> **TIP**
> Try coconut oil to remove your eye makeup. It works amazingly well, and without the chemicals!

Shea Nut Butter

Like coconut oil, shea nut butter melts at normal body temperature. Unlike coconut oil, it absorbs easily into your skin. But there are lots more reasons to try this handy butter, like the way it hushes common skin complaints such as psoriasis, eczema, and sunburn. Or the way its vitamins A and E provide moisture alongside a healthy dose of antioxidants to protect the skin from sun damage. It even reduces the appearance of stretch marks, which is a blessing in itself.

Cocoa Butter

Settle down: there's no chocolate to be found in cocoa butter. But once you get over that disappointment, this guy won't let you down.

Derived from the cacao bean, cocoa butter is an antioxidant-rich fat that helps tighten and firm things up as well as even out skin tone. Cocoa butter happens to be rich in vitamin E, too, so it's great for general moisturizing and soothing.

Emollient Enhancers

While the oils listed above work beautifully all by themselves, they can also be enhanced with any of the following.

Jojoba Oil

If you're prone to breakouts, then jojoba oil really is the gold standard for you.

Extracted from the seeds of the jojoba plant, jojoba oil is similar to sebum (the oil your own skin produces), but it goes one step beyond to dissolve sebum blockages in your follicles. It is, in other words, an awesome pore cleanser. It's also a natural emollient that soothes and softens skin while imparting enviable moisture.

Because it's expensive, jojoba is best added in small amounts to your carrier oil of choice.

Sea-Buckthorn Oil

This seed oil is rich in fatty acids and soothes irritated skin. It also provides the handy benefit of moisturizing while fighting acne on the chest and back. Since body acne usually requires you to choose between moist skin with blemishes and dry skin with zapped zits, sea-buckthorn oil is kind of like a really good mediator.

Aloe Vera Gel

With seemingly magical healing ability, aloe vera is used to treat wounds, burns, and frostbite. But it works on other skin conditions, too, such as psoriasis, eczema, rosacea, and even herpes.

Those just looking for a good, soothing moisturizer will appreciate aloe vera as well. The gel feels almost cool to the touch, and the aloe plant is highly regarded for its anti-inflammatory properties. So if you live anywhere hot, this is a must-try.

Scented Sidekicks

The sense of smell is a powerful thing. Study after study reminds us that nothing evokes memory or inspires attraction quite like scent, so make your moisturizer all your own. Mint refreshes you, lavender relaxes you, and grapefruit just makes you feel happy. But pick whatever your heart, er, nose, desires. Simply add a few drops of your favorite essential oil—be it lemon balm, angelica, cinnamon, or whatever—and rub yourself up good. Or better yet, get someone else to do it for you ...

Scented Oils and Butters

Sure, picking out a single oil and getting shinier than a brand-new penny is straight-forward enough. But how are you supposed to choose that over, say, a basil-and-grape blend by your favorite perfumer? Fear not, dear reader, for I've developed a few winning moisturizer blends so that you can be beautiful, healthy, and elegantly scented with the best of them.

Zen Out Body Oil	½ cup (125 mL) apricot oil 4 drops lavender oil (for a tension-reducing, sleep-promoting calm) 2 drops ylang ylang (to balance hormones while calming and moisturizing) Mix oils and store in a jar at room temperature.
Energizing Body Oil	½ cup (125 mL) extra virgin olive oil 1 Tbsp (15 mL) jojoba oil 4 drops rosemary (to fight acne while stimulating the senses) 2 drops peppermint (to uplift and energize) Mix oils and store in a jar at room temperature.
Buh-Bye-Blemish Body Butter *(Great for acne, eczema, and psoriasis)*	1½ cups (375 mL) coconut oil ¼ cup (60 mL) sea-buckthorn seed oil 1 Tbsp (15 mL) aloe vera gel 3 Tbsp (50 mL) jojoba oil 6 drops lavender oil Melt the coconut oil and mix in the remaining oils. Store in a jar at room temperature.

So Good I Could Eat You Whipped Body Butter

(You'll smell and taste SO good!)

½ cup (125 mL) coconut oil (solid)
½ cup (125 mL) cocoa butter (solid)
¼ cup (60 mL) almond oil
4 drops vanilla essential oil
3 drops cinnamon essential oil

Mix all ingredients in a bowl and whip using an electrical mixer until it forms a light, whipped consistency. Store in a jar, and use all over your body!

Minty Fresh Foot Scrub

½ cup (125 mL) almonds
½ cup (125 mL) oats
1 cup (250 mL) raw cane sugar
¾ cup (175 mL) almond oil
1 Tbsp (15 mL) raw honey
6 drops peppermint essential oil

Grind almonds and oats in food processer until fine. Mix with cane sugar, almond oil, raw honey, and peppermint essential oil until well combined. Store in a jar at room temperature.

13. Kitchen Beautician: Face

If you think your body takes a beating with all the food you eat, exercise you don't do, and skin ailments you endure, consider for a moment what your face undergoes. It's like the register of your emotions, your lifestyle, and your diet. It's where late nights or lots of laughs or too many frowns show up first. And, as such, it's what we attack daily with makeup, serums, masks, and facials in order to retain some control over putting our best face forward.

Sometimes we can be a little too harsh on our face; we ought to give it a little more TLC. True beauty comes from within. But if you're already nourishing your skin from the inside out, there are a few things you can do from the outside in to allow your vibrant beauty to beam right through.

Exfoliate

A great practice in healthy skincare is to exfoliate. It's like taking off your coat at a party and revealing the gorgeous sequined cocktail dress you're wearing. The coat may keep you warm, but the dress is what makes you shine.

Exfoliating does much the same thing for your face. It sloughs off the dull, dead skin cells to prevent pores from clogging and to brighten and even the skin tone. This, you see, is the equivalent of a shimmering gown—it's your best face.

Exfoliating has other perks, too. Besides making you look more fully awake and glowing, it loosens old, stale sebum and washes it away so that new sebum can flow to the skin. (This, of course, helps prevent acne.) And all that gentle scrubbing and sloughing increases blood flow to the skin, which encourages cellular renewal—the closest thing we can get to recapturing the skin of our youth!

And, if you look at it from the perspective of your skincare regimen, exfoliating helps maximize the efficacy of your cleanser and moisturizer. They don't waste time and effort sitting on old skin cells but rather pour all their power directly on the freshest face you've got. One to two times per week is all it takes! So, whether you need to slough off a late night or replenish your skin after a stressful week—or just need to look your best for Friday night—we've got you covered. Here are some edible exfoliants.

Acid Wash—AHA

Natural exfoliants are gentle abrasives that loosen and remove dead skin cells. Many of these fall into the alpha hydroxy acid (AHA) camp, and are mainly derived from fruit and sometimes from dairy (as with lactic acid). AHAs are the darling of chemical peels and over-the-counter skincare products, since they attract moisture as they dissolve the stuff that keeps dead skin cells hanging on to your skin tighter than a woman holding a pair of Jimmy Choos at a sample sale. AHAs do other appreciable tasks as well, like producing collagen, treating acne, and evening out skin tone. The goal, of course, is to wipe away—or at least diminish—wrinkles and fine lines to make the skin look younger and healthier. Which makes you look younger and healthier. Which is something most of us can get on board with.

While all acids work more or less the same, each has its quirks. Below are the types of AHAs and what makes them special.

Types of AHA	Benefits	Food Sources
GLYCOLIC ACID	Reduces fine lines and wrinkles; can lighten age spots and discolored skin; treats acne.	Most commonly found in sugarcane and beet sugar. Other sources include pineapple, cantaloupe, oranges, lemons, and limes.

Types of AHA	Benefits	Food Sources
LACTIC ACID	Reduces fine lines and wrinkles; can lighten age spots; stimulates the production of collagen.	Fermented milk products, such as yogurt, buttermilk, and sour cream
CITRIC ACID	Amazing for reducing the appearance of age spots, acne scars, and small wrinkles; evens out skin tone; eliminates oily skin.	Lemons, limes, grapefruit, and oranges
MALIC ACID	Great for sensitive skin; evens out skin tone; reduces fine lines and wrinkles; tightens pores; reduces symptoms of rosacea; treats acne.	Most commonly found in apples. Other sources include apricots, cherries, gooseberries, lemons, pineapples, and raspberries.
TARTARIC ACID	Treats acne; has antioxidant and antibacterial properties.	Most commonly found in grapes—the kind used to make wine, no less, and consequently my favorite! Other sources include cranberries and bananas.

Raw Cane Sugar

Ever wonder how the dead skin cells hang on to your skin despite being, well, dead? It's because of the stale, dried-out oils that hold them in place like glue. Well, the glycolic acid in raw cane sugar doesn't mess around with any of that—it just pries them off so that you can wash them away.

Coconut Sugar

Coconut sugar buffs away dead skin cells, while its rich mineral content—potassium, magnesium, zinc, and copper—destroys bacteria and brightens your complexion.

Raw Honey

With antibacterial properties that prevent and treat blemishes, raw honey also pulls moisture to the surface of the skin like a magnet. And, as with all exfoliants, it helps loosen those pesky dead skin cells.

Sea Salt

Not to be totally snobby, but there's a (HUGE) difference between sea salt and table salt. Sea salt is always preferred, as it contains minerals required to nourish the skin. And, as you might guess, it acts as a gentle, natural abrasive.

Coffee

Oh, coffee. Unfortunately, the most useful state of coffee is on your skin and not necessarily in your body. In fact, its anti-inflammatory, antioxidant properties are really quite wonderful when applied to your face, since they reduce puffiness and soothe and tone the skin.

Oatmeal

This stuff is as soothing on your skin as it is when eaten for breakfast. It's an anti-inflammatory and a natural moisturizer, so while it calms the skin, it also infuses it with moisture.

Strawberries

These bright red beauties have lots of qualities to recommend them, like vitamin C to strengthen collagen and vitamin E to moisturize. Even the seeds are useful. They contain healthy fats—including omega-3s—for soothing moisture.

Almond Butter

Loaded with vitamins A and E, almond butter shields the skin from sun damage, moisturizes, and puts the brakes on aging. Oh, and it softens and firms the skin, too, which never hurts!

Lemon

Besides smelling heavenly, lemon is a great way to dry up oily skin and diminish the appearance of age spots. It also evens skin color and tone.

Expert Exfoliator Concoctions

Ready to tap the power of all these yummy exfoliants? I thought so! Apply the following to your face. (You can also use these on your body—allowing every inch of you to benefit!)

So Long, Puffy Face Scrub

(This works as a cellulite scrub, but it does wonders for the face as well! It softens, moisturizes, tightens, and brightens skin while reducing puffiness.)

⅓ cup (75 mL) coffee granules
¼ cup (60 mL) extra virgin olive oil

Mix the ingredients together in a bowl, and then rub the concoction on your face with circular motions for a minute or two. Let sit for about 10 minutes before rinsing off.

TIP

You can substitute used coffee granules from your coffeemaker for the coffee granules listed in the recipe. Recycling never looked so good!

The Fountain of Youth Scrub

(This scrub can be used as cleanser.)

½ cup (125 mL) strawberries
½ cup (125 mL) oats
1 Tbsp (15 mL) camu camu powder
1 Tbsp (15 mL) raw honey
3 Tbsp (50 mL) Greek yogurt
2 Tbsp (30 mL) pumpkin seed butter

Add all ingredients to a food processer, and process until well combined. Massage onto your face and let sit until it starts to feel firm. Wash off with lukewarm water.

Berry Oily-No-More Scrub

(This scrub helps rein in an oily complexion, and can be used as cleanser.)

½ cup (125 mL) raspberries (to strengthen collagen and moisturize)
¼ cup (60 mL) coconut sugar
3 Tbsp (50 mL) fresh lemon juice

Purée raspberries, and then mix in remaining ingredients. Massage onto damp, clean skin with circular motions for one to two minutes, and then rinse off with cool water.

The Almond Joy

(This one is SOOO tasty!)

1 banana
¼ cup (60 mL) almond butter
3 Tbsp (50 mL) almond oil (or extra virgin olive oil)
2 Tbsp (30 mL) raw honey

Mash up banana, and then mix in remaining ingredients until well combined. Massage onto damp, clean face with circular motions. Let sit for five minutes, and then gently wipe off with a damp facecloth and wash with lukewarm water.

Cleansers

Washing your face—daily!—is the most important rule when it comes to healthy skin-care. Cleansing in the morning and before bed is essential for keeping skin cells clean and unclogged, getting rid of all the environmental stress, and keeping skin youthful and healthy looking.

While many of the exfoliators listed above also cleanse your face, here are gentler remedies to use on a daily basis.

Oil-Be-Gone Cleanser *(Note: If you have dry skin, replace grapefruit juice with extra virgin olive oil; otherwise, this may be too drying.)*	2 Tbsp (30 mL) lemon juice 1 Tbsp (15 mL) grapefruit juice 2 Tbsp (30 mL) raw honey 1 Tbsp (15 mL) Greek yogurt Add all ingredients to a bowl and whisk until well combined. Rub onto face and rinse right away with water.
Hydrating Cleanser	2 Tbsp (30 mL) oats 2 Tbsp (30 mL) Greek yogurt 1 Tbsp (15 mL) extra virgin olive oil 1 tsp (5 mL) raw honey Add all ingredients to a bowl and whisk until well combined. Massage onto face and rinse with lukewarm water.
Oh-So-Sensitive Skin Cleanser	½ apple 3 Tbsp (50 mL) aloe gel ⅓ cup (75 mL) green tea (steeped) ½ avocado Add all ingredients to a blender and blend well. Massage onto face and rinse with lukewarm water.
Everyone's a Greek Goddess Cleanser *(For all skin types)*	2 Tbsp (30 mL) Greek yogurt or buttermilk 2 Tbsp (30 mL) raw honey 1 tsp (5 mL) extra virgin olive oil Whisk until well combined. Rub on your face and then wash off immediately.

Toners

If you think toners are a waste of time and money, think again. They're like the trainers at the gym: yes, you can exercise on your own, but if you hire a trainer, you're going to get much better results. Toners decongest and minimize pores, balance skin pH, and wipe away the last remnants of oil, makeup, and dirt that washing couldn't get to. Oh, and they impart a youthful glow—provided you have the right toner. Any of the following ingredients can be used on their own as a toner, or you can whip up one of the recipes I've included afterward.

Chamomile Tea

Just as it calms you before bedtime, chamomile tea soothes your skin by reducing inflammation and irritation. It's also a natural antiseptic. Steep the tea and, using a cotton pad, apply it directly to the skin.

Cucumber Juice

Thanks to its silica content, cucumber increases collagen production while toning and firming the skin. Juice it with the skin on, and then apply with a cotton pad. If you don't have a juicer handy (or don't feel like cleaning it), slice the cucumber and wipe those on your skin instead.

Apples

Apples do double duty as an exfoliant and a toner. They tighten pores, clean up excess oil, and boost collagen production. Juice the apple with the skin on, add a tiny bit of freshly squeezed lemon, and use a cotton pad to apply in an upward-and-outward direction.

Apple Cider Vinegar

This bad boy is an antiseptic, so it's great for blasting acne-breeding bacteria. In addition, it increases blood circulation and regulates the skin's pH. It's also awesome for oily skin. Just make sure you use the unpasteurized kind. That's right, the one with the gooey bacterial starter floating around on the bottom. And be sure you DILUTE IT WITH WATER before you apply it to your face. This stuff doesn't mess around. Use three tablespoons of water (or more if your skin is dry) for every tablespoon of vinegar.

Lavender Oil

Lavender oil is great for acne, since it has antiseptic, antifungal, and anti-inflammatory properties that help prevent and treat breakouts. It also helps treat eczema and psoriasis and reduce wrinkles. If none of those apply (lucky duck), you might like it for its soothing properties—lavender oil minimizes redness and soothes irritations.

Rosewater

Who doesn't want to smell like a rose? And if you have dry skin, redness, or puffiness, anti-inflammatory, emollient-rich rosewater is just the answer. Mix a quarter cup of water with three drops of rose oil, or muddle rose petals with pure water. That's right. It's like a mojito, but way better for your skin.

Green Tea

Antioxidants are awesome. But green tea takes them to a whole new level—it has more antioxidants than vitamins E or C! Green tea also contains caffeine, which is an anti-inflammatory that helps smooth the skin. When using steeped green tea, you can apply it directly to your face with a cotton pad. And the stronger the brew, the better.

Lemon

Good for oily skin and combating acne, lemon juice isn't just for exfoliating. It also balances pH and destroys bacteria. And if you have age spots, lemon juice can help lighten them, too. Combine juice of half a lemon to a half-cup of water, and use a cotton pad to rub evenly onto your face. You can leave this on for the day, or you can apply fresh lemon juice directly on your face with a makeup brush. Leave that on for five minutes, and then rinse.

Expert Toner Concoctions

Juicy Age-Defying Toner	1 apple 1 cucumber ¼ cup (60 mL) brewed green tea Juice the apple and a 4-inch (10-cm) piece of cucumber, keeping the skin on. Mix with green tea, and apply to your face with a cotton pad.
The Bliss-Trip Soothing Toner *(Great for calming inflamed skin!)*	¼ cup (60 mL) chamomile tea 3 drops rose oil or ¼ cup (60 mL) rosewater 2 drops lavender oil Mix ingredients, and apply to your face with a cotton pad using upward, outward strokes.
Shine-No-More Oily Skin Toner	½ cup (125 mL) apple juice, freshly squeezed 2 Tbsp (30 mL) apple cider vinegar Juice apple with skin on, and mix in apple cider vinegar.
The Moisture-Magnet Toner	¼ cup (60 mL) rose petals ¼ cup (60 mL) fresh basil ½ cup (125 mL) pure water 3 drops lavender oil Add rose petals and basil to boiled water that has slightly cooled. Let steep until cooled completely. Strain liquid into a jar, add drops of lavender oil, and mix.
Cool as a Cuke Skin-Lightening Toner	1 cucumber 3 drops lavender oil Juice one cucumber with the skin on, and add lavender. With a cleansing pad, gently apply the toner to your face using circular motions. You can also pour the liquid into a spray bottle and use it as a hydrating spritzer.

Moisturizers

It seems as though we're always in search of the perfect moisturizer, trying all sorts of concoctions just to achieve the ideal state of dewyness. It doesn't have to be so hard! These oils all serve as excellent daily moisturizers.

Extra Virgin Olive Oil

This is my all-time favorite moisturizer: it works wonderfully all by itself! And it can address a wide variety of skin ailments, thanks to its antiviral, antibacterial, antioxidant, antifungal, and anti-inflammatory properties, all without losing any of its hydrating punch. While its vitamins A and E fight off free-radical and UV damage, its naturally occurring squalane helps restore and retain lost moisture. Fine lines, meanwhile, are no match for it, as it helps repair, renew, and regenerate skin cells. Add a drop of sea-buckthorn oil for added anti-aging benefits.

> **TIP**
> Try EVOO as an eye-makeup remover! It works great as an eye serum, too, as it helps reduce the appearance of lines. Just make sure you're using a pure, high-quality EVOO so that it absorbs without a smeary, greasy mess.

Almond Oil

Almond oil is similar to EVOO, so if you prefer a milder scent, give this a try. Its abundant vitamin E protects skin from UV damage, while also rejuvenating and deeply moisturizing. Almond oil boasts emollient properties, too, which help smooth and soften skin.

Sea-Buckthorn Seed Oil

Whether you're looking to minimize wrinkles, eliminate acne, or calm irritated skin, sea-buckthorn seed oil has the solution. Its fatty acids (including omega-3s) work to soothe and reduce inflammation while also serving as an extremely effective moisturizer. But where sea-buckthorn really stands out is in the anti-aging arena. Its rich supply of antioxidants combines with its essential fatty acids to treat skin conditions, acne, wrinkles, and even wounds. Add to both facial and body moisturizers for anti-aging benefits.

Jojoba Oil

Jojoba works in a similar way to the sebum your body produces, but takes it one step further: it actually dissolves blockages in the hair follicles. (This, obviously, helps out in the acne department.) Jojoba is also a natural emollient, so it softens and moisturizes even as it excavates your pores.

Coconut Oil

If you're looking to firm up skin, coconut oil's cell-strengthening properties are worth trying. Be aware, though, that it doesn't penetrate as deeply into the skin as EVOO does.

Water

Nothing screams aged skin like dehydrated skin. Hydration is key to a flawless, glowy, youthful complexion. Proper hydration reduces the appearance of wrinkles, eliminates dryness, and helps with elasticity. Aim to drink half your body weight in ounces each day.

Green Juice

The juice from watery veggies, such as cucumber and celery, provides the same benefit as water, plus the added value of vitamins, minerals, and nutrients that cleanse the skin and reduce inflammation and puffiness. When juicing cucumber, keep the skin on, as it's rich in silica—an important mineral that strengthens collagen and improves skin elasticity.

Want Glowing Skin? Just Mask!

The best way to get instant results is to use a mask. The right ones can help moisturize, hydrate, regenerate, and rejuvenate skin—and that means you'll look glowingly good. Here are some of my faves:

Glowing Pumpkin Mask

½ cup (125 mL) pumpkin purée (contains vitamin A, which protects against UV damage; vitamin C, which increases collagen production, preventing and reducing the appearance of wrinkles; and zinc, which adds brightness, soothes, and moisturizes)

1 banana (moisturizes and revitalizes)

¼ cup (60 mL) yogurt (exfoliates and hydrates; contains alpha hydroxy acids to even skin tone, get rid of dry skin, and prevent wrinkles)

1 egg white (tones and tightens saggy skin, maintains its elasticity)

2 Tbsp (30 mL) pumpkin seed butter (high in fats for moisture, and high in zinc to combat acne and to pump up the glow factor)

Add all ingredients in blender and blend. Let sit on your face for 10 to 20 minutes, then wash with lukewarm water.

Yo-Vo Skin Glow Anti-Aging Mask

1 avocado, ripe (vitamin E hydrating, prevents wrinkles, protects skin from sun damage)

½ cup (125 mL) yogurt (contains lactic acid, a derivative of the alpha hydroxy acids used in chemical peels; helps treat mild wrinkles and evens skin tone—unglues proteins holding dead skin cells in place)

¼ cup (60 mL) papaya (papain enzyme dissolves old surface skin cells; can help reduce fine lines, wrinkles, and age spots)

Add all ingredients in blender and blend. Let sit on your face for 10 to 20 minutes, then wash with lukewarm water.

Banana-Not-Chemical Peel

¼ cup (60 mL) buttermilk (contains alpha hydroxy acid, which rejuvenates skin and is often used in professional peels)

1 avocado (high fat content; antioxidants vitamins A and E soften the skin)

½ banana (potassium revitalizes the skin)

1 kiwi (high in antioxidants, vitamin C, and antioxidant vitamin E)

Blend all ingredients in blender, rub onto skin, and let it sit for 20 minutes. Then wash off with lukewarm water.

Kiss and Tell

Nothing is sexier on a mouth than moist, gunk-free lips. So forget glittery glosses, gooey sticks, and chemical-laced balms. All you need is the right scrub and a good, natural gloss.

Sweet 'n' Spicy Lip Scrub

1 tsp (5 mL) raw honey
½ tsp (2 mL) ground cinnamon
¼ tsp (1 mL) cayenne
toothbrush

Mix ingredients together and apply to lips with your fingers. Leave it on for a few minutes, then scrub your lips with a wet, clean toothbrush. Wipe your lips dry with a damp towel, and apply lip balm.

Honey-Do Lip Balm

coconut oil

extra virgin olive oil

raw honey

Mix four parts coconut oil with four parts extra virgin olive oil and one part raw honey. Keep in a small container, and apply to lips for an über-moisturizing treatment.

High-Shine Lip Gloss

vitamin E oil (1 capsule)

Pop open a vitamin E capsule and spread the oil directly on your lips. It makes the shiniest lip gloss ever! If you want a sexier, pouty look, add 1 to 2 drops of cinnamon or peppermint essential oil to increase your lips' fullness.

Plump and Sexy: 2-in-1 Lip Balm and Exfoliant

2 Tbsp (30 mL) coconut oil

2 Tbsp (30 mL) EVOO

2 drops cinnamon essential oil

1 Tbsp (15 mL) strawberry juice (no seeds)

Melt coconut oil and stir in EVOO, cinnamon oil, and strawberry juice. Pour into a small container and use as needed.

Turn this balm into a lip exfoliator by mixing raw honey with EVOO, cinnamon, and cayenne. Let it sit on your lips for 10 minutes, then wash it off with a wet, clean toothbrush. Follow with lip balm.

PLUMPERS BEWARE!

Think you have to use a store-bought lip plumper to get great full lips? Not so! Cinnamon and cayenne are irritants that increase blood flow to the lips, making them look plumper and rosier! Honey, meanwhile, exfoliates and moisturizes. And scrubbing with a clean, wet toothbrush exfoliates and increases circulation—which translates to a fuller mouth.

Traditional lip plumpers, meanwhile, are full of not-so-hot ingredients like the following:

- **Methylparaben.** Carcinogens just to look beautiful.
- **BHT.** An agent that interferes with the immune system.
- **Dimethicone.** Use of this chemical has been restricted by the Cosmetic Ingredient Review Board due to the dangers it poses for damaged skin. It also rates as a high hazard (earning a 9/10 score) on the Environmental Working Group's list.

Beauty Bite

It's one thing to have your age revealed by a wrinkle or two. It's another thing alto-gether to have yellow teeth give it away. So restore your mouth to its pearly splendor with this natural remedy. The breath freshener recipe will make your mouth taste as good as it looks!

Teeth Whitener	4 strawberries 1 tsp (5 mL) non-aluminum baking soda 2 drops mint essential oil Mash up strawberries in a bowl and then stir in the baking soda and mint. Dip your toothbrush into the mixture and brush away all those stubborn stains!
Breath Freshener	**Star ingredient:** Cinnamon sticks Nix those candied mints in favor of cinnamon sticks! Cinnamon is antibacterial, so not only will it immediately freshen breath, it will also kill odor-causing bacteria. Break off a small piece of cinnamon stick and suck on it like a mint. Or, if you want to wash and go, mix one tablespoon of ground cinnamon with water and gargle with it like a mouthwash.

14. Kitchen Beautician: Hair

Don't you just love those shampoo commercials where women have the super-shiny, lustrous hair that bounces exaggeratedly with every step they take? Like, come on, unless you've got some souped-up hydraulic system attached to your scalp, whose hair really bounces like that? Nonetheless, those commercials work, since we ALL want that hair! Only problem is, many shampoos and hair-care products are laced with harsh chemicals and irritants that, in the long term, can cause more damage than good.

Hair's Anatomy

Each strand of hair grows out of a hair follicle, which is housed in the dermis—right below the skin's surface. The follicles are attached to the sebaceous gland, which produces sebum, the oily substance that moisturizes hair. (And when the sebaceous gland gets overzealous in production, you end up with greasy hair.) The hair that lies within the follicle beneath the skin is alive; that's where hair growth is stimulated. The hair that extends beyond the surface of the skin is not alive: it's made of keratin, which is pretty much a hard (and dead) protein. This part is called the shaft.

The hair shaft is made up of three layers:

1. The medulla is the innermost layer of the shaft; it's where some of the pigment for your hair color is stored.
2. The cortex is the middle layer. This makes up most of the hair shaft; it holds keratin bundles and color pigment. It also determines how strong your hair is.
3. The cuticle is the outermost layer. This part looks a lot like fish skin—the cuticles overlap like scales—and it can make your hair look shiny (when the scales are nice and flat) or dry and damaged (as if the fish has been electrocuted).

DID YOU KNOW?

Straight hair tends to be shinier than curly hair because it's easier for the sebum to travel down the shaft and moisturize the entire strand. But straight hair has its pitfalls, too. Specifically, it gets greasier faster.

Dry Hair Demystified

Whether we've seen it or lived it, we all know what aesthetic destruction dry hair can cause. It totally sucks. It gets frizzy, looks brittle, and devastates the overall appearance of whoever's wearing it. Here's why your hair can be lacking luster.

1. Cuticle damage
   - The cuticle is designed to protect the inner layers of your hair from damage and to prevent moisture from seeping out. Once the cuticle becomes damaged, moisture and natural oils from the hair escape, causing hair to become dry and dull looking.
   - The obvious cause is the abuse we inflict on our hair. I have naturally curly hair, so I myself am victim to this every time I tug on my locks to straighten them. Our trusty hot tools (flat irons, curling irons, blow dryers) do quite the number, yet they're impossible to live without. And they're not the only or worst cause of haylike hair. Harsh shampoos, hair dyes, chemical hair treatments, overstyling, chlorine exposure, and UV rays are all damaging.
2. Impaired sebum production
   - Sometimes the sebaceous gland just isn't producing enough sebum. This can be the result of a hormonal imbalance, thyroid issues, a lack of healthy fats in the diet, or generally poor nutrition.

Just as they can do to your skin, poor diet, stress, lack of sleep, bad habits (smoking!), and environmental toxins can make your hair look aged, dry, and dull. A healthy lifestyle coupled with proper nutrition is key to keeping your hair shiny and "bouncy" *au natural.*

The foods you eat feed your hair follicles. The healthier the foods, the healthier your hair follicles, the healthier your scalp, and the healthier new hair growth. Here are some key nutrients to feed your hair from the inside out.

Protein

Proteins are the building blocks for hair growth. In fact, 97 percent of hair IS protein—hardened protein, but protein nonetheless. So getting enough protein in your diet helps strengthen the hair follicle as well as the shaft.

Omega-3 Fatty Acids

Want shiny, lustrous hair? Bust out those fats. There are a ton of health reasons for adding more omega-3s to your diet, of course, but one of the best (superficial) reasons is the quality of your hair. Omega-3 fatty acids are essential for nourishing hair follicles. Not only do they reduce inflammation and balance hormones—which can bog down follicles and slow hair growth—they also add amazing moisture to hair, upping its shine, luster, and elasticity. In fact, they help alleviate all manner of hair disappointments, whether it's dry, damaged hair or flaky scalp. Some evidence also suggests that omega-3s might help mitigate hair loss.

Best foods for protein AND omega-3s:
- Oily fish
- Whole eggs
- Nuts (walnuts and almonds)
- Seeds (sacha inchi, pumpkin, hemp, chia)

Biotin (Vitamin B7)

Biotin (vitamin B7) is the heart and soul of healthy hair. Since it's an abundant mineral found in a variety of sources, biotin deficiencies are rare, but signs include hair loss, hair breakage, brittle hair, and even brittle nails. If you're looking to strengthen your tresses, ignite hair growth, or just feel confident that bad hair won't plague you, stock up on foods rich in biotin for that added insurance.

Foods high in biotin:

- Swiss chard
- Egg yolks
- Carrots
- Almonds
- Peanuts
- Bananas
- Salmon

Silica

Good for preventing wrinkles AND for strengthening hair, silica is a beauty junkie's dream. This trace mineral strengthens connective tissues, tendons, cartilage, muscles, hair, and nails. It can also help prevent hair loss.

Foods rich in silica:

- Leeks
- Green beans
- Chickpeas
- Strawberries
- Cucumber (their skin, anyway)

Vitamins A, C, and E

These antioxidant powerhouse vitamins come to the rescue again, this time to nourish your mane. Here's where they shine:

- Vitamin E promotes follicle growth and prevents UV damage.
- Vitamin C helps strengthen protein bonds and supports a healthy scalp and hair follicles. A vitamin C deficiency can lead to breakage.
- Beta carotene is the healthiest way to get vitamin A, which prevents dry hair. (Your body converts beta carotene into an appropriate amount of vitamin A.)

Some foods containing vitamins A, C, and E:

- Kale
- Asparagus
- Sweet potatoes
- Strawberries
- Avocados

See Chapter 10, pages 117–119 for more.

Iron

Iron is the pack mule of your body, helping to carry oxygen—not to mention other nutrients—to your hair follicles. Low iron levels or anemia can actually lead to hair loss! This usually affects premenopausal women.

Foods high in iron:
- Chickpeas
- Lentils
- Chlorella
- Shellfish
- Sea veggies (kelp, nori)

Silver Fears

Copper

While premature graying is largely attributable to genetics, a copper deficiency could be another factor. Copper is what gives hair its color, and a deficiency could lead to salt-and-pepper tresses before your time. To avoid spending too many hours in your color tech's chair, try adding more copper-rich foods!

Foods rich in copper:
- Crimini mushrooms
- Sesame seeds
- Cashews
- Quinoa
- Miso
- Chickpeas
- Turnip greens
- Swiss chard

Lock-Loss Monsters

Thinning hair is hard for men, and even more terrifying for women. Pinpointing the cause, however, is like finding the proverbial needle in a haystack: there are SO many factors to consider. From genetics to stress, hormonal imbalances to radiation, and disease to poor diet, the possibilities abound. And when it comes to diet, a deficiency in any of the above nutrients can be a contributor, although it's typically more than ONE thing. Like a complicated updo, everything is interconnected.

But in addition to the nutrients listed above and an overall healthy diet and lifestyle, one nutrient does stand out: zinc.

Zinc

This trace mineral does a lot of things. It supports the immune system, encourages new cell growth, and supports the sebaceous gland, providing hair with moisture and shine. But it's a zinc *deficiency* that can lead to hair loss.

It all starts with the enzyme 5-alpha-reductase, which converts testosterone into DHT, a stronger and more active androgen. While some guys may consider this a good thing, in excess it's not. Testosterone and DHT are important sex hormones that serve many functions in the body. But when DHT is too high relative to other hormones, it can lead to harmful effects like bad acne, prostate issues, *and* hair loss.

But this is where superhero zinc comes into play. Zinc acts as a 5-alpha-reductase *inhibitor*, limiting the production of DHT. What's great here is that zinc actually *increases* testosterone, yet inhibits its conversion to DHT. So for men (and women) who are worried about potentially losing their sex drive, think their testicles will shrivel up and dry out, or are stressing to think their interests will shift from bro-bonding over Monday night football to glitter and *Gilmore Girls*, there's no need to get your panties in a knot, sweetheart. None of that will happen. With enough zinc in your life, you might just be able to have your cake and keep your hair, too!

Foods high in zinc:

- Oysters (lobster, crab)
- Wheat germ
- Sesame seeds
- Roasted pumpkin seeds
- Crimini mushrooms
- Spinach
- Summer squash
- Cocoa powder
- Miso
- Maple syrup

DIY Hair Remedies
Foods to Wear on Your Hair

AVOCADO	High in fats and vitamin E—strengthens and moisturizes
BANANA	Moisturizes and conditions, while potassium strengthens hair
EGG	Rich in protein and fat—strengthens and moisturizes damaged hair
EXTRA VIRGIN OLIVE OIL	Rich in fats and vitamin E for deep conditioning
ALMOND OIL	Rich in fats and vitamin E for deep conditioning, plus B vitamins help to nourish scalp
GREEK YOGURT	Lactic acids help to cleanse and remove dirt and buildup

(Continued)

HONEY	Locks in moisture
LEMON	Can get rid of oily, greasy hair, but make sure to dilute as it can dry out hair
APPLE CIDER VINEGAR	Adds shine while detangling and cutting through grease
GREEN TEA	Contains tannic acids to cut through grease

TIP

Once a week, after washing your hair, try giving it a quick rinse with apple cider vinegar, then rinse out with water. It will cut through all the buildup and make hair super shiny.

Expert Hair Concoctions

If you're looking for a place to start, here are some great combos to tame your tresses.

High-Gloss Locks *(for dry hair)*	1 avocado 3 Tbsp (50 mL) almond oil 1 banana ¼ cup (60 mL) Greek yogurt Mash all ingredients into a bowl, then massage into clean, damp hair and let sit for 15 minutes before washing out.
No-More-Breakage Conditioner *(strengthens brittle hair)*	3 eggs 1 avocado 2 Tbsp (30 mL) extra virgin olive oil Add egg whites and yolks to a bowl and give them a good whisk. Scoop out the flesh of a ripe avocado and mash it right in along with the oil, mixing well (or add ingredients to a blender). Massage into clean, damp hair and let sit for 15 minutes before washing out. Eggs and avocados are the perfect protein-and-fat duo to treat damaged hair and prevent breakage. They help strengthen keratin bonds and add moisture back to dry, damaged hair. They also help prevent frizziness and boost shine. Win-win.

Deep Conditioner	extra virgin olive oil or almond oil (Both are rich in vitamin E and fats to moisturize and hydrate hair.) With damp hair, massage oil directly onto the scalp and then work all the way to the ends. Let sit for 20 to 30 minutes. Then wash hair. This provides an awesome deep-conditioning treatment and adds luster. Sometimes I do this before bed, then wrap my hair in a towel and wash it out in the morning.
Flaky Scalp	3 Tbsp (50 mL) almond oil 1 tsp (5 mL) lemon, freshly juiced Whisk ingredients in a bowl, then massage onto scalp. The almond oil will moisturize and hydrate, while the lemon will get rid of dry, dead skin cells. Massage for minimum of 5 minutes (it can stay in hair for 15 minutes), then wash out.
Oily Hair	green tea (contains tannic acids, which can help cut through grease) Steep 4 tea bags in 2 cups (500 mL) of boiling water, then let cool. Add contents to spray bottle and saturate hair from root to halfway down the shaft, let sit for 10 minutes, then rinse out. Other options that work: ½ cup (125 mL) apple cider vinegar + 1 cup (250 mL) water ¼ cup (60 mL) fresh lemon juice + 1 cup (250 mL) water Apply using same method as above.

PART 4

The Food–Health Connection

Feel amazing every day with foods to improve digestion, boost immunity, get rid of pain and inflammation, improve bone health, keep your ticker ticking, fight menopause, and beat the monthly PMS woes!

My intention in writing this book—and in doing what I do—is to promote wellness. My goal is to educate people in how to live a more vibrant, fulfilled life by making simple lifestyle changes to maintain health and become even healthier. For many, unfortunately, it's only once their health takes a turn that they look seriously at their eating habits. They may learn that they have high cholesterol, metabolic syndrome, or even cancer—and then they start to make changes. But these health problems can be prevented and treated by making smart, easy decisions every single day.

At around the time I was about to leave my investment career behind, I decided to go on a "healthy adventure" holiday in the Florida Keys. What I thought would be a leisurely yet active vaycay—scuba diving, hikes, swimming with dolphins, and enjoying raw, plant-based meals prepared by Chef Chad Sarno—ended up being something rather more than that. And it essentially changed my life.

After the plane landed in Miami, I shared a shuttle bus with about six others who were heading to the same retreat. A man in his mid-sixties sat beside me; he was from L.A., he told me, and was traveling with his wife. "So, what made you decide to take this trip?" I asked him as we drove from island to island through gin-blue waters. "Well," he began, sitting up straighter, "a year ago I was diagnosed with stage four lung cancer." He went on to explain that after multiple rounds of chemo and radiation therapy, there was nothing left for the doctors to do. He was frail and ill and had been given four weeks to live. And yet here he was a year later, telling me his story. "How did you do it?" I asked, curious. "I just changed my diet and my lifestyle and used alternative treatments," he said with a peaceful energy.

To my amazement, I soon came to realize that nearly all of the 150 people who attended this "healthy adventure" had been able to reverse cancer, heart disease, diabetes, or some other serious health deterrent. I'd made the trip because it suited my healthy lifestyle; it was a way of life for me to eat clean and exercise. But most others had come to the retreat because of a *forced* lifestyle change. Many had been successful in fighting and even reversing what ailed them; but still, theirs had been a reactive approach to illness rather than a proactive approach to wellness.

After I'd attended a week of lectures from experts around the world, listened to success stories, and celebrated health (and of course swam with those dolphins and indulged in gourmet raw food), at the very end a dinner was held with a panel of experts who debated health issues and answered questions. I got up and posed one of my own: "I know so many people who've been diagnosed with cancer or heart disease, and they all approach it with conventional medicine. They get better, then they go back to their old ways and get sick again. But here I've been witnessing dozens upon dozens of people who've been cancer-free for 10 to 20 years. One guy even cleared his clogged arteries through diet and lifestyle changes! How do I take this message about real health and make it mainstream? How do I do my part in promoting wellness so that people want to feel their best and healthiest every day?" The answer? "Sign up for the health educator course that starts next week in West Palm Beach." Done. I signed up, packed up my Toronto life, and went back to school so that I could do what I was meant to do: educate and promote wellness.

Einstein was right when he said you can't solve a problem with the same consciousness that created it. Sometimes things have to change. And in order to create change, there'll be periods of discomfort. This is a good thing! You can feel your absolute healthiest every day—and it's NEVER too late. No matter where you are in your life, in your health, and in your habits, I'll meet you right where you are.

I hope you feel inspired. Be well.

15. Tummy Troubles

I love the sound of popping bubble-wrap ... but not when it's coming from my stomach! Rumbles, grumbles, and bloating, oh my! Not the most attractive thing, especially when accompanied by a six-inch expansion in waist circumference.

Many amazing things are going on in that tummy of yours. It's where the magic happens. Food gets broken down and nutrients get absorbed. Your health, your thoughts, your weight—everything we talk about in this book is connected not just to *what* you eat, but to *how* you assimilate your food and nutrients. Remember, 80 percent of your immune system resides in your gut. Listen to what it's telling you, and it will thank you by keeping you feeling your best!

Let's take a look at the two most common digestive issues—an underactive stomach and an overactive stomach.

I'm Bloated: Underactive Stomach

An underactive stomach is one of the most common digestive complaints. Many people confuse it with an overactive stomach and take antacids as a result—which makes the condition even worse! An underactive stomach is one that doesn't produce enough hydrochloric acid (HCl). This acid is released in the stomach to break down food, including fiber and plant roughage. The enzyme pepsin, which is used to digest protein, is activated only in the presence of HCl.

HCl also works to protect the body from harmful microorganisms like bad bacteria, parasites, and viruses. It encourages the production of enzymes and the absorption of vitamins and minerals. In particular, calcium, iron, and zinc require adequate levels of HCl in the stomach in order to be metabolized and absorbed.

HCl naturally declines with age. However, the following factors also aggravate the condition:

- Diet high in red meat
- Dairy products
- Refined and processed foods
- Drinking too much fluid with meals
- Poor food combining
- Not chewing your food
- Emotional stress
- Eating too quickly

The symptoms of HCl deficiency can include:

- Excessive gas, belching, or burping after meals
- Constipation
- Stomach bloated after eating
- Halitosis
- Feeling too full after a heavy-meat meal
- Heavy, tired feeling after eating
- Nausea after taking supplements
- Dry skin, acne
- Undigested food in stool
- Poor absorption of nutrients/malnourishment

How to Combat an Underactive Stomach

1. Take digestive enzymes. Take four or five digestive enzymes immediately before a meal. This helps break down food and assimilate nutrients. *Try to purchase digestive enzymes that contain HCl.*

2. Slow down. Don't eat when rushed, anxious, or stressed. This will only aggravate the condition.

3. Chew your food! **The digestion of carbohydrates begins in your mouth. Amylase, which breaks down carbs, is secreted through your saliva gland. So the longer you munch away on your food, not only will you be breaking down the particles into smaller pieces, making it easier for your body to digest, but you'll be kick-starting the digestive process right in your chomper! See those teeth? They aren't there just to look pretty ... use those pearly whites and chew, chew, chew till your food is liquid!**
4. Don't drink with meals. **Drinking with meals flushes away those precious digestive enzymes. Drink at least 30 minutes before or two hours after meals for optimal digestion.**
5. Take a spoonful of apple cider vinegar. **Acidic foods like apple cider vinegar can help stimulate HCl. Try taking one tablespoon before a meal or add to salads. If you take apple cider vinegar with your meals and your symptoms dissipate, it's because you have low stomach acid. If they worsen, you have high stomach acid (see the next section on an overactive stomach).**
6. Try an elimination and rotation diet. **Food sensitivities can cause inflammation of your intestinal tract, impeding the digestive process and preventing the assimilation of nutrients—and causing serious bloating. Try cutting out major allergens (such as wheat, gluten, dairy, and soy) for a minimum of two weeks and then slowly add these foods back in, one by one, taking note of how you feel. I guarantee that during that two-week window you'll feel fab and your tummy will feel tight!**
7. Practice food combining. **Different foods digest at different rates. Melon may take only 30 minutes to digest, whereas a steak can take four hours! Follow the simple principles below and you should notice your symptoms improve.**

Food Combining

Proper assimilation of food requires the use of digestive enzymes. Different types of food require different digestive enzymes. The human body isn't designed to digest more than one type of food in the stomach at the same time, nor can it manufacture all the necessary enzymes simultaneously. Some foods, such as melon, digest in less than 30 minutes, whereas nuts can take up to four hours. Eating these types of foods together causes stress to your digestive system.

Here's how food types translate into different digestive times:

Protein	Starch	Vegetables and Leafy Greens	Fruit
~4 HOURS TO DIGEST	~3 HOURS TO DIGEST	~2.5 HOURS TO DIGEST	~2 HOURS TO DIGEST
• Nuts • Seeds • Fish/meat • Milks (nut, hemp)	• Grains • Beans and legumes • Winter squash • Potatoes, sweet potatoes, and yams	• Sprouts • Leafy greens • Cucumber • Peppers • Summer squash • Broccoli • Cabbage • Cauliflower • Corn • Root vegetables (carrots, beets, parsnips)	• All fruit, including tomatoes • Melons take 15 to 30 minutes to digest and should not be combined with any other fruit

Some results of poor food combining:

• Bloating
• Weight gain
• Indigestion
• Poor assimilation of nutrients
• Lack of energy
• Toxic waste buildup

Combinations to *avoid*:

• Starch + protein—creates various gases in your system, including sulfur
• Starch + fruit—creates fermentation and alcohol
• Protein + fruit—produces a variety of toxic byproducts

Combinations to *follow*:

• Leafy greens and vegetables + proteins
• Leafy greens and vegetables + fats
• Leafy greens and vegetables + starches

- Fruit and sweet foods should be eaten alone
- Avocados combine well with almost everything (protein, fruit, vegetables, leafy greens) but do not combine well with starch

Burn, Baby, Burn: Overactive Stomach

An overactive stomach occurs when your body produces too much HCl. Typically, this may be associated with an ulcer or lesion in the intestinal lining.

Here's how to tell if your tummy is overacting:

- Stomach pain one hour after eating or at night
- Burning sensation in stomach
- Pain aggravated by worry/tension
- Hiatal hernia, gastritis, gastric ulcer
- Nausea, vomiting
- Sensation of acidity in abdominal area
- Lower back pain
- Blood in stool

The causes of an overactive stomach can include a diet rich in spicy foods, caffeine, alcohol, tobacco, sugars, and nitrates, and a long-term use of aspirin. One of the best foods to treat an overactive stomach? Aloe vera. See page 127 for more on this tummy-calming food!

Foods to Aid Digestive Health

Whether your stomach is overactive or underactive, here are a few key foods that will help it return to a happy, healthy state of being.

Ginger

You might think of ginger as a common spice in Indian or Asian cooking, but don't be fooled by its boring beige color—ginger is anything but bland! This powerful herb, spice, nutritional supplement, and medicinal healer has been used all over the world since ancient times for much more than just spicing up dishes (and cookies).

Ginger's effects as a digestive miracle worker are by far its most impressive qualities. For thousands of years Chinese doctors have used ginger to manage nausea, vomiting, diarrhea, and stomach upset. Your mom was onto something when she made you drink flat ginger ale for an upset tummy. Ginger helps relieve indigestion, gas pains, diarrhea, and stomach cramping by increasing the production of digestive fluids and saliva. The relief ginger provides from nausea caused by morning sickness or motion sickness is by far its most highly acclaimed action in the body. Studies have shown that its anti-nausea properties are significantly more effective than Dramamine in curbing motion sickness.

DID YOU KNOW?

A double-blind randomized trial done at Thammasat University in Thailand compared the effects of one gram of ginger in capsule form taken daily and 100 milligrams of dimenhydrinate (Dramamine) on 170 women experiencing nausea and vomiting during pregnancy. The results showed that ginger is equally effective in the treatment of nausea and vomiting during pregnancy, and has fewer side effects.[59]

Ginger has many other health properties. It's a known diaphoretic, meaning it causes you to sweat, and so it's perfect for helping break a fever and detoxifying the body when excess toxins are present. As a natural anti-inflammatory, it's often used as a therapeutic natural remedy for sufferers of arthritis and rheumatism. Ginger also has properties that stimulate blood circulation, remove toxins from the body, cleanse the kidneys, and strengthen bowel function. Its ability to protect against symptoms of the common cold and flu also make it a fantastic preventative measure when your immune system needs a boost. On top of all that, ginger lowers cholesterol and acts as an antioxidant and antihistamine, improving allergy symptoms. Ginger root is also useful for respiratory problems, helping to rid the lungs of phlegm.

TIP

Ginger is believed to have aphrodisiac powers—and is even mentioned in the *Kama Sutra.*

HOW TO USE

In his book *Perfect Digestion,* Deepak Chopra recommends a drink of ginger and lemon to kindle the digestive fires while helping tone the digestive tract. Consuming ginger in the form of tea, either fresh or dried, is an easy and delicious way to get your digestive juices flowing. Ginger in cooking isn't necessarily enough to ignite that flame, so if you need more support, try a ginger capsule daily. This all-around health booster will work wonders for your digestion and assimilation (and maybe even your libido!).

Licorice

Licorice is best known for giving that distinct, much-loved taste to its popular candy counterpart, but most people remain unaware of what a powerful herb licorice root is in supporting whole body health. This naturally sweet and delicious herb has been used for medicinal healing in China since ancient times, and is considered to be among the most important healing herbs in the practice of traditional Chinese medicine. It got its name from the Greek word for "sweet root," and has been used for thousands of years as a flavoring and an intense sweetener.

Licorice's "demulcent" action is the reason it's praised as a wonder herb to help calm and support digestive health. It does this by coating the mucous membrane with a soothing film that helps alleviate pain and inflammation while protecting the integrity of the stomach and intestinal walls and supporting smooth digestive tract function. A form of licorice, deglycyrrhizinated licorice (DGL), is a natural supplement often used to treat ulcers (both gastric and duodenal) with great success. Licorice is believed to promote the healing of the digestive tissues in cases of ulceration by stimulating the protective lining of the stomach. When taking it as a supplement, be sure to take it only in the DGL form, as the glycyrrhizin has been removed (hence the term *deglycyr-rhizinated*). Glycyrrhizin can cause negative side effects like high blood pressure.

In recent years, herbalists have also been using licorice to combat adrenal weakness, which can be caused by a combination of stress and poor diet. The herb contains a natural hormone that stimulates increased production of cortisone and aldosterone, helping the body to better cope with excess stress and exhaustion while boosting energy levels at the same time. Licorice root is also considered an "herbal alterative": a cleansing stimulant that's effective in removing toxins and wastes from the body. It promotes cleansing of the colon and is also used to purify the liver, which is the body's center for detoxification.

HOW TO USE

Thinking of heading down to the corner store for some licorice laces? Think again! There are much more effective ways you can add licorice to your diet without the empty calories. Licorice can be taken regularly for the maintenance of healthy digestion in tea, or in the form of DGL capsules for therapeutic purposes. If you think licorice could work to help you balance your digestive processes, bear in mind that contraindications include those with high blood pressure, as well as women who are pregnant or nursing. Otherwise, let this nutritious, tasty herb do its thing!

Kale and Hemp-Seed Salad *(page 301)*

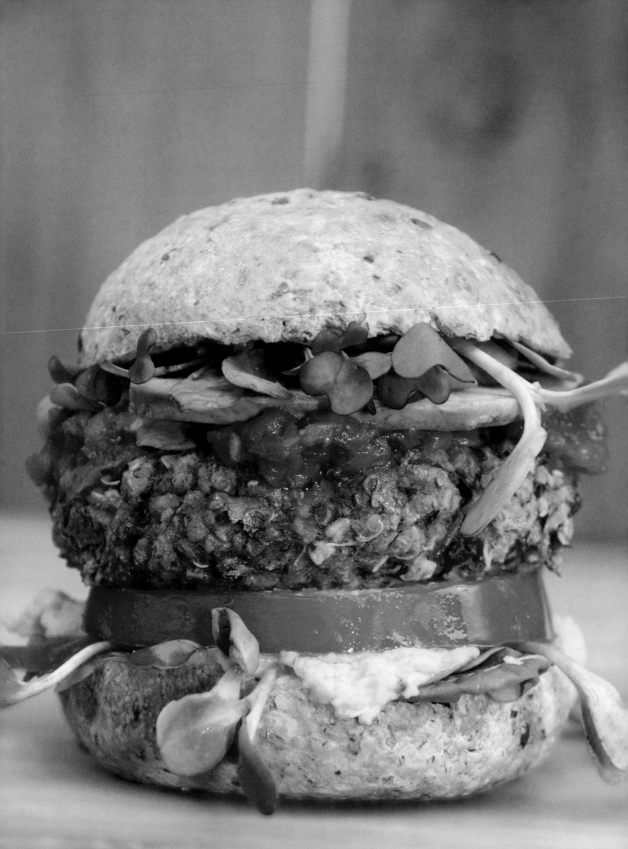

Quinoa Bean Burger *(page 308)*

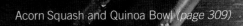
Acorn Squash and Quinoa Bowl *(page 309)*

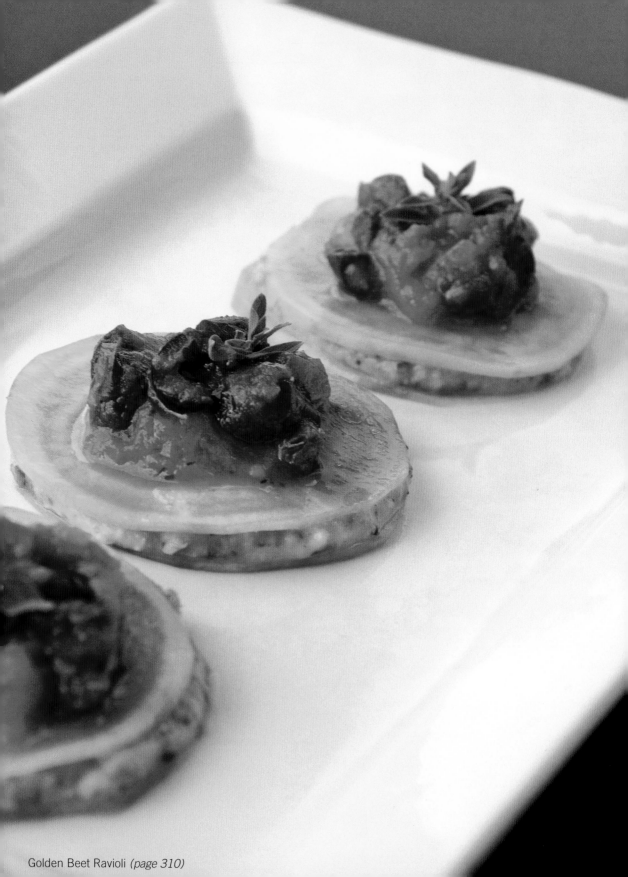

Golden Beet Ravioli *(page 310)*

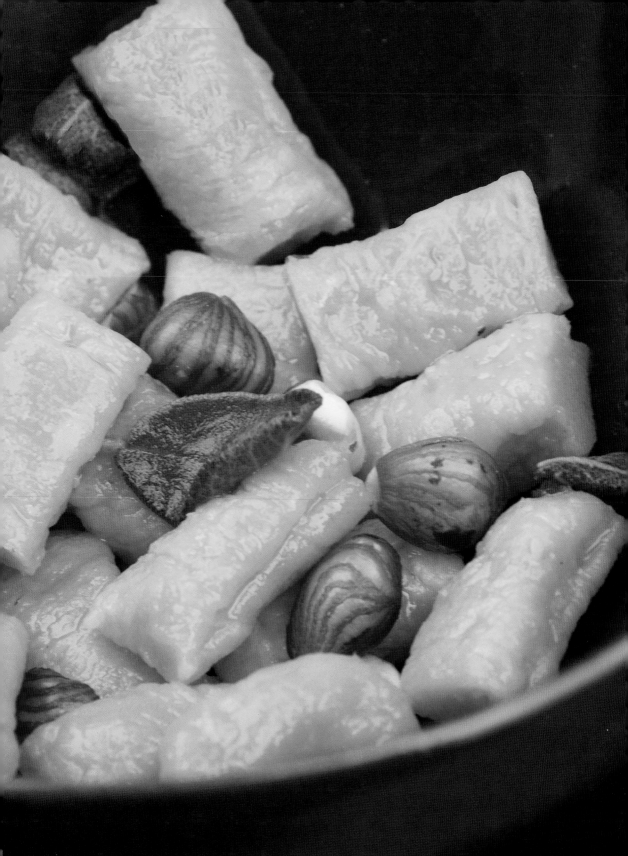

Sweet Potato Gnocchi *(page 312)*

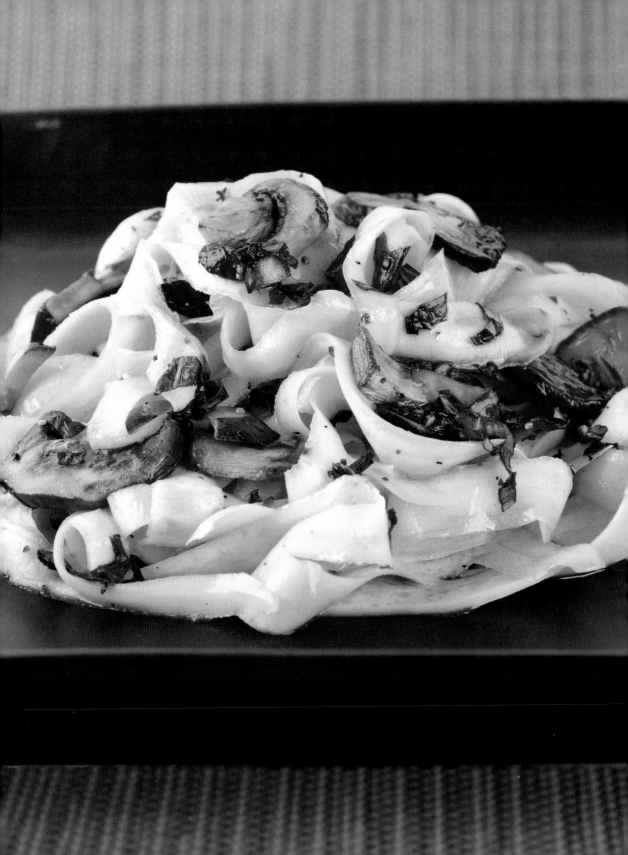

Mushroom and Zucchini Fettuccini *(page 314)*

Peggyfied Pizza Party *(page 315)*

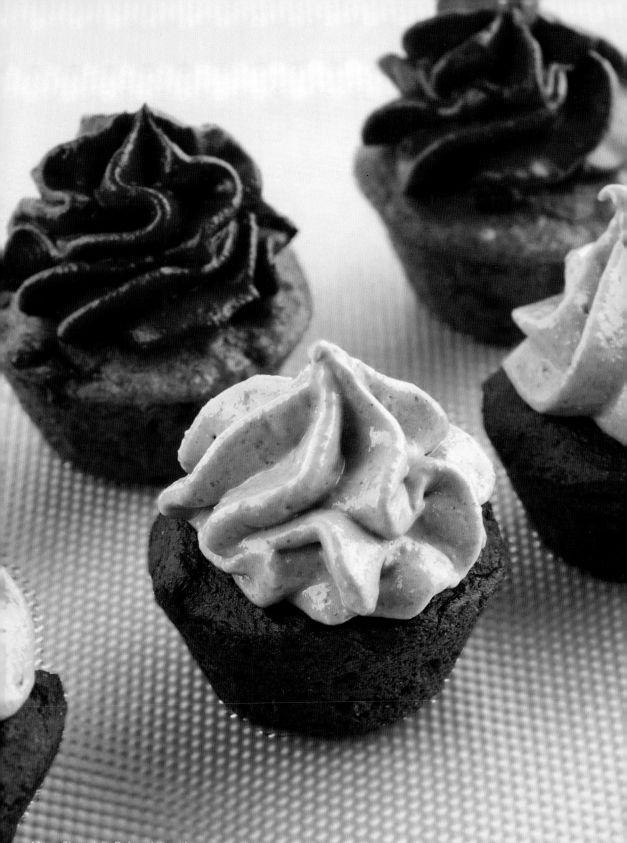

Maca Chocolate Babycakes with
Cherry Cashew Frosting *(page 320)*

Apple Cider Vinegar

Vinegar is a pretty typical culinary condiment. Apple cider vinegar, however, is produced slightly differently from other vinegars and has many more health benefits than your run-of-the-mill supermarket vinegar. Apple cider vinegar is made by crushing organic apples to produce a liquid. Sugar and yeast are added to this liquid, which is then matured in wooden barrels (which help to boost fermentation much more than in other distilled grocery store vinegars). The process turns the sugars into alcohol, which is then converted (by an acetic acid–forming bacteria) into vinegar.

When the vinegar is "mature," a dark, cloudy scum called the "mother" of vinegar forms on top of the cider. This scum is actually composed of bacteria and yeast cells that have died. I know—totally gross. Although it doesn't sound very appetizing, natural vinegars that contain the mother have extremely high levels of enzymes and minerals that other vinegars do not. It's a natural bacteria-fighting substance that contains many vital nutrients and minerals to support a healthy body. And it's why apple cider vinegar is believed to have so many health benefits. Forget how it's made and reap the benefits.

You'd be surprised at some of the things apple cider vinegar is used for! Some of the more common are weight loss, acne, yeast infections, constipation, and diarrhea. Heading out on the town? It's also used to combat bad breath, body odor, and cellulite. It's even suggested for diabetics to help regulate blood-sugar levels.

One of the most commonly acknowledged uses for this powerful vinegar is in balancing acid levels in the stomach to facilitate proper digestion. As we age, it's common for our bodies to produce less stomach acid. This decrease in hydrochloric acid can lead to digestive problems, especially sensations of heartburn and stomach upset. Although heartburn is commonly accepted in the medical world as a problem of excess acid in the stomach, acid reflux can also result from diminished stomach acid.

HOW TO USE

By taking two to three tablespoons of apple cider vinegar in water before every meal, you can enhance stomach acid production and increase digestive enzyme function. This vinegar can also improve assimilation and nutrient uptake while helping to rebalance the gut ecology and having an overall alkalinizing effect on the body. And like many healthy-but-not-necessarily-tasty remedies, you can always take it as a shooter if that helps it go down!

Peppermint

This leaf works magic in a mojito, or in mint chocolate-chunk ice cream ... or in a creative combo of the two, if that's how you roll! And you might want to save a few leaves to work their magic on your tummy, post nosh. Peppermint tea is recognized around the world for its wide range of medicinal benefits in the body, but it's most loved and appreciated for the wonderful effect it has on our digestive system.

Apart from its distinct and delicious taste, peppermint's herbal properties include anti-spasmodic, antiseptic, and anti-emetic (relieving vomiting) effects; it also acts as a nerve tonic to relax the central nervous system. As well, peppermint is an effective carminative, meaning that it helps soothe the stomach and intestinal wall, relaxing and calming our digestive tract and relieving cramping.

The active ingredient in peppermint leaf is menthol, a volatile oil with very powerful therapeutic properties. Menthol acts as a mild analgesic, relieving nausea, vomiting, travel sickness, and morning sickness. Bloated? Its relaxing effects on the muscles surrounding the digestive system help relieve gas (in a way that won't clear the room). It also promotes digestive function by stimulating the release of bile and the flow of digestive juices in the stomach and intestines. In fact, peppermint oil can even play a role in treating more severe digestive disorders, such as ulcerative colitis, Crohn's disease, and irritable bowel syndrome.

And don't think peppermint tea is just for digestion! It's good for what ails you if you want to strengthen your immune system, jack up your vitamin C, get rid of a pounding headache, or just chill after a long day.

HOW TO USE

Make yourself a soothing peppermint tea or blend some peppermint with chocolate hemp milk for a nutritious and delicious minty smoothie. Or go straight to the source and chew on some leaves to freshen breath and aid digestion.

TIP

If you're feeling constipated, try combining peppermint tea with a magnesium supplement to get things moving again!

Kombucha

This living health drink has been used for thousands of years to balance and harmonize the body. Kombucha is a fermented tea that's been called the Tea of Immortality and the Elixir of Life. But just how does kombucha support total health and vitality?

The kombucha culture is a mushroom, often called the "mother," or SCOBY, which stands for symbiotic culture of bacteria and yeasts. The culture is placed in black or green tea, turning the sweet tea into a delicious, naturally bubbly beverage packed with vitamins, minerals, enzymes, and health-promoting organic acids. As the kombucha culture digests the sugar, it produces a range of organic acids, including glucuronic acid and lactic acid. It also produces B vitamins and vitamin C, as well as amino acids and enzymes. On top of all these health-supporting nutrients, the SCOBY itself contains a plethora of probiotic microorganisms to support all body systems.

The probiotics present in the SCOBY are one of the main reasons kombucha is such a fantastic digestive tonic. Probiotics are good bacteria that keep our digestive system balanced. As a probiotic, kombucha aids the stomach in the breakdown and digestion of food, preventing acid reflux and relieving constipation. The good bacteria and yeast present in the drink reduce bad bacteria and parasites in the gut, which is why kombucha can be effective in the treatment of candida, an increasingly common overgrowth of yeast in the body.

The synergism of stomach acid and fermented kombucha is thought to cause the formation of an alkaline substance in the digestive tract, which aids in the proper functioning of all body organs, particularly the spleen, intestines, gall bladder, and pancreas. Impressive, but that's not all. This power drink is often used for its energy-boosting properties; it can also improve metabolism and support healthy weight loss, and it has detox properties.

Other health properties include antibiotic, antifungal, and antiviral characteristics, which allow our bodies to fight off bacteria, viruses, and all other foreign invaders they come up against. Kombucha is thought to improve hypertension, allergies, chronic fatigue, and especially arthritis. There are even those who believe it has a part to play in the treatment of HIV and cancer.

HOW TO USE

You can find kombucha bottled and ready to drink in the fridge of most health food stores. Enjoy with a meal or on its own. You can make fun cocktails with it, or a kombucha float using my Banana Walnut Ice Cream recipe on page 334. If you're feeling adventurous, you can make kombucha at home: it takes approximately two weeks to ferment, so get brewing! Its funky fermented taste may take a little getting used to, but the physical and mental effects are highly addictive. Drink responsibly.

TIP

Kombucha not only gets rid of belly bloat, but also makes for a great hangover remedy.

16. Immune Boosters

Our bodies work hard. We stay up too late, push ourselves at work, and don't always get the right foods in our diet. And sometimes we complain about not looking as great as we'd like in certain pairs of jeans. We often take for granted how hard our bodies are working for us every second of the day—and so we need to give them some love.

Since we're continually exposed to foreign organisms like bacteria, viruses, parasites, fungi, and microbes, our bodies' defense systems are constantly kicking some serious microorganism ass. Take your saliva, for example. It's not just for the joy of eating, digesting food, and smooching. It's actually part of your first line of defense for keeping pathogens out of your body. A healthy immune system is geared up to keep those harmful invaders away! But if our defense mechanisms are compromised, we might be in for some trouble. Health issues arise when the immune system is unable to stop a disease in its initial stage.

How the Immune System Works

Here's a look at how hard your body is working for you.

First Line of Defense

Pathogens, like viruses, bacteria, or microorganisms, first have to get into your body to do their damage. Your body comes equipped with plenty of barriers to keep the bad guys out—including your skin, mucus, saliva, tears, and vaginal fluids. Keeping these barriers strong and healthy is an important first step in achieving a good immune health. Remember, your body is a temple—make it a fortress!

Second Line of Defense

This is the defense system that kicks in once a pathogen slips through those outer barriers and enters the body. If the first line fails, your body has a whole host of other defenses just waiting in the wings.

As soon as a pathogen enters the body, an inflammatory response occurs. It's a protective measure to prevent the spread of injury and initiate healing. There are two kinds of inflammation: acute and chronic.

- Acute inflammation is short-term and typically the result of an injury. Our body sends neutrophils to deal with acute inflammation. These are cells that destroy pathogens at the acute phase of injury.
- Chronic inflammation is the kind that lasts longer than a couple of weeks, stressing the immune system and potentially leading to disease if left untreated. This is when you need your macrophage cells, the ones that not only destroy pathogens but also present them to lymphocytes, which are cells that support the immune system.

Other invader-kicking members of the second line of defense:

- Natural killer (NK) cells. As the name suggests, these cells "naturally kill" viruses and malignant cells.
- Fever. Yes, it's true. The body promotes healing by increasing its metabolic temperature.

Third Line of Defense

If the pathogens make it this far, your immune system kicks into full throttle to get those invaders out of your body and eliminate the threat. In the second line of defense the macrophage cells presented the pathogens to lymphocytes: the godfather of defensive cells. There are two types of these lymphocytes, and they tag-team to give you the best protection possible:

- T-cells are created in the thymus gland and destroy pathogens.
- B-cells are created in bone marrow and are responsible for antibody production.

Let's say you've been hit with a stomach flu. It's crossed your first line of defense because it's now in your body and has created an inflammatory response. You're all mucus-y and fevered-up. So the second-line, bad-boy macrophage cells attack the invader and present them to the third-line lymphocyte cells. Here, the T-cells will work hard to destroy the flu bug and the B-cells will create specific antibodies against it. Go team.

The antibodies/immunoglobulins (Ig) created by the B-cells are proteins that fight against particular antigens, such as your stomach flu. If it's the first time you've been hit with this particular strain of flu, the B-cells will create a specific antibody against it. Not only that, but these suckers will store these antibodies for future use! So, if you get hit with the same virus again, the B-cells will evaluate and pull the appropriate fix from the file. Bet you didn't know your body was so smart.

Key Nutrients That Boost Your Immune System
Vitamin D

Who doesn't love that sun-kissed glow? Even the thought of it can make you feel healthier. Well, look no further. If you want to keep your immune system ready and raring to go at a moment's notice, give it a little sunshine! Studies show that people with low blood levels of vitamin D have significantly higher incidences of the cold or flu. Even more research suggests that vitamin D can be just as (if not more) effective as the flu shot (plus, hitting the beach is way more fun). Adequate levels of vitamin D in the bloodstream are essential for activating the immune response and defending against disease-causing microbes. Essentially, vitamin D is required to turn on an antimicrobial protein that fights against foreign invaders. It also helps prevent inflammation brought on by the flu.

The best way for your body to get vitamin D is through direct sunlight, which contains UVB rays. UVB helps your body manufacture its own vitamin D in the perfect amount by converting cholesterol in the skin to D3. But if, like me, you live in the northern hemisphere and relish the entire five minutes of sunshine you may get during the winter months, direct sunlight just won't cut it. And if that trip to Cabo isn't on the radar this year, it's important to get your vitamin D through other means.

Vitamin D can be found in some fish oils, milk and dairy products, and egg yolks. However, vitamin D from food sources doesn't supply us with adequate amounts, which is why it's best to take a supplement during winter months. Although government guidelines hover around 200 IU per day, research suggests that at least 2,000 IU per day is necessary to ensure normal blood levels.

TIP

The vitamin D rule of thumb? Generally, you need 35 IU per pound of body weight.

Antioxidant Vitamins A, C, and E

I've already gone on about how amazing antioxidants are for reducing stress and making you look and feel fabulous. They are just *that* awesome. They'll also keep your immune system strong and healthy by protecting it from the harmful effects of free-radical damage, which leads to disease. Each of the following vitamins has its own unique function.

Vitamin C is a powerful antioxidant that not only helps get rid of a cold or flu, but is essential for preventing it in the first place. Vitamin C increases the production of antibodies and white blood cells, which are key in fighting against infection. In particular, it increases levels of the antibody interferon, which coats cell walls and prevents the entry of viruses.

Since your body doesn't manufacture or store vitamin C, you need to add it to your daily routine. Fruits and vegetables are excellent sources. Camu camu berries are one of the world's highest plant-based sources of vitamin C (and can also be found in supplement form). Other excellent sources include goji berries, red bell peppers, strawberries, broccoli, Brussels sprouts, kiwi, lychees, and parsley. And believe it or not, these ALL trump oranges in the amount of vitamin C they contain.

> **TIP**
> Next time you're feeling run-down, swap out your O.J. for a VegaTini (see page 288). It has over 60 times the amount of vitamin C, along with other immune-boosting and anti-inflammatory nutrients.

Vitamin E is essential for healthy immune function. It's required for the production of immunoglobulins, the immune-cell antibodies that destroy all those pathogens that try to do us harm. They're like your own personal bodyguard, standing by to protect you. So give 'em some vitamin E love, and they'll love you back!

Beta carotene, which your body converts into vitamin A, also enhances the functioning of your immune system. It works by increasing the number of immune-boosting cells, including natural killer cells. These are required for normal T-cell metabolism and the production of antibodies, which prevents entry of pathogens. Keep building that fortress.

Probiotics

Probiotic literally means "for life." Probiotics are live bacteria culture, and yes, you're supposed to eat them. These live microorganisms, classified as *good* bacteria, help fight off all the *bad* bacteria (foreign, disease-causing microorganisms). Eighty percent of our immune system resides in the gut, and to keep it strong we need to keep our intestinal system healthy. Probiotics help improve immune function by increasing the number of T-lymphocytes (the virus-fighting white blood cells we call T-cells) and natural killer cells, thereby giving you more ass-kicking friends. Who can't use more of those? Probiotics prevent the overgrowth of yeast, mold, fungal colonies, and other not-so-cool microorganisms, which are the precursors to diseases such as cancer and heart disease. They also treat yeast infections, vaginal infections, and candida.

Probiotics also improve digestion and help your body assimilate the precious vitamins and nutrients within your food. After all, you're not only what you eat, but also what you *assimilate*! You could be eating extremely well, but if you don't have a good digestive system you could be missing out on all the good stuff.

Probiotics are naturally found in fermented foods like miso, coconut kefir, yogurt, sauerkraut, kimchi, kombucha, and fermented soy sauce. So make friends with bacteria —the good kind—and watch your immune and digestive systems flourish!

Beta Glucans

Beta glucans are polysaccharides that can activate the immune system and prevent infections. They modulate white blood cells and keep them in a highly prepared state to attack any threat to our immune system. Think of it like this: the local radio station announces that your fave band is doing a secret show somewhere in the city tonight, but you have to keep listening for clues. The radio DJ (aka the beta glucan) is making sure you (aka your white blood cells) are in a high state of excitement, constantly checking for the clue to where the concert (the immune threat) will be. Once you hear it, bam! You go into party mode, and your white blood cells go into attack mode.

What's also great about beta glucans is that while they activate the immune system, they don't cause overstimulation, which can lead to autoimmune disease.

Beta glucans can be found in baker's yeast (the bran in grains such as oats and barley) and also in mushrooms, especially the shiitake, maitake, and oyster varieties.

Foods That Boost Your Immune System
Mushrooms

Who knew these delicious pizza-toppers could boost your immune system and prevent diseases such as cancer? All mushrooms are rich in beta glucans, those polysaccharides that are among the strongest immune-boosting compounds around. They have strong anti-tumor properties, activate the immune system, and regulate disease-fighting white blood cells so that they're ready to attack whatever comes their way. It's kind of like a military boot camp for immune cells.

Mushrooms are rich in minerals, vitamins, polyphenols, and sterols that keep our immune system healthy and strong. They're also one of the few foods that contain vitamin D. (However, because the amount of vitamin D in mushrooms is small relative to the daily required intake, it's still best to supplement.) In addition to their pathogen-fighting power, mushrooms are beneficial in preventing cardiovascular disease.[60] They help prevent white blood cells from building up and sticking to blood vessels in an inflamed environment, narrowing blood flow.

Here are some of the top mushrooms containing medicinal (not to be confused with magical!) properties:

AGARICUS BLAZEI MURILL (ABM)	Native to Brazil; widely cultivated in Japan; known as the "Mushroom of God." And rightly so! These contain the highest concentration of beta glucans compared with all other 'shrooms. They're also higher in protein, which helps support the immune response and stimulate macrophage activity.
SHIITAKE	Contain lentinan, a type of beta glucan that stimulates the production of white blood cells, has reported anti-cancer benefits, increases cancer patients' quality of life, and reduces the rate of cancer reoccurrence. These mushrooms also lower cholesterol and can prevent heart disease.

(Continued)

MAITAKE	Immune-boosting and cancer-fighting abilities. Studies show they can block tumor formation in mice.
REISHI	Increase production of interleukins—cytokines that regulate immune response and inflammatory reactions and inhibit tumor formation. They contain strong anti-inflammatory, antioxidant, antibacterial, and antiviral properties. These mushrooms increase interferon production, which blocks viruses from spreading. They also protect against radiation.
WHITE BUTTON	Researchers at Tufts University found these mushrooms to boost the immune system by increasing production of proteins that fight disease-causing pathogens.[61] They also increase the maturation of dendritic cells, which produce T-cells and fight against microbial invasion and tumor development.
CRIMINI MUSHROOMS	Beneficial in slowing estrogen-dominant breast cancer growth. Criminis are an excellent source of CLA (conjugated linolenic acid), which blocks the enzyme that feeds estrogen production, which feeds breast tumor growth.[62]

DID YOU KNOW?

Crimini mushrooms are baby Portobello mushrooms that haven't grown to full maturity. They also belong to the *Agaricus bisporus* family as white button mushrooms.

HOW TO USE

Mushrooms seem to make everything taste better! Add them to pizza, pastas, sauces, salads, and soups, or make my Mushroom, Chard, and White Bean Crostini (recipe on page 296). You can purchase them fresh or dried. Rehydrate the dried mushrooms by soaking in water, and use the soaking water in sauces or as a soup stock.

Aphanizomenon Flos-Aquae

Can algae help you cut down on sick days? Yep. *Aphanizomenon flos-aquae* (AFA) is a blue-green freshwater algae that's been around for, well, forever. It's one of the most primitive life forms on earth, and among the most nutrient-dense foods around. AFA embodies a plethora of vitamins (including B vitamins and antioxidants A, C, and E), minerals, trace minerals, phytonutrients, amino acids, and essential fatty acids. It also has antiviral, antibacterial, anti-inflammatory, antioxidant, and anti-cancer properties. Start adding this tiny superstar to your diet.

Phycocyanin is what gives AFA its blue pigment; it constitutes up to 15 percent of the alga's dry weight. Whereas the green pigment rejuvenates and strengthens blood through its rich chlorophyll content, the blue pigment strengthens immune function. Phycocyanin's antioxidant properties allow it to act as a free-radical scavenger, preventing disease, inhibiting inflammation, and revving up stem cell production. The blue pigment is also a COX-2 inhibitor—and since the COX-2 enzyme is dominant in many breast cancer cells, it's suggested that phycocyanin can result in reduced tumor growth.

DID YOU KNOW?

A study conducted by McGill University researchers concluded that human consumption of AFA leads to rapid changes in immune-cell "trafficking," or migration. Just two hours after consuming one and a half grams of AFA, 40 percent of the immune system's natural killer cells migrated from the bloodstream to the tissues to work their magic. The AFA also resulted in higher T-cell, B-cell, and monocyte subset counts.[63]

AFA is rich in carotenoid antioxidants, including beta carotene, lycopene, and lutein, which help prevent disease and reduce inflammation. And it's an excellent source of EPA and DHA (omega-3 derivatives), which help reduce inflammation, stabilize and strengthen cell membranes, speed up healing, and assist in the production of pathogen-fighting antibodies and bacteria-eating white blood cells. Seriously, this blue piece of goo is packed with so many nutrients you'll be wondering where it's been all your life.

AFA's rich mineral profile includes iron, which is required for the production of antibodies and immune response, as well as zinc, which increases natural killer cell activity, augments macrophages activity, and assists in the reproduction of DNA (and not just because it also boosts your libido!). It also helps detoxify the body, eliminate heavy metals, and balance blood-sugar levels.

And check this out. AFA is one of the highest natural sources of phenylethylamine (PEA), the natural mood elevator and antidepressant that's also found in chocolate. Known as the "love molecule," it stimulates mood, the sense of overall well-being, and the same euphoric feeling and feel-good chemicals that the body naturally produces during those beginning stages of falling in love. PEA also improves attention span, concentration, memory, and the stabilization of mood swings.

Astragalus

Astragalus is another super-nutritious food that might not be on the display rack at your local grocery store, but it's totally effective when it comes to boosting your immune health. A perennial plant native to China, astragalus has been used in traditional Chinese medicine for thousands of years to strengthen the body and prevent disease. Isn't it amazing how some of the world's healthiest foods are totally under the radar in the Western world? Stock up on this ancient plant, and your friends will be begging you for your stay-well secret!

The root is the medicinal part of astragalus; usually harvested after four years, it contains antiviral, antibacterial, and anti-inflammatory properties, helping prevent disease and boost the immune system. It's also used to prevent colds, treat diabetes, lower blood pressure, and prevent liver damage.

Similar to maca and ginseng, astragalus is an adaptogen, meaning it increases your body's response and resistance to stress. Stress is a leading cause of a suppressed immune system. You know how when you're stressed out and run off your feet and you *finally* get to take a vacation? Then, dang! You're sick in bed for a week, with the worst possible timing. All the stress you were under was eating away at your immune system. Stress causes inflammation and weakening of the adrenal glands, increases cortisol levels, disrupts sleep, and impairs immune function. Stress also slows down and impairs the digestive process, which means nutrients don't get absorbed and there's more toxicity of undigested food particles (which makes you feel gross and bloated, which gives you one more thing to stress about, and the vicious cycle continues). The adaptogenic properties of astragalus help reduce your body's stress response rate, strengthen the adrenals, and reduce cortisol levels, all of which increase immune function. It also helps bring your body into a natural balance and state of homeostasis.

Astragalus is rich in the flavonoid quercetin, which has high antioxidant properties and can help prevent certain forms of cancer. In addition, the root increases phagocytosis and interferon production (trust me, these are good things), promotes T-cell maturation, and increases IgA levels. The root is also rich in the minerals zinc, magnesium, silica, and iron, all of which support immune function.

DID YOU KNOW?

A clinical study conducted by researchers in China suggested that supplementing astragalus with chemotherapy could inhibit the development of tumors, decrease the toxic effects of the chemo, and boost the immune function and quality of life in cancer patients.[64]

HOW TO USE

So how do you get your hands on this ancient root? Astragalus, commonly taken in supplement form, can be found in most health food stores. Traditionally in Chinese medicine, the roots of the plant were boiled and the liquid was used as a remedy, often combined with other herbs and adaptogens such as ginseng. But heads up: those with autoimmune diseases shouldn't take astragalus. For everyone else, consult with your health practitioner on a dose that's best for you. Check out the next chapter for more on autoimmune diseases.

Miso

Who knew your favorite sushi starter would be so good for you? Miso has a salty, buttery consistency, and—aside from being a culinary staple in Japan for centuries—its health benefits trump its culinary applications (although it is super tasty). Miso is usually fermented soy, although it can also be made from fermented rice, wheat, or barley, or a combination of these. The soybean paste is mixed with salt and fermented using a live active (remember, this is good!) bacteria culture or a B12-synthesizing bacteria. Miso is high in protein, B vitamins, immune-boosting minerals, and probiotics—our "friendly" bacteria.

Miso is also a rich source of zinc, which is one of the most immune-boosting minerals around. Zinc improves immune function, speeds up the healing of wounds, increases natural killer and macrophage activity, and is required for the reproduction of DNA and most enzymatic processes in the body. As well, miso is rich in copper and manganese, which help make up the powerhouse antioxidant superoxide dismutase (dare you to say that five times fast), which in turn is essential in fighting free-radical damage and disease.

Because a bacterial form of B12 is often used in the fermenting process, miso may provide a good source of vegetarian B12 as long as it's unpasteurized. B12 is essential for a healthy immune system and disease prevention.

TIP
Use unpasteurized miso to ensure that the B12 is still intact.

HOW TO USE
Whip up an easy-peasy Creamy Crimini Miso Soup (see page 298 for recipe). It takes no time at all and does wonders for your health. It's always great to have a simple bowl of miso soup before meals to aid digestion. Miso makes an excellent salt substitute in dishes, marinades, sauces, and dressings.

Hemp Seeds

These, creamy, tiny little seeds pack a big nutritional punch. Hemp seeds are produced from the hemp plant, aka *Cannabis sativa L.* But don't get too pumped: they're THC-free, and no, you can't smoke them. Very different plant.

Both hemp seeds and the oil extracted from them are considered to be the perfect balance of essential fatty acids found in nature. These fats are crucial for proper brain function, heart health, and digestive function, and support almost all other body systems. They're a rich source of insoluble fiber, helping to cleanse and lubricate the digestive tract. They're also rich in plant-based protein, including all nine essential amino acids, and are high in key nutrients like B vitamins, vitamin C, calcium, magnesium, phosphorus, potassium, and iron ... just to name a few.

Besides all these wicked health benefits, hemp seeds play a key role in keeping the immune system primed. About half of the seed consists of a globulin known as edistin, which helps enhance the body's natural immunity. The protein from the globulin helps give the boot to any infecting agents that may be present in the body. And these little powerhouses are rich in chlorophyll, which also detoxifies the body.

Not to be outdone by our other immune-boosting foods, hemp is one of the highest sources of gamma linolenic acid (GLA), an essential fatty acid that plays a key role in reducing disease-causing inflammation. In addition, the omega-3s and omega-6s present in hemp seeds have a slight negative charge, allowing them to carry harmful and toxic substances to the intestines, the lungs, the kidneys, and the surface of the skin, where they can be expelled.

HOW TO USE

The creaminess of the tiny seeds makes them an easy addition to any meal. Throw a tablespoon in your morning cereal, afternoon salad, or soups. Sprinkle on top of vegetables or blend into your smoothie. You can also use hemp butter as a nut-butter substitute, hemp oil in dressings, and hemp milk as a delish milk alternative. The little seeds blend nicely into a chocolate macaroon crust in my Cocoa Mocha Torte; check out the recipe on page 326 and I guarantee you'll be jonesing for more.

17. Putting Out Fires: Pain and Inflammation

I recently did some damage to my knee (as I describe in the next chapter), so I know a little bit about pain! The whole episode did sideline me long enough to write a book, but still, I wanted to heal, stat! After all, as Christian Louboutin famously said, "High heels are pleasure with pain. If you can't walk in them, don't wear them." I wore them, and I was determined to wear them again.

Determination, it seems, pays off, because I got the pain and inflammation under control as quickly as possible. I'll share what I did to speed up my recovery, but I'm not going to lie. I still have wires in my knee joint from the surgery, and over a year later, runs, jump squats, lunges, and walking up and down stairs in heels all hurt like crazy and cause my kneecap to swell up. It makes me realize how much I took my joints for granted before. Yet it also drives me to preserve my joints by controlling inflammation.

Now, whether it's a broken bone, headache, back pain, athletic injury, arthritis, muscle ache, broken heart, or sore feet caused by dancing the night away in stilettos, we all know what pain feels like. And many of us turn to the medicine cabinet when it strikes, relying on Advil or some other non-steroidal anti-inflammatory drug (NSAID). But it doesn't have to be that way. Aches and pains aren't cosmic payback for playing too hard, but rather symptoms of inflammation. And doesn't it make sense to treat the condition rather than the symptoms? Yes, it does.

How Inflammation Happens

Inflammation is kinda like your body's own emergency response team. As soon as you suffer an injury or an invasion by pathogens, viruses, or bad bacteria, your Pattern Recognition Receptors (PRR) sound the alarm. Your body's defense team gets the call, and immediately blood vessels begin to widen to ensure that blood plasma can carry your fighter cells to the crime scene as quickly as possible. Those fighter cells prevent the injury or pathogen from spreading, protect the neighboring cells from injury, and destroy the pathogen that started the fuss in the first place. But while they're working, the increased blood flow results in swelling, warmth, redness, and tenderness at the injury site.

As this inflammatory response happens, pain receptors amp up their sensitivity so that you don't keep using whatever's been injured. This prevents further damage while the rescue crew works away at the scene. It's a lot like an "Under Construction: Visit Again Soon" sign. If you step beyond the scaffolding, you might get a bump on the head. Likewise, if you keep using the injured area, ouch! Those pain receptors will prick you to keep you in line. It's their way of saying, "Dummy, it's injured! Why are you trying to use it? Leave us alone, and let us fix the problem, will ya?" It pays to listen to your body (and to read construction signs). Otherwise, how else will you begin to heal?

Acute vs. Chronic Inflammation

You know how at parties there's sometimes a person you want desperately to avoid in conversation but who always seeks you out anyway? It can go one of two ways. You can have a painfully dull but quick chat and then be rescued by a friend. Or, you can end up seated next to the person at dinner for the duration of the night. Inflammation is like that. In the case of *acute* inflammation, the inflammatory response is short-lived. This usually happens after injuries, sprains, burns, cuts, bites, and infections. Once these things heal, the inflammation is no longer necessary, and it's business as usual.

Chronic inflammation is another story altogether. That's when ongoing, systemic, low-grade inflammation doesn't go away. It stays through dinner and beyond. It just sucks. And it taxes the immune system, throwing it into overdrive and potentially leading to diseases like arthritis, asthma, irritable bowel syndrome, diabetes, Alzheimer's, cancer, heart disease, obesity, and even depression. I know—it's depressing just to think about.

But what's really fascinating is this: every disease is preceded by inflammation. Every. Single. One. Cancer doesn't become cancer without inflammation first. Same goes for heart disease. And there isn't an obese person who doesn't have a fire in his belly—literally, there's inflammation in the fat cells—that can eventually develop into diabetes.

So if you can imagine an ongoing fire in your body, think about what happens to your internalized response system. Compare it to running, if you will. Your response system is more of a sprinter than a marathon runner, and when you, with lifestyle and dietary choices, force it to keep chugging along, it's eventually going to get mad and fight back. (Wouldn't you do the same if someone forced you to run 26.2 miles with no prep?) The problem is that we may not even be aware this is going on until the inflammation develops into something worse.

Set Fire to the Pain: Why Inflammation Happens

Your body may be resilient, but it's also really sensitive. If you don't believe me, take a look at this list of inflammatory triggers.

Stress

Put simply, stress is the cause of all inflammation. It can be nutritional, mental, emotional, or physical, but stress is always the cause of an inflammatory response. A broken bone places physical stress on your body, for example, while mental and emotional stress is the stuff of systemic inflammation. Since the latter is what leads to disease, I devoted an entire chapter to its management. (See Chapter 2.)

It's a simple equation, really, and one worth remembering:

$$Stress \rightarrow Inflammation \rightarrow Disease$$

So what makes stress the head honcho in the inflammation department? It begins with the stress hormone cortisol, which helps control the immune system's response to injury and invasion. It helps, in other words, to regulate inflammation. But too much stress in the body reduces cortisol's effectiveness and results in immune cells not getting the whole message. This in turn leads to out-of-control inflammation. Research out of Carnegie Mellon University suggests that chronic psychological stress is associated with the body losing its ability to regulate the inflammatory response. "Runaway inflammation" goes on to encourage the development of disease.

Dr. Sheldon Cohen, the psychology professor on this study, concludes that, due to this runaway inflammation, people who suffer from unusually high or sustained psychological stress are more likely to get a cold. He goes on to suggest that the symptoms of a cold (runny nose, mucus, and cough) are symptoms of inflammation, not symptoms of the virus itself.[65]

This is huge, because it turns the whole concept of virus and symptoms on its head. If he's right, our tendency to relieve "cold symptoms" with over-the-counter meds that dry up runny noses and soothe sore throats is entirely misguided. Suddenly a cold is a cry for help from your body, not an inconvenience to be ignored. And this puts a certain degree of power back in your hands. You can choose to squelch symptoms and get on with your day, or you can try to fix the root problem (i.e., stress).

But colds are only one mild example of the manifestation of stress. Because stress suppresses cortisol's ability to regulate inflammation, it can run rampant on any weakness in the body, resulting in afflictions like cardiovascular disease, allergies, arthritis, and autoimmune disease. Nothing, in other words, you want to deal with.

NO REST FOR THE IMMUNE SYSTEM

What's your brain like with no sleep? Irritable, confused, and likely to mess up, right? Well, that's a lot like your immune system when chronic stress causes systemic inflammation. Because your immune system is so overworked, it gets confused and starts to attack your body's own (healthy) tissues. This is why stress and inflammation contribute so significantly to the development of autoimmune diseases, including rheumatoid arthritis, multiple sclerosis, inflammatory bowel disease, and lupus. So give your immune system a break and learn how to relax.

Lack of Exercise

Heads up, couch potatoes! Your sedentary ways are about to catch up with you. I know, I know. Everyone's got a good reason why you should exercise. Hear me out!

A direct correlation exists between sedentary behavior and systemic inflammation.[66] Inactivity increases fat storage and throws off levels of leptin, the hormone that regulates hunger. (This creates a vicious circle of overeating, increasing fat storage even more.) A surge in fat storage then promotes inflammation and increases the risk for metabolic syndrome, which is a group of risk factors, such as obesity, that in turn increases the risk of heart disease, stroke, and type 2 diabetes.[67] Not a happy ending.

But that's not all. Sedentary behavior also exacerbates joint pain.

Still, you CAN have too much of a good thing. Moderate exercise can help keep inflammation—and all its ugly consequences—at bay, but TOO MUCH exercise can lead to the same problem of inflammation. When you physically stress your body during a workout, inflammation helps it heal muscles and tissues. This in itself is fine. But if you over-train, don't rest sufficiently between workouts, and don't refuel with proper nutrition, you'll find yourself in the same state of chronic inflammation that will further stress your body and affect cortisol levels. That's why fueling up on the right nutrient-dense foods before and after a workout can boost recovery time and heal inflammation. It also explains why the foods you eat can be just as, if not more, important than the workout itself.

Food

Pain and pleasure—such is the experience of food. Champagne? Wonderful in a glass or two; not so much after five. Chocolate cake? Yes, thank you! Just stop after one slice. You get the idea: food can be used for good and evil, especially when it comes to inflammation. Nutritional stress is in fact one of the largest contributors to inflammation. It can also aggravate pain, especially that of the joints. So before you put that fork in your mouth, take a look at the following.

FOOD SENSITIVITIES AND ALLERGIES

You know how conspiracy theorists warn that someone may be watching you without you knowing it? Well, food allergies and sensitivities are much the same way. There are a number of foods you could be eating right now, blissfully unaware that you have an allergy or sensitivity to them. (Well, maybe not so blissfully. More on that in a minute.) And of course, different people are affected by different foods.

If you have a type 1 food allergy, of course, you'll know it. This is the kind of immediate-onset allergy that lands you in a hospital. Within a couple hours of eating the offending food your immune system will form IgE antibodies to attack, and you'll suffer hives, diarrhea, swelling, throat closure, or anaphylactic shock. It's the most serious type of allergy, but not that common: it affects only 2 to 5 percent of the population.

Food *sensitivities* (or delayed-onset food allergies) are different. Like a type 1 food allergy, a food to which you have a sensitivity will trigger an immune response, but in the form of IgG antibodies and histamines that attack the food as a foreign invader or toxin. This leads to inflammation, which can appear as headaches/migraines, hives, bloating, brain fog, fatigue, irritable bowel syndrome, or weight gain. Where it gets tricky is in the timing. These symptoms can appear up to several DAYS after ingesting the wrong food. And if you can't even remember what you had for breakfast, good luck trying to recall what you ate two days ago. As a result, plenty of people never identify the culprit, and the ongoing inflammation can lead to the complications outlined above. By the way, when I say "plenty," I mean plenty. Food sensitivities may be less of an emergency than a type 1 food allergy, but they're extremely common and affect millions of people!

The most common food sensitivities include milk/dairy, wheat, gluten, soy, eggs, corn, shellfish, peanuts, Brazil nuts, and cashews. But these are by no means the only options. Food sensitivities, as I mentioned, are extremely broad, and in my experience, a food that you eat and crave regularly is often the problem.

Be aware that food sensitivities can be harder to detect via blood work than an IgE type 1 allergy test. You can try figuring it out at home, though. Here are the two best ways:

1. Elimination-and-rotation diet. **Start by eliminating common allergens for at least two to three weeks. See how you feel. If your symptoms subside, reintroduce each food, one at a time, for a one-week period. If your symptoms return, you'll know what the troublemaker is.**

2. Food diary. **Log what you eat and how you feel. After a few weeks, a pattern will emerge revealing which foods trigger reactions—even if they happen days later.**

FOOD FEELINGS

Since food sensitivities are, well, sensitive, you could easily go years without realizing you have one. That migraine, after all, could be the result of flying next to a two-year-old for nine hours. Or it could be the cheese ravioli served on the plane (another reason to pack your own airplane food!). Common food-sensitivity symptoms include headaches/migraines, hives, bloating, brain fog, fatigue, mood imbalances, irritable bowel syndrome, fluid retention, runny nose, congestion, joint pain, eczema, psoriasis, acne, and weight gain. If you get any of these on a regular basis, try one of the identification methods listed above.

FOOD ADDITIVES

Food additives exist for many (mostly superficial) reasons. They extend shelf life, lower calories, make a food look better—the list goes on and on. Even "whole" foods aren't always safe: the Citrus Red 2 dye is used to impart that sun-kissed glow to Florida oranges!

Many food dyes, flavor enhancers, artificial sweeteners, and pesticides are treated as toxins in the body, subsequently promoting inflammation and its array of symptoms. Cut them out where you can!

NIGHTSHADE VEGGIES

When it comes to nightshades, there's some good news and some doubt. Nightshades belong to the Solanaceae family and include tomatoes, potatoes (except sweet potatoes and yams), eggplants, goji berries, and all peppers and chili peppers except peppercorns. Some studies suggest that nightshades particularly aggravate joint pain in those who are sensitive. They can trigger flare-ups and aggravate symptoms in those who suffer from arthritis, for example. Yet other studies suggest that certain nutrients—like lutein in tomatoes—can help REDUCE inflammation. The same goes for capsaicin in chili peppers: when applied topically, it can also reduce pain and inflammation. What's a person in pain to do?! Well, if you're suffering from joint pain, try cutting nightshades out of your diet. I've cut them out completely when I've had injuries, but since I also tightened up on a lot of other things to reduce pain and inflammation, I can't be sure if there was a direct effect. It won't hurt to try, though!

> ### TIP
> The pro-inflammatory property in potatoes is located in the skin, so peeling it (and the underlying green layer) will significantly reduce its inflammatory properties. (The flip side: it'll also reduce key nutrients.)

OMEGA-6 LINOLEIC ACIDS

Yes, omega-6 fatty acids are considered "essential" since our bodies can't make them on their own, but modern North American diets overdo it. These fatty acids produce molecules that lead to inflammation when they're not balanced by enough omega-3 fatty acids. (Omega-3s reduce inflammation.) The optimal ratio is two parts omega-6 to one part omega-3. A typical North American diet, however, follows a ratio that's more like 20 to 1. The results are inflammation, allergies, cognitive issues, and a whole host of other problems. That's why it's critical to add more omega-3s to our diet and make a conscious effort to reduce the amount of omega-6s we eat.

Omega-6 linoleic acids are typically found in plant-based oils, such as cottonseed, peanut, canola, sunflower seed, vegetable, wheat germ, grapeseed, soybean, sesame seed, and safflower. These oils are also found in almost all packaged foods, including tomato sauce, salad dressing, bread, crackers, cookies, pasta, dried fruit, breakfast cereals, baked goods, and condiments.

> **DID YOU KNOW?**
> Stress, exercise, and food are the major contributors to inflammation, but they're not the only ones. Other factors include environmental toxins, heavy metals, insulin resistance, free-radical damage, and consumption of refined and hydrogenated oils.

Nature's NSAIDs: Ways to Prevent Pain and Inflammation

While Advil and other NSAIDs are common household staples, they don't need to be. Here are some ways to cure your aches and pains in the kitchen, and kick Advil to the curb. Ciao, Advil.

Omega-3 Fatty Acids

Omega-3 fatty acids are an anti-inflammatory powerhouse.[68] Like omega-6s, they're essential, meaning we must get them through food. UNLIKE omega-6s (unfortunately), most of us aren't consuming enough![69] It takes some effort to switch this ratio around, but it's well worth it. EPA and DHA are omega-3 derivatives, and both help reduce and control inflammation. EPA competes with particular omega-6 derivatives (one being arachidonic acid, or AA) at a cellular level, so by incorporating more omega-3s into your diet, you can push inflammatory compounds out of their seat. Both EPA and DHA are essential for reducing chronic inflammation and preventing both autoimmune diseases (lupus, Crohn's, rheumatoid arthritis) and inflammatory diseases (heart disease, aging, depression, osteoarthritis, cancer).

Food sources of omega-3s:

- Fish (wild salmon, Spanish mackerel, halibut, sardines)
- Seeds (sacha inchi, chia, hemp)
- Walnuts
- Algae (chlorella, spirulina, phytoplankton)

Gamma Linolenic Acid

Gamma linolenic acid (GLA) is another type of omega-6 fatty acid—but a good type in terms of inflammation. Unlike the pro-inflammatory omega-6 linoleic acid (LA), GLA is anti-inflammatory. Plus, omega-3s help to boost the effectiveness of GLA.

Food sources of GLA:

- Hemp seeds
- Evening primrose oil
- Black currant seed oil

Bromaline

Effective in treating and preventing pain and inflammation, bromaline is a protein-digesting enzyme found in pineapple. This is a handy little enzyme for treating indigestion; plus it acts as a systemic enzyme to help reduce both chronic and acute inflammation.

Specifically, this means bromaline can help you out if you're suffering from ulcerative colitis (a bowel condition involving swelling and ulcers), swelling of the nose and sinuses, or inflammation stemming from infection or injury. It's also effective against joint pain. One study found that, in the case of arthritis and knee pain, a combination of bromaline, trypsin (a pancreatic enzyme), and rutin (a plant substance found in foods like buckwheat, tea, apple peels, onion, and citrus) can be just as effective as prescription painkillers.[70] Rutin, by the way, contains quercetin, an anti-inflammatory antioxidant. Double points!

Bromaline is not without its drawbacks, though. It may act as a blood thinner, so if you're taking any related medications, check with your doctor about taking a bromaline supplement.

TIP

Papain, derived from papaya, is another systemic enzyme like bromaline that helps reduce pain and inflammation, especially when it's related to injuries.

Curcumin

Curcumin, an active component found in turmeric, is one of the most powerful disease-preventative compounds around! And that's not hyperbole. Its amazing anti-inflammatory and analgesic (painkilling) properties directly inhibit the COX-2 enzyme to reduce pain and inflammation, whether it's related to injury or symptoms associated with rheumatoid arthritis and inflammatory bowel disease. It's so powerful, in fact, that it's as effective as the anti-inflammatory medicine cortisone.

I told you curcumin is amazing, and I meant it. The stuff can actually inhibit cancer cell growth, reduce amyloid plaques in the brain to decrease the risk of Alzheimer's, and help prevent heart disease, arthritis, and autoimmune diseases. Its strong antioxidant property even protects against free-radical damage. See? Amazing.

Vitamin D

Doesn't the sunshine always make your feel better? Well, there's some science to back that up![71] A direct correlation exists between lack of sunshine and chronic pain—and vitamin D, the superstar sunshine vitamin, may help mitigate the discomfort. As reported in the *Journal of Immunology*, researchers suggest that patients with chronic inflammatory diseases (such as asthma, arthritis, and prostate cancer) who are vitamin D deficient may benefit from vitamin D supplementation.[72] According to this controlled study, vitamin D reduces the presence of inflammatory indicators like cytokines IL-6 (interleukin 6) and TNF (tumor necrosis factor alpha). Cells supplemented with vitamin D exhibited a much lower inflammatory response to a particular virus than non-supplemented cells. Other studies show that lower rates of vitamin D are also linked to higher rates of asthma,[73] and that vitamin D can inhibit the growth of breast cancer cells.[74] So get outside! (Or take a supplement.)

Magnesium

Not only does magnesium help to relax muscles and nerves—thereby aiding in stress relief—but studies show that an uptake of magnesium can also reduce inflammatory markers, such as C-reactive protein (CRP), TNF, and IL-6. Plus, it helps to reduce the inflammation of arterial plaque, reducing the risk for heart disease.

Vitamin K

As perhaps the dark horse of the anti-inflammatory group, Vitamin K has some surprising benefits. A study published in the *American Journal of Epidemiology* revealed that higher blood levels and dietary intake of K1 correlated with lower levels of 14 different inflammation biomarkers.[75] K1 also displays protective effects against osteoporosis and cardiovascular disease, both of which are inflammatory diseases. Taking a supplement of 10 milligrams per day is recommended.

Antioxidants

Antioxidants are perhaps the greatest multitaskers of all time, and among their many benefits are their enviable anti-inflammatory properties. These guys put the brakes on free-radical damage that, as a result of oxidative stress, can otherwise ignite the inflammatory process to speed up aging and disease.[76]

> **TIP**
> Is your diet going nowhere? It could be due to inflammation, which actually prevents weight loss. Try following an anti-inflammatory diet—not only will it reduce aches and pains, it could also reduce your jean size!

Food Fight: What to Eat to Reduce Pain and Inflammation

Whether you have chronic or acute inflammation, these foods can help! Here's what to put in your grocery cart.

Turmeric

This spice earns the gold for both reducing inflammation and pain and preventing (and possibly even treating) inflammation-driven diseases such as dementia, cardiovascular disease, diabetes, and cancer. Turmeric, the ginger-family plant whose curcumin compound earned rhapsodies from me earlier in this chapter, is native to tropical South Asia. In addition to its curcuminoids, which may help prevent rheumatoid arthritis and reduce inflammatory mediator production, turmeric has some anti-cancer properties. Chronic inflammation leads to the production of DNA-damaging and carcinogenic nitrates, and turmeric shows promise in reducing the number of nitrates produced.

Turmeric powder is a beautiful color—a rich, sunny orange-yellow that has earned it its "Indian saffron" nickname. The underground stems of the plant are what harbor the valuable compounds, and curcumin can be extracted for supplements.[77]

HOW TO USE

Turmeric powder is often used as a spice in South Asian and Middle Eastern dishes, and in beverages like healing Ayurvedic teas. You can use turmeric as a substitute for saffron in savory dishes, as it imparts an earthy flavor. Finally, if you can't stomach the idea of mustard not being yellow, look for turmeric added to it (and other foods) as a natural colorant.

Ginger

Like turmeric, ginger is derived from the rhizome (underground stem) of a plant in the same family as cardamom and galangal. As a result, you'll find it cultivated in similar places—South Asia (especially India), the Caribbean (particularly Jamaica), East Africa, China, Australia, and other tropical countries.

Besides being pretty, palatable, and exotic, ginger is super useful! It inhibits prostaglandin production, which in turn reduces inflammation. Ginger may also help reduce pain and leukotriennes (which are major inflammation mediators) in people with inflammatory rheumatic disorders. Its 6-gingerol compound, meanwhile, may spell good news for people suffering from allergic asthma: the compound shows signs of reducing pulmonary inflammation. In addition, ginger is great as a digestive tonic, and helps to alleviate nausea.[78]

HOW TO USE

Ginger makes a pungent addition to many dishes, particularly in Asian and Indian cuisine. It can also be steeped to make ginger tea, or juiced as an addition to vegetable/fruit juices. When dried and ground into a powder, ginger can add flavor to drinks and to baked goods like cookies and cakes.

TIP

Leftover ginger should be stored in the refrigerator or freezer.

Hemp Seeds

You may not get high off hemp seeds, but they can still make you feel pretty darn good. Hemp seeds are rich in omega-3 fatty acids, which have an anti-inflammatory effect that may benefit those suffering from rheumatoid arthritis, psoriasis, asthma, inflammatory bowel disease, and atherosclerosis. It may also help improve chronic inflammatory ear, nose, and throat (ENT) disorders like external otitis, laryngitis, pharyngitis, sinusitis, and tonsillitis.[79]

If you're worried that using hemp will get you in trouble with your company's drug screening, don't be. Although it's a cannabis plant and related to marijuana, it's virtually void of tetrahydrocannabinol (THC), marijuana's primary psychoactive ingredient. What it does have a lot of is eco-friendliness. Growing hemp requires no herbicides and minimal pesticides. You benefit, the earth benefits, we ALL benefit!

> **HOW TO USE**
> Eat the seeds raw (they have oils that don't handle heat well), or use the extracted oil blended into dips (like hummus), salad dressings, or smoothies. Whole hemp seeds have a mineral-rich outer shell; the bare seeds are referred to as dehulled hemp seeds, hulled hemp seeds, hemp hearts, shelled hemp seeds, or hemp nuts.

Chlorella

What can a single-cell green algae do for you? Well, you can check out Chapter 1 on energy to get the full rundown, but for those who need help for inflammation, a chlorella supplement may be the answer.

Chlorella has shown promise in studies on inflammation. The chlorella-11 peptide, for example, is a component that can slow down the progression of thermal injury–induced inflammation. Chlorella has also shown signs of inhibiting inflammation by decreasing the production of reactive oxygen and increasing antioxidative processes. In English, that means its antioxidant power is good at getting inflammation under control. Plus, it's super high in chlorophyll and omega-3 fatty acids, which also help keep inflammation under control.[80]

Wild Salmon

Salmon is like the homecoming queen of omega-3s—it's popular, likable, and has a good reputation. The last of these is well earned. In addition to its omega-3 content, salmon is high in selenium (shown to exhibit anti-inflammatory properties in people with inflammatory diseases) and cobalamin (vitamin B12). In high doses, cobalamin has also been shown to reduce inflammatory responses.

But which type of salmon should wear the proverbial crown? The best choice is fresh, wild King or Chinook salmon. They not only are the best-tasting of the group; they also have the highest omega-3 content. (Sockeye salmon has a high omega-3 content, too.) But remember to get WILD, never farmed.

Atlantic salmon should be avoided, since it's farmed and may have been fed astaxanthin and canthaxanthin pigments to get its flesh just the right shade of orange. Farmed salmon in general is to be shunned. (It contains more toxins like PCBs and may contain antibiotics.) So-called organic salmon, meanwhile, is a bit of a ruse: there is no USDA organic standard for salmon, so the label just means the fish was farmed.[81] Wild salmon is the way to go.

Pineapple

Endless sunsets, balmy breezes, palm trees rustling as waves roll up the beach—pineapple evokes the best of an idyllic tropical vacation. And for good reason. This seedless, tropical fruit is indigenous to Central America, South America, and Jamaica.

The fact that pineapple is a rich source of bromaline only adds to its appeal. The protein-digesting enzyme reduces the production of cytokines and leukocytes, both of which are pro-inflammatory. Pineapple juice supplementation has even been shown to help reduce colon inflammation and abnormal cellular growth in mice with chronic colitis. Studies show that it's also effective in reducing the pain and inflammation associated with musculoskeletal injuries, in addition to arthritis, bursitis, and tendonitis. Plus, it might even help with bruising!

Inflammation caused by allergic airway disease and allergic asthma may also respond to bromaline, meaning pineapple can become one sweet solution to a number of ailments.[82]

HOW TO USE

Check for a yellow skin and pleasant aroma when you select a pineapple, and get ready to peel and dice. The core is inedible and should be discarded before sinking your teeth into the soft, juicy fruit. Pineapple is best eaten raw in order to preserve the enzymes, especially bromaline. Eat it by itself, toss some in a salad, use it in a sweet-and-sour recipe, or employ some as a garnish for dinner or drinks!

Tart Cherries

If inflammation means your life isn't a bowl of cherries, consider eating them. The anthocyanins in tart cherries may help reduce inflammation and associated pain, while the juice can do that and more. Marathoners, take note: tart cherry juice helps reduce muscle damage and oxidative stress after strenuous exercise.[83]

DID YOU KNOW?

A study conducted by researchers at Oregon Health and Science University found that two cups of tart cherry juice per day significantly reduced inflammation markers and may help those suffering from osteoarthritis.[84]

HOW TO USE

You can try tart cherries raw, but they're really sour! However, they're delish blended into a chocolate smoothie or enjoyed dried. They're typically used in pie fillings, sauces, preserves, and relishes. For most effective results, use the juice—and make sure it's pure tart cherry juice with no additives.

Tart cherries, also known as sour cherries, are smaller than sweet cherries. They're grown in Eastern Europe as well as in Michigan, Utah, New York, Washington, Ontario, and British Columbia.

Green Tea

Green tea, black tea, white tea—which is your cup of tea? Well, if you have inflammation, invest in some green.

Made from the leaves of the *Camellia sinensis* plant, green tea leaves are immediately dried to prevent fermentation and minimize oxidation. (Oxidation turns the leaves black and, you guessed it, they make black tea.) Dried whole leaves can be ground into powder to make matcha tea.

So what does all this have to do with inflammation? All green tea polyphenols can, generally speaking, inhibit inflammatory responses. And the main antioxidant compound in green tea, epigallocatechin gallate (EGCG), inhibits the pro-inflammatory activities of neutrophils. That means it's time to start brewing!

HOW TO USE

Green tea bags and loose-leaf green tea can be steeped in water for drinking, and matcha tea powder can be added to dessert recipes for things like ice cream and cake, but beware—its green tea flavor will seep into the end result. Matcha tea and supplements make the most use of its polyphenols, particularly EGCG.[85]

Herbal, Homeopathic, and Topical Treatments

Devil's Claw

Foods aren't the only ones to heal inflammation! Devil's claw, an herb, is a natural pain reliever. Grown in South Africa, Namibia, and Botswana, the plant is a favorite for treating joint pain, back pain, and arthritis. Unlike arnica, devil's claw can be used in tea, as a capsule, or in a tincture. Just be sure to check with your health practitioner before taking it—the plant can interact badly with blood-sugar medications, and those with gallstones or ulcers should steer clear of it.

Eggshell Membrane

You know—that piece of skin that separates the egg from its shell? Yep, that. Now
before you go wasting your time peeling it off hardboiled eggs, its most effective (and
efficient) form is as a supplement. It helps reduce inflammation and alleviate chronic
pain within a week. And it's true: believe the marketing hype. When I started taking
it, given what was going on with my knee, I noticed a HUGE difference within DAYS!
I love this stuff! While research surrounding eggshell membrane is relatively new,
studies show that it helps reduce joint pain in people with osteoarthritis and joint and
connective tissue disorders. It contains joint-healthy nutrients like collagen (which
strengthens and builds connective tissue), hyaluronic acid (the fluid that lubricates
joints), and a usable form of glucosamine (more effective than that found in shellfish).

Arnica

Arnica, a plant used in creams and ointments for topical use, is another natural pain
reliever. It helps soothe pain and inflammation and heal wounds, being particularly
effective for acute sprains and injuries. As a rule it's not safe to take orally, although
some oral homeopathic remedies contain extremely diluted amounts of it.

Cayenne Pepper

It may be counterintuitive, but heating things up with cayenne pepper can actually
help inflammation. Cayenne's active compound, capsicum, can stop the formation
of the pain-causing COX-2 enzymes and inhibit inflammation. Studies also show that
when used topically, it can be effective in increasing range of motion and reducing
shooting pain.

18. Bone Appétit

When it comes to our health, we usually take a lot for granted—until something stops working. And that "we" includes me. In 2011, right before I started writing my first book, *Must Have Been Something I Ate*, I broke my knee. I'd just flown in from Vancouver after signing my book deal, and I went straight to the studio of a talk show where I'm a regular guest. As I was getting ready, I rattled off my schedule to the makeup artist, saying, "How am I going to write a book with my crazy schedule?! I need a break ... I need a BREAK!" And lo and behold, the ol' universe was listening.

Minutes later I was running backstage, full throttle, to get on set in my five-inch stilettos when a curved metal gap in a tiny lift on the floor that shouted "Caution" in bright yellow caught hold of the top of my foot and yanked me down. The first thing to soften the blow on the cold, hard concrete was my right kneecap. And I got my "break." I shattered my patella in four pieces, damaged my cartilage, tore off my patella ligament, and ultimately needed major reconstructive knee surgery. I've now learned to ask the universe for a "vacation." One that includes a beach.

After my fall, totally paralyzed by pain, I lay face-planted on the floor for a good 90 seconds before I could muster the energy to call for help. Even then my attempts to scream came out as soft whispers—"*help ... help ... help*"—that no one could possibly hear. Moments later my producer stumbled upon me. She put me in a chair, insisting I go see a doctor, but being all sassy, I was like, "Oh, I'm fine. I just need a few minutes to regroup." So they reordered the segments to give me some extra time and I sat there with ice on my knee joint, watching it grow from the size of a tennis ball to the size of a soccer ball. Finally I staggered up, threw my stilettos back on (I'm five-one; I need them to see over the table), and using the counter as support, I STILL did my segment! No one (including me) knew that my knee was smashed. I totally deserved an Emmy for that performance. It's called adrenaline (see Chapter 2).

What hurt MUCH more than the physical pain was the fact that I had a full leg cast—from hip to ankle—for weeks! Ms. Independent and Extremely Active became Ms. Totally Useless. I needed help getting places and doing everyday tasks, like getting in and out of a bathtub. But the worst part for me, the part that was sheer torture, was the fact that the cast meant no running! I'd see people running along the street and would yell out, "Do you know how lucky you are?! Do you?!?!" Okay, so the lack of endorphins pumping through my body due to lack of movement left me a little crabby. But the simple things we take for granted, like going for a run in the morning, walking the dog, climbing stairs, dancing, or just sitting on a toilet, make life pleasurable. And all of these things require healthy bones.

Since I had to spend weeks and weeks doing not much more than sitting, I had time to contemplate my situation. And what I struggled with the most was this question: if I was so healthy and in such great shape, why wasn't I strong enough to prevent such damage to my bones? The answer, along with the scoop on how to keep our bones healthy and strong, became this chapter.

Bone Basics

We all know that without our bones we'd be slumped piles of mush. Bones support and protect our organs (What's a brain without a skull? What's a heart without a rib cage?) and bolster our body segments and muscles. Tendons connect muscles to bones and allow us to move the entirety of our joints—unless you haven't been to yoga lately, in which case the ability is more theoretical than practical. But at least the possibility exists!

What a lot of people don't know, however, is that bones also help keep us healthy and produce most of our red and white blood cells. That's why osteoporosis is just one of many problems you'll face if you suffer bone loss. Others include suppressed immune function, lack of energy, inflammation, digestive issues, and weight gain.

But what exactly is a bone, anyway? It all starts with collagen. Yep, that good stuff that keeps your skin looking young and some lips pouty. Bone collagen is a protein that hardens into bone tissue with deposits of minerals, specifically calcium and phosphorus, so that the final product is roughly 50 percent bone collagen, 50 percent minerals.

Unfortunately for us, 100 percent of bone mass peaks between ages 20 and 30, which means childhood and adolescence are crucial times for building healthy bones. Adults have to focus on preventing bone loss. Yes, this is one more reason to envy the young, but who has time to do that when you're busy arranging a diet and lifestyle that protects the bones you've got? Bone loss can begin in your early thirties—sometimes earlier—so preserving bone health needs to be a priority. Osteoporosis *can* be prevented. It's reversing it that's more difficult.

TIP
Healthy bones are desirable all on their own, but for those of us who need a little extra incentive, look to your skinny jeans. Having higher bone density actually burns more calories, while bone loss can lead to weight gain. So keep those bones strong and your body in shape!

Osteoporosis

Sometimes life just isn't fair. The mean girl with great hair gets the guy. Your colleague gets the promotion. That cute party dress you were saving up for is stocked in every size but your own. Osteoporosis is kind of like that. You think that if you get enough calcium and exercise a decent amount, you can stave off a condition in which bones lose so much mass and tissue that they become brittle, fragile, and way too breakable. But it turns out calcium intake isn't the problem. And that leaves many people with an osteoporosis diagnosis wondering where exactly they went wrong.

One of the problems with osteoporosis is that it creeps up on you without warning. One day you're running marathons. The next you trip over your sneakers and end up with a busted knee. There are no big signs or symptoms until you're in the hospital with a fracture caused by an otherwise minor bump.

The other problem is a fundamental misunderstanding. Osteoporosis should not be associated with a lack of calcium *intake*. North Americans have one of the highest calcium intakes in the world,[86] and yet more than 20 million of us are affected by osteoporosis.[87] In fact, North America also has the world's highest incidence of osteoporosis! The real causes have to do with protein intake, acid-alkaline balance, hormonal balance, exercise, and a diet that leads to calcium and other mineral *loss*.

The Skeletal Situation

Getting your bones in tip-top shape is more than just a matter of eating the right foods and popping a daily supplement. It's not a puppet show, it's a Broadway show with lots of action happening behind the scenes to get the star—your skeleton—into the spotlight. Let's pull back the curtain to see what's going on.

Calcium and Bone Loss

Of all the minerals in the human body, calcium is the favorite. It's the most abundant, making up 1.5 to 2 percent of our total body weight. And while 99 percent of calcium cozies up in our bones and teeth, it's the prodigal 1 percent that resides in our blood and tissues that gets top priority. Yep, blood and tissues trump their skeletal sister's bony bottom because their needs must be met first.

Normal blood calcium levels are 10 milligrams per 100 milliliters. If this balance isn't maintained through a proper diet, the parathyroid hormone will draw calcium from our bones to meet the blood and cellular requirements, resulting in bone calcium loss.

> **TIP**
>
> Beware of calcium supplements! A German study found that the risk of having a heart attack almost doubled among calcium supplement users compared with non-users, as the supplement form of calcium may potentially contribute to blood vessel calcification.[88] So it's best to get your calcium intake through food, as it doesn't have the same effect.
>
> Iron inhibits the absorption of calcium, so avoid consuming calcium with iron-rich foods.

So you should just guzzle a liter of milk to offset the leaching, right? No. In fact it's the worst thing you can do for a number of reasons. Calcium is absorbed in the small intestine, but at decreasing rates. Children absorb approximately 50 to 70 percent of calcium through dietary sources, while adults absorb only 30 to 50 percent. That continues to decrease as people age, and eventually you may absorb just 15 percent or less of the calcium you ingest. The ultimate irony? More is not better. The more calcium you consume at a single time results in *less* calcium being absorbed. Absorption is highest in small doses—less than 500 milligrams at a time. So ultimately it's best to eat a variety of bone-building foods throughout the day.

But before you condemn the small intestine as an ageist saboteur in your quest for calcium absorption, spread the blame around. Factors like the acidic condition of your intestines, exercise, your vitamin D and magnesium levels, your age, your estrogen levels, and your protein and fat intake all affect your calcium absorption as well.

Here are some great plant-based sources of calcium:

Food Source	Calcium (mg) per ¼ cup	Magnesium (mg) per ¼ cup
Blackstrap molasses	708	174
Sesame seeds	560	126
Almond butter	168.8	189.5
Almonds	94.5	95.8
Amaranth flour	75	110
Navy beans	30.8	30.8
Rhubarb	26.3	3.7
Turnip greens	26.3	4.3
Figs	26	13
Kale	22.6	5.7

Many herbs and spices are also bone-building. Here are a few examples:

Food Source	Calcium (mg) per ¼ cup	Magnesium (mg) per ¼ cup
Dill seed	848	143.4
Ground cinnamon	562	33.6
Thyme	226	89.6
Fresh peppermint leaves	136	44.8
Garlic	61.5	8.5

Protein and Bone Loss

In North America we're obsessed with high-protein diets. "Protein, protein, protein" is all we hear. And it's absolutely a very important macronutrient. Proteins form the building blocks of our cells, repair tissue, encourage new cellular growth, provide energy, support the immune system ... the list goes on. However, both the type and the amount of protein we consume significantly affect bone health.[89]

Put simply, eating a lot of protein isn't good for you. More and more research is revealing that the more protein you consume, the more calcium is excreted in your urine. In fact, if you double your required protein intake, you'll lose 50 percent more calcium through your urine. Stick to a normal or plant-based diet, however, and your calcium levels will settle back to where they should be. In other words, if you're looking to increase your calcium levels, you need to decrease your protein consumption.

If this has you panicking about your pant size, take a deep breath. You can lose weight without the crutch of a high-protein diet. In fact, a Purdue University study concluded that older women who consumed high-protein diets and meat products lost more weight through bone density than those who consumed normal protein diets and no meat products.[90]

What about dairy products? Milk is super high in protein—as noted above, a key factor in calcium loss. And cow's milk not only leaches calcium from bones, but also is acid forming. Acid-forming foods pull calcium from your bones in order to neutralize blood pH, leaving your body with a calcium deficit. A study published in the *American Journal of Epidemiology* concluded that the consumption of dairy products (particularly in the early years) is associated with an increased risk of hip fractures in old age.[91] Hmmm. If milk really did a body good, my bones should have been rock solid. As a child and an adolescent—i.e., in my peak bone-building years—I consumed ridiculous amounts of milk. I would go through cartons a day. And yet my bones still managed to fail me.

As with most things, though, protein isn't an all-or-nothing game. It turns out that having too little protein in your diet can lead to bone loss, too. Or, if you can't give up your carnivorous, dairy-consuming lifestyle and decide to just consume more calcium to offset your high-protein habit, you face one of two possibilities. You either don't absorb enough to make a difference, or you absorb so much that you face a host of risks, like a buildup of plaque in your arteries.

So what's a skeletally aware person to do? The key here is the type and quality of protein. Plant-based proteins are alkaline forming and contain necessary minerals, such as calcium and magnesium, that essentially come as an all-in-one package. Leafy greens and vegetables, such as kale and broccoli, are rich in magnesium, which helps the body absorb their calcium, and they're an excellent source of vitamin K, which delivers calcium to the bones rather than having it hang around in the bloodstream or calcifying in the arteries and joints. They're also alkaline forming, which further contributes to bone health.

Sources of plant-based, bone-building proteins:

- Hemp seeds
- Sacha inchi seeds
- Chia seeds
- Sesame seeds
- Chlorella (high source of chlorophyll and magnesium, supporting bone health)
- Pumpkin seeds

Now, I'm not trying to tell you to never eat ice cream or cheese again. I'm Greek, so feta is a staple in my family's diet and I love goat cheese. However, treat dairy products as you would a piece of chocolate cake. Enjoy them as a treat, but don't rely on them to boost bone health.

The Acid-Alkaline Balance

Balance is something we're always striving for in all aspects of life. Your blood is no different. For optimal health and survival, blood needs to maintain a pH of 7.4, which is slightly alkaline, and the body works constantly to stay around that number. What it has to work with in maintaining that balance, however, is up to you. (Stay with me here. I'm getting to my point about how it relates to bones.)

Once a food is digested, it falls somewhere along the pH scale of acid to alkaline. The important thing isn't the pH of the actual food, but the pH effect that the food has on your body. Once the food is digested, its byproduct, or "ash," can leave your body in an acidic or alkaline state. Hence, when a food is digested, it can be either acid forming or alkaline forming.

Predicting a food's ash isn't exactly intuitive. When you think of a lemon, for example, would you guess it'd be acid or alkaline forming? Many would guess the former, since it's an acidic fruit, but the digested lemon, or ash, is actually alkaline forming. I know, so tricky.

The mineral content of the ash is what determines which camp it falls into. Acid-forming foods leave a high residue of phosphorus, chloride, and/or sulfur, which subsequently create acids in the body, thereby earning the title "acid forming." Alkaline-forming foods, meanwhile, leave a high residue of calcium, magnesium, and potassium, which are alkaline minerals. Here's a chart to help you out with some common foods:

Alkaline-Forming Foods	Neutral (or Almost Neutral) Foods	Acid-Forming Foods
• Green vegetables and lettuces (especially asparagus, broccoli, spinach, parsley) • Garlic • Ginger • Lemons and limes • Onions	• Raw honey • Raw sugar • Sprouted lentils • Raw goat cheese • Bananas • Carrots • Mushrooms • Quinoa	• Artificial sweeteners • Chocolate • Peanuts • Wheat/White flour • Beef • Pork • Shellfish • Processed cheese

• Olive oil • Herb teas • Mangoes • Papayas • Grapefruits	• Avocados • Wild rice	• Beer and soft drinks • Cow's milk

So what does all this have to do with bone health? Acid-forming foods essentially put your body (and blood and bones) in a deficit state. Because your blood needs to maintain a pH of 7.4 for health, and your body is slightly acidic as a result of an acid-forming diet, it will pull alkalizing minerals from wherever it can to neutralize blood pH. Calcium is one of those minerals. And guess where the greatest keeper of calcium is? Aha, that's right, smarty-pants, your bones. And the result: bone loss.

Think of it as a balloon filled with oxygen. The balloon represents your bones, and the oxygen inside the balloon represents the calcium that makes up your bones. Now imagine that the oxygen in the outside environment suddenly and dramatically decreased. We all know we need oxygen for survival. What would we do to ensure our oxygen needs are met? We'd start inhaling the oxygen from our balloon to survive. The balloon would lose oxygen, becoming limp and losing strength and mass. That's what happens to our bones in an acidic environment: they lose bone-mineral density.

Now when we consume alkaline-forming foods, our bodies don't need to work so hard to maintain blood pH. That means they don't need to tap into the mineral reserve in our bones, which ultimately preserves bone health. Alkaline-forming foods, then, are like the properly oxygenated environment in our example. They let you keep your balloon intact.

Exercise

We know exercise is good for your heart, your waistline, and your mood. And if that weren't enough, it turns out exercise is good for your bones, too.

Just as weight training provides muscle-building resistance, contracting muscles create resistance and tension against bones, which ultimately increases their density. Both aerobic exercise and resistance training do the trick when it comes to building bone density, but as you might guess, resistance training is most effective.

Since exercise also gets your heart pumping, it improves the circulation of calcium and increases absorption as well. So strap on your sneakers and hit the gym. Just don't overdo it, since continued overexertion can affect hormonal balance, eventually leading to bone loss. Which brings me to the next section ...

Hormonal Balance

When I was in my twenties—the prime age for bone building—I thought I was the healthiest person around. (Oh, how cruel hindsight can be.) I had a career in investments and worked insane hours, with the corresponding stress levels. So to blow off excess steam, I'd work out any spare second I got. I'd get up at 5 A.M., run anywhere between 5 and 20 kilometers (depending on my training schedule and what I was training for), fuel up with a small bite or shake, then hit the gym for weight training—all before 8 a.m. Conveniently, the gym was in the same building where I worked, so I'd shower, get ready for work, and head straight upstairs for my morning meetings. At lunchtime I'd head back down to the gym and teach or participate in a fitness class, whether it was kickboxing, skip-and-sculpt, or boot camp. Then after work I might go for another run, take a boxing or yoga class, or play a sport like Ultimate Frisbee. If I got out of work before 7 p.m., I'd do two of the above.

I probably spent a minimum of six hours a day working out. That, coupled with stress (and copious amounts of wine), threw my hormonal system completely out of whack. My body-fat percentage was too low, so I wasn't producing enough estrogen. As a result, I didn't have my period for seven years, and I became borderline osteopenic, meaning my bone-mineral density was lower than normal, which can be a precursor to osteoporosis.

At the time, I thought I was doing everything right. My raw-foodie diet was as clean as could be: it was loaded with raw veggies, greens, superfoods, sprouted nuts, seeds, grains, smoothies, green juices, and shakes. I got enough protein and knew exactly how many nutrients I was getting each day. I didn't know what effect stress was having on my body and hormonal system, so I certainly didn't know how to manage it through diet. All I knew was that I was superfit, overworked, and kinda happy with the fact that I didn't have the inconvenience of my period. It was awesome, actually. My doctors, however, felt differently. When they suggested that since I wasn't getting my period I should go for a bone density test, I laughed. "Are you kidding me?" I asked. "My bones are so strong! Do you know how much I work out?" Never did I imagine that low estrogen levels could have such a damaging effect on my bones. But lo and behold, at age 28 I was diagnosed with low bone density.

Here's what happened. Stress—both mental and physical—causes the adrenal glands to release the stress hormone cortisol. But when cortisol is produced in excess as a result of chronic stress, a lot of bad things begin to happen, including suppressed immune function, blood-sugar imbalances, elevated blood pressure, and in my case, loss of bone density. Not only that, but excess cortisol disrupts other hormones like estrogen and testosterone, inhibiting them from functioning at optimal levels.

In the presence of low estrogen levels—something that typically results from menopause, chemotherapy, or in my case amenorrhea caused by over-exercise—bone density is reduced. Since estrogen is required to prevent bone loss, postmenopausal women are at the highest risk for bone fractures.

Given that I was pretty far away from menopause at the time, my diagnosis totally took me by surprise. But it spurred me on to make some serious changes in my life, part of which included quitting my job and studying to become a nutritionist.

While you probably don't need to quit your job to boost your bone health (well, maybe you do, but that's a different conversation), you probably do need to chill out a little more (see Chapter 2 on how to combat stress), exercise a *healthy* amount, eat healthfully, and limit wine and alcohol consumption to a reasonable degree. Your bones depend on it.

TIP

Think twice before you buy another round for the gang. Alcohol can reduce your body's calcium absorption and inhibit liver enzymes that help convert vitamin D to its active form.

Other Factors Responsible for Bone Loss

We've looked at some of the behind-the-scenes stuff that affects how well calcium is absorbed and maintained. Now it's time to look at some additional sneaky suckers that undermine bone health.

What Accelerates Bone Loss	What Preserves Bone Health
• Acid-forming foods	• Alkaline-forming foods
• Alcohol	• Dark leafy greens
• Soft drinks	• Veggies
• Caffeine	• Exercise
• Meat and dairy products	• Sunshine
• Stress	• Hormonal balance
• Diets high in protein, phosphorus, and salt	• Magnesium
• Oxalic acids	• Vitamin D
• Smoking	• Vitamin K
	• Silica

TIP

If you're taking a multivitamin supplement with a high dose of vitamin A (1.5 milli-grams or more), throw it out! A high vitamin A intake is linked to bone loss and an increased risk of hip fractures. The best way to get your antioxidant vitamin A is through food, especially beta carotene, which your body converts to a healthy amount of the vitamin.[94]

Bone-Building Nutrients

Some things are inherently lovable. Pudgy babies, furry puppies, and, if you're a skeleton, certain vitamins and minerals. Here are a few of your bones' favorite things.

Magnesium

Everyone stresses over getting enough calcium—and yet calcium deficiency is extremely rare. However, it's been estimated that roughly 75 percent of the North American population is deficient in magnesium. And magnesium has a lot going for it.

Magnesium is vital to all enzymatic activity in the body. That means it does things like make calcium more absorbable, help maintain proper pH balance in the body, and (with some help from vitamin B6) dissolve calcium phosphate stones that build up from excess dairy intake. It also works with calcium to help regulate heart and muscle contraction and nerve conduction. Plus, if your system is a little backed up, magnesium can help alleviate constipation and get you regular again.

So how can you load up on this unsung mineral hero? Good sources include green leafy veggies like kale and collards, whole grains, and orange juice.

Vitamin D

If magnesium is calcium's silent partner, vitamin D is its best friend. This handy vitamin is essential for absorbing both calcium and phosphorus from the digestive tract. It also helps maintain normal blood calcium levels, which, as we've seen, is crucial for cardiac function and bone health.

Unfortunately, for most people in North America, getting enough vitamin D can be tricky. That's because UVB rays stimulate our bodies to make the vitamin, and most people living north of the Sunbelt just don't get enough sun exposure. (Not to mention that prevalent sunscreen use and growing concern over sun damage encourage people to shun the sun.) If you do venture into the blaze, make sure to take calcium within the first couple of hours in order to maximize absorption and utilization. Otherwise, consider taking a daily supplement.

Vitamin K

Typically touted for its blood-clotting benefits, vitamin K is also vital for optimal bone health. That's because it transports the calcium from your blood to your bones, acting as a glue that makes bone-enriching calcium stick. Studies have shown that vitamin K helps prevent bone fractures even in those who are already experiencing unwanted bone loss.

There are two types of vitamin K: K1 (also known as phylloquinone and phytonadione) and K2 (also known as menaquinones).

K1 is a fat-soluble vitamin that, in conjunction with vitamin D, helps bones absorb calcium. (Studies have shown that vitamins K and D, which are known to team up for bone metabolism, work synergistically on bone density as well.) Ninety percent of dietary vitamin K is K1, with women requiring 90 milligrams daily and men needing 120 milligrams daily.

K2, meanwhile, provides the remaining 10 percent of dietary vitamin K, and also helps shuttle calcium to the bones. But K2 is also a bacteria-synthesizing vitamin and stays in your body longer. It helps prevent calcium from hanging around in your bloodstream, thereby preventing calcification in your tissues and arterial plaque from forming. Basically, K2 drives calcium to your bones and away from places it shouldn't be (bloodstream, joints, arteries, and tissues). K2 synthesizes and is colonized in your gut, so a healthy gut means healthy bones.

Good sources of vitamin K:
- Cabbage
- Broccoli
- Cauliflower
- Spinach
- Kale
- Turnip greens and other dark leafy greens

Fermented foods, such as natto, contain higher sources of K2, but all vitamin K–rich foods promote bone health.

Silica

Silica is an important mineral that's beneficial to bone health and connective tissues. Although I speak about it a fair bit in the beauty chapter, it plays the same role for your bones and connective tissues as it does for your skin and hair. This workaday mineral is required for bone formation as well as for the synthesis and stabilization of collagen. It also helps to heal bones at the onset of fractures—and I know firsthand that it works!

Good sources of silica:
- Leeks
- Green beans
- Garbanzo beans
- Strawberries
- Cucumber
- Mango
- Celery
- Asparagus
- Rhubarb

Bone Appétit! (Redux)

Can you really eat your way to healthier bones? Of course! Here are some bone-building foods that your skeleton will thank you for.

Sesame Seeds

Sesame seeds come from the tiny pods of the sesame plant, which typically grows in tropical regions. The sesame seed has one of the highest oil contents of any seed, and it makes a creamy, delicious tahini in its blended/buttered form.

Besides being tasty and a good source of fiber, sesame seeds have an enviable assortment of essential minerals like magnesium, vitamin B1, manganese, zinc, selenium, and copper. Many of these are critical for proper bone mineralization, red-blood-cell production, enzyme synthesis, hormone production, and regulation of the cardiac and skeletal-muscular activities. Copper, for example, supports bone and blood-vessel health, while zinc aids in the production of collagen. This is important in light of a study published in the *American Journal of Clinical Nutrition*, which found a correlation between a low dietary intake of zinc and osteoporosis at the hip and spine.[95]

Sesame seeds are also an amazing source of calcium; in fact, ounce for ounce, they significantly trump milk in the amount of calcium they provide. Plus they're rich in magnesium, which helps with the absorption of calcium.

HOW TO USE

Sesame seeds are most nutritious when the entire seed is used. They add texture to baked goods and a nutty flavor to sushi rolls, stir frys, and salads. When the seed is crushed, as in tahini, hummus, or sesame butter, its nutrients are more easily digested. When left whole, the seeds don't break down as well during digestion. Toasting sesame seeds, meanwhile, has been shown to slightly elevate calcium levels.

Kale

If ever there were a food to eat in abundance, it would be dark green leafy vegetables, which protect and strengthen bones.

Which brings us to kale, a form of cabbage with green or purple leaves that's high in magnesium, vitamin K, and an absorbable form of calcium, all while being an alkaline-forming food. And did we mention that it's also a good source of vitamins A and C, fiber, iron, folic acid, amino acids, antioxidant flavonoids, and lutein? What's not to love?!

Kale and spring greens provide about 150 milligrams of calcium per 100 grams of raw weight.

Figs

Figs are among the richest fruit sources of calcium. One cup of figs contains just as much calcium as a cup of milk. Plus, they're one of the richest fruit sources of magnesium, which, again, helps with the absorption of calcium. Figs are also a source of vitamin K. Vitamin K helps create bone-forming cells (required for strong, healthy bones) and helps deliver calcium from your blood to your bones so that it sticks.

Figs are also a great source of vitamins C and B6, manganese, fiber, and potassium. In fact, the fruit's potassium may also help reduce calcium loss due to a high salt intake.

Almonds

Almonds are a great little bone-building snack! They act as a mediator for a positive calcium balance, providing the perfect amounts of magnesium and calcium.

Almonds are one of the alkaline-forming nuts that help contribute to bone health. Plus, these nuts contain stress-busting nutrients, which also contribute to a positive calcium balance (meaning calcium stays in your bones!).

Broccoli

This green nutritional giant isn't called a superfood for nothin'. In addition to being loaded with vitamin K and absorbable calcium, broccoli is an alkalizing food that's been linked to greater bone density and reduced bone loss in postmenopausal women.

Wild Salmon

It's versatile, it's easy to get—and it's amazingly good for you. Yes, wild salmon is a good meal choice for lots of reasons. It's rich in bone-building vitamin D (which is difficult to get from many food sources), plus it contains calcium, omega-3 fatty acids, magnesium, selenium, and potassium, which are also bone building!

Studies suggest that a diet rich in omega-3 polyunsaturated fatty acids from sources like wild salmon may help increase bone formation and minimize bone mineral loss.[96] And because it contains the vitamin D–calcium combo, it can also decrease bone loss and the incidence of nonvertebral fractures in men and women who are over the age of 65, and at greatest risk.[97]

19. I ♥ You

How can you not be head over heels in love with your own heart? It's one of the most vital organs in the body! It pumps oxygen- and nutrient-rich blood through every single cell, keeping you alive and vibrant.

Just as your heart touches, by way of its function, every part of your body, your body has a strong impact on your heart, too. Your lifestyle, diet, behaviors, and even your thoughts all affect your heart. Think about what happens at the merest suggestion of reuniting with the love of your life. Your heartbeat speeds up, pitter-patters, and you feel joy (and blood) racing through every inch of your body. And that's just at the *thought* of it. Imagine how all of the other lifestyle factors come into play!

One thing to note is that the most important love in your life is, well, yourself! After all, you want to make sure your own heart is in tip-top shape before you go giving it to someone else. Love your heart and it'll love you back. Here are some heart-healthy tips to keep your ticker ticking—and lovin'!

How Our Ticker Ticks

If you think *you* work hard, compare your job with that of the heart. It pumps about 2,000 gallons of blood per day. And while that's impressive enough on its own, it's also more profound work than most of us do. (Don't get defensive; it's just true. When was the last time paper-pushing kept someone alive?) This process is the heartbeat, and as pretty much everyone knows, it sounds something like this: "lub-dub, lub-dub."

In a nutshell, the heart supplies our trillions of cells with life-giving oxygen and nutrients by pumping blood through its arteries. (Arteries take blood away from the heart.) This is the "lub" or systole stage, where the ventricles in the heart contract, pushing blood out to the rest of the body. The systolic measure of your blood pressure (the top number) measures the pressure of this blood as it flows out of the heart and against the walls of your arteries. Our veins then carry deoxygenated blood back to our lungs for a refill before chugging back to the heart. This is the "dub" or diastole stage, when the ventricles of the heart are relaxed to allow blood to flow back. The "dub" is measured as the diastolic rate of your blood pressure (the bottom number).

While this cycle, which happens roughly 60 times per minute, seems relatively straightforward, it's the body's most important function. It gives life! And yet heart disease is still the leading cause of death in North America. Canada's Heart and Stroke Foundation categorizes cardiovascular diseases as diseases and injuries of the cardiovascular system, which includes blood vessels in the heart and throughout the body. A stroke is the result of a lack of blood flow to the brain and is also considered a form of cardiovascular disease.

DID YOU KNOW?

In Canada, every seven minutes a person dies as a result of cardiovascular disease.[98] In the U.S., the statistics are even grimmer: cardiovascular disease kills someone every 38 seconds.[99]

Cardiovascular Disease: The Players

The term "cardiovascular disease" is a tidy one that encompasses many factors. Here are some of the contributing players.

Blood Pressure 101

Blood pressure is the measure of the "lub" and "dub" cycles of the heartbeat. You'll remember that the pressure of the "lub" is the top number of the ratio, or the systolic measure. The "dub" is the bottom number, which measures the diastolic rate.

You know how when you're stressed or anxious about something and can feel your heart pounding in your chest? Typically, that's because your blood pressure is rising. There's more pressure in the systolic stage when the ventricles are pushing blood out of your heart, causing more pressure against artery walls. So if your blood pressure is normally 120/80, it might bump up to 140/80 because of the extra stress or "pressure" placed on your heart. Periodic changes in blood pressure during the day are completely normal. For example, if someone nearly runs you over while you cross the street and scares the daylights out of you, your blood pressure will definitely rise, but that doesn't mean you have high blood pressure.

It's when your diastolic pressure is high that you really should begin to worry. The diastolic number measures how much pressure there is when the heart is relaxed. People with high diastolic pressure are at higher risk for heart failure and stroke.

Chronically high blood pressure is classified as hypertension, and the risks it carries are very real. Hypertension can damage blood vessels and the organs to which they deliver blood. Eventually this can cause stroke, heart attack, and even things like kidney failure, dementia, and erectile dysfunction.

> ### TIP
> Determine what your own "normal" blood pressure is. For most people, it can range from 90 to 120 (systolic) and from 60 to 80 (diastolic). Your medical history, family history, and exercise habits will all help determine what "normal" means for you.

Atherosclerosis

Atherosclerosis is an inflammatory disease in which the artery walls are hardened with a thick plaque made up of fat, bad cholesterol, and other debris. As plaque builds up, blood has a harder time flowing through the narrowed arteries. It's like trying to get water through a clogged drain. Because it takes longer to get oxygen and nutrients to your cells and organs, they become starved of vitality—while blood pressure rises, along with the risk for heart attack and stroke.

And then there's the issue of blood clots. Narrowing arteries make it easier for clots to get jammed in there and block blood flow, which is life-threatening. Pieces of the plaque could also break off and block smaller blood vessels elsewhere in the body. Unhealthy fats, bad cholesterol, smoking, being overweight, inactivity, and stress all promote inflammation, which is the underlying cause of atherosclerosis and what makes symptoms worse.

OXYGEN DELIVERY

Oxygen is the most important element: we must get it to every cell in our body for optimal health and survival. Carried through our blood, oxygen delivers nutrients and vitality to our cells. When delivery is less than optimal, our organs and cells are compromised, and disease ensues.

Cholesterol

Though it's been much maligned by popular culture, cholesterol is actually useful to our bodies. This fatty, waxlike substance in your bloodstream and cells is used to make cell membranes, hormones, and other bodily components. The problems arise when you have too much of it—especially the bad kind. That can lead to plaque buildup in the arteries, which puts you at risk for coronary disease and, later, heart attack and stroke.

TYPES OF CHOLESTEROL

Here's what goes into cholesterol; its varying makeup determines whether it's the "good" or "bad" kind.

LDL (low-density lipoprotein). **This is the "bad" kind that can clog arteries and raise your chances of having a heart attack or stroke.**

HDL (high-density lipoprotein). **This is the "good" kind that helps kick LDL out of your body, clean out your arteries, prevent blockages, and reduce your risk for cardiovascular disease.**

Triglycerides. **This is a fat that's both made in your body and ingested through food (typically sugar, refined grains, and alcohol). Triglycerides are kind of like the bad seed in a group of friends—the one kid who drags the rest down, and before you know it, everyone has a bad rap. Well, high triglyceride levels often lead to a high total cholesterol with lots of LDL and a little HDL. Not good.**

TIP

Those who are diabetic should avoid foods containing cholesterol.

CAUSES OF HIGH CHOLESTEROL

Speaking of high cholesterol, it's important to note that high blood cholesterol is not caused by dietary cholesterol. Sound confusing? Bear with me.

Cholesterol comes from two sources: 75 percent of blood cholesterol is made by your liver and other cells, and 25 percent comes from the foods you eat. So while some foods do contain dietary cholesterol (like eggs and shellfish), high dietary cholesterol does NOT equate to high blood cholesterol levels. What do cause high blood cholesterol are obesity, smoking, inactivity, stress, diabetes, sugar, animal-based saturated fats, trans fats, and processed foods. So even though those whole-wheat crackers promise with a bright yellow label on the box that they have zero percent cholesterol, they'll raise your blood cholesterol a heck of a lot faster than scrambled eggs for breakfast.

DID YOU KNOW?

There's a direct correlation between high cholesterol and erectile dysfunction. If heart health isn't enough of a reason to get cholesterol levels in check, maybe this is!

Fats

The dreaded F-word. Fat. For decades now we've been inundated with fat-free and low-fat varieties of some of our favorite foods, eliminating the guilt factor in simple indulgences. But with the rise of fat-free consumption over the past several years also comes the rise of obesity, heart disease, diabetes, and an increasingly overweight society. Could it be that fat-free foods are in fact making us fat? Yep. While it's tempting to think you can eat fat-free cake bars all day without busting out of your pants, the fact is you can't. Advertisements lie; your waistline doesn't.

This is how it works. When you suck out the fat from something—milk, cake, whatever—it becomes dull and tasteless, so manufacturers pour in sugar to compensate for it. And sugar stored as fat is much worse (and much harder to shed) than regular old fat itself. Plus, any excess sugar not burned as energy gets converted by the liver into triglycerides via a process called lipogenesis. This leads to elevated blood triglycerides that contribute to heart disease (and obesity).

Sugars like these come from carbohydrate-rich foods, particularly those with refined and hidden sugars. Dietary fat, on the other hand, is essential for the absorption of fat-soluble vitamins (A, D, E, and K) and for the regulation of hormones. It can even, ironically enough, curb hunger, since it takes a while to digest and therefore increases satiety.

But how's this for some amazing news: some fats actually improve heart health, prevent disease, alleviate depression, and fight weight gain. Which ones? I'm glad you asked!

THE GOOD

Omega-3 Fatty Acids. Omega-3s (ALA—alpha-linolenic acids) are an essential fatty acid, meaning that our bodies can't make it, so we have to get it from food. There are all sorts of reasons to gobble up omega-3s—your body loves them, and your heart is no exception. Omega-3s, particularly DHA and EPA (omega-3 derivatives), are critical for improving heart health, reducing the risk of heart disease, and reducing inflammation. They do this by way of some seriously good housekeeping: omega-3s clean out cholesterol and fatty deposits from the body, lower lipid levels, and improve circulation. They also reduce blood clotting and, as a result of all of the above, lower blood pressure.

The best plant-based source of ALA is found in sacha inchi seeds; other food sources include chia seeds, hemp seeds, and walnuts. Our bodies can convert ALA into EPA and DHA, but the conversion amount isn't guaranteed. Direct sources of DHA and EPA are fatty, cold-water fish (such as salmon, mackerel, anchovies, and sardines) or a good-quality fish oil.

TIP
Omega-3 oils are extremely sensitive and will become rancid with exposure to oxygen, heat, and/or light. (And by rancid, I don't mean just bad. I mean they'll convert to really bad trans fat.) So store any such oils in dark bottles and keep them refrigerated.

Monounsaturated Fats. Monounsaturated fats are less temperamental than omega-3s: at least they don't go rancid as easily! These fats tend to decrease the risk of cardiovascular disease by lowering bad cholesterol levels and increasing good cholesterol levels.

Monounsaturated fats tend to be liquid at room temperature. Good sources include olives, olive oil (including extra virgin), avocados, nuts (such as almonds, hazelnuts, and pecans), and seeds (such as pumpkin and sesame).

THE OKAY (IN MODERATE QUANTITIES)

Saturated Fats. **Contrary to popular belief, saturated fats aren't all that bad. In fact, a little bit can actually be GOOD for you!** Our bodies need saturated fats to help absorb omega-3 fatty acids and calcium, to improve our immune function, and to strengthen our cell membranes and protect them from viruses, bacteria, and harmful microorganisms.

Short-chain fatty acids (found in butter) and medium-chain fatty acids (found in coconut oil) have antimicrobial properties that help fight fungal infections and candida. And because they're small and medium chains, these fats don't require the full digestive process; they're typically absorbed in our small intestine, making them easily converted into energy.

But wait! There's more good news. These fats are also extremely stable and can withstand high heat, making them GREAT for cooking! Just be mindful that a little goes a long way in terms of flavor and satiety, so don't throw in a whole stick of butter when a pat will do.

Omega-6 Polyunsaturated Fats. **Although omega-3 fatty acids are also polyunsaturated fats, they get a free pass.** (That's why they're listed above in the Good group. Think of them as the teacher's pets.) The other polyunsaturated fats that should sometimes be used with care, and at other times avoided altogether, are omega-6 fatty acids. (Think of these guys as average students who need tutors from time to time.) You'll find them in vegetable oils like safflower, sunflower, corn, soy, and cottonseed. And although, like omega-3s, omega-6 fatty acids are "essential," most people today consume too many of them relative to their omega-3 intake.

Why does the ratio matter? Well, as in any class, you want more star students than average ones. In the case of these essential fatty acids, having the wrong ratio (too many omega-6s, too few omega-3s) can disrupt the production of important prostaglandins and result in inflammation, high blood pressure, irritation of the digestive tract, depressed immune function, premature aging, cancer, heart disease, and weight gain. Yep, it's that bad. So avoid omega-6s where you can, and opt instead for foods that contain a natural balance of omega-3 and omega-6 fatty acids, such as free-range eggs, hemp seeds, and nuts.

THE UGLY

Trans Fats. THIS is the fat that *deserves* the F-word! It's the worst of all fats and should be avoided at all costs. Trans fats are created when unsaturated fats are heated at high temperatures with the addition of hydrogen atoms in a process called hydrogenation. They're treated this way in order to make liquid fats solid at room temperature, which lengthens the shelf life of food products. (Never mind that it *shortens* the shelf life of our own health.) Trans fats increase the risk for developing cancer, diabetes, and heart disease. They also increase bad cholesterol and decrease good cholesterol, all while raising total blood cholesterol levels.

Sadly, trans fats can be hard to avoid. You'll find them in baked goods (cookies, crackers, cakes, piecrusts, etc.), fried foods (french fries, nachos, doughnuts, chips, etc.), margarine, shortening, microwavable popcorn, peanut butter, candies, cake mixes, and pancake mixes.

Where things get tricky is in products labeled "trans fat free." Why? Because they contain trans fats! Crazy! This happens because government standards allow manufacturers to market a product as trans fat free if the amount of trans fats is less than 0.5 grams per serving. So the manufacturers simply reduce the "standard" serving size on package nutrition labels, which bumps the product into the realm of acceptable levels. But don't be fooled. Trans fats accumulate in your body to negatively affect your overall health. If a product's ingredient list includes the words "partially hydrogenated" or "shortening," it has trans fats, and you should steer clear!

JUST TO RECAP ...

Fats should make up around 20 to 30 percent of your total daily caloric intake. So if you consume 2,000 calories per day, roughly 400 to 600 of them should come from fats, most of which should be made up of omega-3-rich seeds (including sacha inchi, chia, and hemp), oily fish, nuts, avocados, olives, extra virgin olive oil, and coconut oil. No more than 10 percent should come from saturated fats.

TIP

Each gram of fat contains nine calories. (To put that in perspective, carbs contain only four calories per gram.) So, to calculate how many grams you should be consuming, divide your total caloric intake by nine. In the example above, 400 to 600 calories is equivalent to 44 to 67 grams. This may seem like a lot, but keep in mind that one tablespoon is approximately 15 grams!

Heart-Healthy Lifestyle Changes

Keeping your cardiovascular system healthy requires more than avoiding trans fats and eating a lot of flax. After all, your heart is busy pumping thousands of gallons of blood. The least you can do is pitch in with a few lifestyle changes!

Reduce Stress

For starters, relax! Chronic stress is linked to high blood pressure, irregular heartbeat, chest pain, and increased risk for heart attack. In a study published in the *Journal of Clinical Endocrinology and Metabolism*, European researchers concluded that those with the highest levels of the stress hormone cortisol had an increased risk for death from heart disease.[100]

Does that stress you out? Try incorporating more stress-reduction practices into your lifestyle, such as yoga, meditation, or simply taking time to breathe mindfully. You can also tap the power of nutrient-dense, stress-busting foods like maca, which is an adaptogen that helps your body deal with stress and manage cortisol levels. See Chapter 2 for more stress-busting info.

Exercise

If you love to run on the treadmill, great. Do it. But if you identify with those who "hate to exercise," it's time to change your tune. There are millions of ways to be active, from zumba to barre classes. Heck, you can even do it in your own home: just pump up the music and bust a move, Gangnam style! Your heart will love you for it. Exercise is a guaranteed way to lower cholesterol levels and raise HDL levels, thereby reducing your risk for heart disease. Not to mention that it's great for reducing stress, lowering your diabetes risk, dropping pounds, and lowering your blood pressure. So go on, shake that booty, and give yourself some love!

Don't Smoke!

If those nasty pics on cigarette packages aren't enough to deter you, I don't know what is. Pretty much everyone knows what your lungs look like after a cigarette, but if you're still in the dark, just imagine a piece of coal. And don't forget you're relying on that piece of coal to get clean oxygen to your heart and cells, something that's kinda tough to do when oxygen has to compete with carbon monoxide. Ha. Quite the pipe dream. Smoking increases plaque buildup in the arteries, and it's one of the top contributors to heart disease–related death. That makes sense when you consider that a single inhalation brings with it around 4,000 different toxic, inflammatory chemicals. Nothing—including your heart—stands to benefit from that.

Limit Salt/Sodium Intake

Don't worry. You don't have to give up the pinch of sea salt at the dinner table or avoid what's naturally occurring in food. That's not where the excess intake of sodium comes from. It's packaged, processed, and canned foods that account for nearly 80 percent of excess sodium intake. Sodium is an important mineral and essential for a variety of cellular functions. However, *excess* sodium can increase your risk of high blood pressure, which increases your risk for heart attack or stroke. The un-bacon-wrapped reality is that the average person consumes DOUBLE this amount per day!

> **TIP**
> What's considered excess sodium? Over 1,500 milligrams per day—which is less than one teaspoon!

Reduce Sugar and Refined Carbohydrates

The devil is in the dextrose. We're talking excess sugar consumption here. As noted earlier, our brains need a bit of sugar, and depending on the intensity of our workouts, it helps fuel those too. However, more often than not, we aren't consuming that red velvet cupcake on our way to crossfit. Not only is excess sugar and refined carb consumption terrible for the waistline; it's also terrible for the heart. Refined sugars and carbs (which convert immediately into sugar in your body) increase triglyceride (fat) levels in your blood. The accumulation of these fats wreaks havoc on cholesterol levels—it lowers the good cholesterol and prevents the elimination of bad cholesterol. Plus, these triglycerides lead to obesity and type 2 diabetes, which further increase the risk of cardiovascular disease.[101]

Heart-Healthy Nutrients

In addition to the omega-3 fatty acids and monounsaturated fats described earlier, here are the key nutrients your heart needs to pump with flair.

Fiber

Fiber does more than keep you regular. It clings to cholesterol like a drowning man clutches a life preserver, absorbs it, and helps your body eliminate it. Not surprisingly, a diet high in dietary fiber—especially soluble fiber—has been shown to help lower blood cholesterol levels. You should aim to get 25 grams of it per day.

Vitamin C

Vitamin C is a powerful antioxidant that significantly helps to reduce inflammatory diseases like atherosclerosis. It does so by reducing C-reactive protein, a compound that promotes inflammation and increases the risk of heart failure.[102] It all goes back to inflammation! (See Chapter 17 on how to reduce inflammation.)

Vitamin C also loves your arteries! In addition to preventing plaque buildup, it helps repair already damaged arteries. And it can help lower bad cholesterol levels to significantly reduce blood pressure. A meta-analysis of 29 human studies concluded that 500 milligrams of vitamin C per day significantly reduced both systolic and diastolic blood pressure.[103] So eat up that kiwi!

Vitamin E

Like its BFF vitamin C, vitamin E is a powerful antioxidant that works to keep the bad cholesterol from hardening the arteries. Vitamin E can also prevent the formation of blood clots, and eating more vitamin E–rich foods helps those suffering from heart disease to reduce their risk of death from it.[104]

TIP

The best way to get your vitamins C and E are with a little fiber. Eating a variety of plant-based foods, namely veggies and fruits, provides a one-two punch in boosting antioxidant and fiber intake.

Co-Enzyme Q10

Also known as CoQ10 or ubiquinone, co-enzyme Q10 is a powerful, fat-soluble antioxidant found in every cell in the body. It's responsible for the production of energy, and is hugely beneficial in the prevention and treatment of heart disease.

Doctors in Japan have been using CoQ10 to treat congestive heart failure since 1974, and there are a number of reasons why. Studies show that it can reduce symptoms of heart palpitations and chest pain, plus it helps reduce inflammation and prevent plaque buildup. The last of these is thanks to its antioxidant properties, which stop LDL from oxidizing and hanging out where it's not wanted (in the arteries). See page 117 for how antioxidants work!

TIP

Not only is CoQ10 amazing for your heart, it also gives your skin some love with its amazing, wrinkle-fighting antioxidant power. And since CoQ10 is fat soluble, it's best to consume it with healthy fats, such as olive oil, avocado, or a small handful of almonds.

Magnesium

Magnesium and calcium are like trapeze artists. Calcium contracts the heart and blood vessels, and then magnesium relaxes them. Calcium needs to be absorbed, and magnesium helps the body do so. But sometimes one person (or mineral, as the case may be) gets all the glory while the other is left in the shadows. (Haven't you ever seen *Beaches*?) Well, magnesium is the one in the shadows.

TIP

It's worth saying it again: a direct correlation exists between the intake of calcium supplements and the risk of heart attack. It's best to get calcium through food, and mainly through plant-based foods at that, since they have optimal calcium–magnesium ratios.

Most North Americans simply don't consume enough magnesium, despite the fact that it's one of the most important minerals in the body. It helps prevent blood clotting and heart disease, *and* it helps relax muscles and nerves—while helping our bodies cope with stress, no less!

Having a magnesium deficiency not only means you miss out on its benefits, but also may mean you incur extra risk. When there's too much calcium in our bodies and not enough magnesium to absorb it, excess calcium can build up as plaque in the arteries. It's time for magnesium to take the spotlight!

Potassium

Just as calcium and magnesium must work as a team, sodium and potassium make for a powerful duet. Good potassium levels are critical for balancing sodium levels, and that applies when sodium is moderate *and* high. Unfortunately, it's MUCH easier to get sodium through the diet than potassium. So make a point of loading up on potassium-rich foods.

Potassium's role is huge: it helps trigger the bear-hug squeeze of the heart that results in a heartbeat. Getting enough potassium through your diet, therefore, helps to ease (and lower) systolic blood pressure.

Foods rich in potassium:

- Swiss chard
- Crimini mushrooms
- Spinach
- Celery
- Fennel
- Yams
- Lima beans
- Papaya
- Avocado
- Beet greens
- Watercress

DID YOU KNOW?

One cup of cooked Swiss chard provides over a quarter of your RDA of potassium (960 milligrams). Plus it's super high in magnesium, which also contributes to a healthy heart!

THE YIN AND YANG OF HEART HEALTH

Your heart has four chambers that divide the work evenly. It's not surprising, then, that its required electrolyte balance mimics this proportion. Calcium, magnesium, sodium, and potassium all provide cellular energy while working in teams to provide optimal balance and health.

YIN	&	YANG
Magnesium Relaxes		Calcium Contracts
Potassium Provides energy inside the cell		Sodium Provides energy outside the cell

---

Eat Your Heart Out

Making your heart happy with your diet means eating a lot of plant-based foods like veggies, leafy greens, fruits, and the heart-healthy fats found in nuts, seeds, and oily omega-3 fish. A glass of red wine now and then helps, too!

Here are the foods your heart loves.

Garlic

While this powerhouse bulb may not be the best thing for your breath, it IS the best thing for your heart! Garlic contains allicin, which is the sulfur-based organic compound that gives garlic its odor. This is the same compound we chatted about in the sex chapter. It helps boost libido by helping your heart lower cholesterol and plaque buildup, allowing blood to flow freely (and quickly)—and a healthy heart directly translates to a healthy sex life!

The superhero quality here is allicin. Allicin increases nitric oxide, a chemical gas used by blood vessel walls to trigger the arteries and surrounding muscles, causing them to relax. The more nitric oxide, the wider the blood vessels become and the less the heart needs to work to pump blood through your body—which has a positive effect on blood pressure and reduces risk of cardiovascular disease.

Garlic's most powerful star quality is that it helps lower cholesterol and prevent blood platelets from building up and forming artery-clogging blood clots. A UCLA study showed that plaque progression slowed by more than 50 percent in those taking garlic extract. And here's the kicker: those who weren't taking garlic were taking prescriptive meds![105]

Garlic is also a great natural antibiotic. It has antibacterial and antifungal properties, and can help protect against the cold, flu, bacterial infections, some cancers—and vampires.

HOW TO USE

As described in the sex chapter, garlic can be minced, chopped, or crushed—it's through this manual process (or some serious chewing) that allicin is formed. Then let the garlic sit for a few minutes to allow the process to happen. As well, since heat destroys allicin, it's best to eat garlic raw. Add some minced, raw garlic to salad dressings, mix with extra virgin olive oil and drizzle over steamed veggies, and perhaps even stuff some in olives!

Sea-Buckthorn Fruit Oil

Red and exotic, sea-buckthorn berry oil just looks like it should have some extraordinary properties. And, for once, reality actually meets expectations!

Sea-buckthorn is native to Siberia and Mongolia, and while you can source nutrients from the entire plant—fruit, seeds, leaves, and even the bark!—the berry flesh is what provides the fruit oil. People have been using the fruit medicinally for centuries, although today you'll likely find this phytonutrient-rich oil in nutritional supplements and skincare products.

While the fruit oil has a lot fewer omega-3 fatty acids than the seed oil, it's still a heart-healthy option. That's because it's high in monounsaturated fats and contains plant sterols, vitamin E, and beta carotene, all of which reduce the risk of heart disease.

DID YOU KNOW?

Research has shown that not only do the monounsaturated fats help prevent coronary disease by lowering blood cholesterol (especially the bad LDL), but they may also help prevent atherosclerosis through other means, including carbohydrate metabolism, blood pressure, and lipoprotein oxidation.

Plus, we've all heard about the benefits of omega-3, 6, and 9, but omega-7 fatty acids haven't been given the attention they deserve! Omega-7s are amazing for slowing down the signs of aging when it comes to your skin, contributing to a clear, flawless complexion. They're also amazing at helping to regulate fat and blood sugar while reducing LDL cholesterol.

Sea-buckthorn fruit oil is generous—it helps out other parts of your body, too! It can protect against a host of maladies, including macular degeneration and prostate cancer, while improving cognitive performance and helping to regenerate damaged skin and mucous membranes. So perhaps this time the reality even *exceeds* expectations![106]

Sea-Buckthorn Seed Oil

There's bound to be some sibling rivalry between the seed and berry oil of the sea-buckthorn plant. While they both improve cardiovascular health and protect against related diseases, they also have their individual advantages.

Case in point: sea-buckthorn seed oil is high in polyunsaturated fats, with a perfect ratio of omega-3 and omega-6 fatty acids. (Remember how important it is to get these essential fats in the right ratio? Sea-buckthorn seed oil nails it.) And while sea-buckthorn berry oil uses the flesh of the berry, the seed oil is extracted from—you guessed it!—just the seeds of the berries.

The omega-3s are what make the seed oil so darn attractive, since getting enough of those (whether through food or supplements) reduces a bunch of unpleasant things like, oh, overall mortality, death from myocardial infarction, and sudden death in patients with coronary heart disease.

The seed oil is also higher in gamma-tocopherol levels, which is a type of vitamin E in which those who have coronary heart disease tend to be deficient. Sea-buckthorn seed oil is also high in vitamin B12, which can help prevent hyperhomocysteinemia, an independent risk factor for atherosclerosis and coronary artery disease. And it contains other important nutrients like vitamin K, phospholipids (brain-boosting fats), and phytosterols, which can lower bad cholesterol.

Like its sister oil, sea-buckthorn seed oil can do other things for you besides save your heart. It can improve gastrointestinal health, for one, and it helps with a number of skin issues such as acne and rosacea. It also has anti-inflammatory and regenerative properties.[107]

Hawthorn

Once you get past the somewhat creepy fact that hawthorns are the sacred trees of Wicca and witchcraft, you can appreciate their berries' more physical benefits. Specifically, the chemical compounds in hawthorn fruits help dilate coronary arteries, which helps reduce blood pressure. They also help prevent congestive heart failure by reducing fluid buildup and improving your heart's ability to pump blood throughout the body.

Hawthorn fruit contains antioxidant-rich bioflavonoids as well. The bioflavonoids are varied and include oligomeric procyanidins, vixtexin, quercetin, and hyperoside. These may improve circulation to the extremities by reducing blood vessels' resistance to blood flow.

Sacha Inchi Seeds (aka Savi Seeds)

Some foods are good for you. Some foods are great for you. And then there are the foods like the unassuming sacha inchi seeds, which are AMAZING for you!

Sacha inchi seeds are found in the eponymous plant's star-shaped green pods. These pods are sun-dried until the seeds are exposed, at which point they're placed inside huge bank vaults and protected by armed guards, because their health benefits are so valuable.

Okay, maybe the situation isn't *quite* so extreme, but sacha inchi seeds ARE that good. They contain heaps of omega-3 fatty acids (more than even wild salmon!), vitamin E, fiber, and more tryptophan than turkey. Plus, they're nut- and gluten-free!

As far as your heart is concerned, the omega-3s are where it's at. These unsaturated fatty acids can reduce the risk of a heart attack by 30 percent or more, AND they reduce inflammation. That's important, because inflammation can damage your blood vessels and lead to heart disease.

Omega-3s also decrease triglycerides, lower blood pressure, reduce blood clotting, boost immunity, and improve arthritis symptoms. Now can you see why they're worth their weight in gold?!

HOW TO USE

Add the seeds to green salads, or munch on roasted seeds for a snack. (You can even get them chocolate- or caramel-covered!) Sacha inchi seeds are also made into powders and oils that you can add to everyday meals.

Chia Seeds

Once a staple of the Aztec diet, chia seeds have overcome some unfortunate merchandising (Chia Pets, anyone?) to re-emerge as a nutritional powerhouse.

Chia seeds come from a plant that's part of the mint family, but the seeds do a lot more than freshen breath. For starters, they're a complete source of dietary protein and provide all essential amino acids, including omega-3s. (Approximately 64 percent of chia seeds' oil is omega-3.) The omega-3s help your body absorb fat-soluble vitamins (including heart-hugging vitamins E and K), among many other things described in this chapter. The seeds are also a good source of fiber, which is another heart-healthy dietary component to pull bad cholesterol and triglycerides from your body, reducing total cholesterol levels.

Since chia seeds are great at stabilizing blood sugar (chia seeds mixed with water form a gel that releases carbs slowly, thereby avoiding an insulin spike), they're useful for more than heart health. And because they can absorb up to nine times their volume in water, they can prolong hydration and help your body retain electrolytes while you implement that all-important lifestyle change: exercise!

Chia seeds are gluten- and cholesterol-free, so they're a good choice for a lot of people!

Olives

If your heart could talk, it just might say "O-live you" when you drizzle olive oil on your salad or nosh on whole olives as a snack. Why the amorous sentiments? Because olives are rich in iron, vitamin E, and fiber as well as being a good source of monounsaturated fat, polyphenols, and flavonoids.

The monounsaturated fat is particularly helpful since it reduces the risk for atherosclerosis while raising good HDL cholesterol. Flavonoids, meanwhile, have anti-inflammatory properties that help reduce your risk for heart disease. Plus, olives' omega-3 fatty acids do all those good things like reduce the risk of blood clots, lower blood pressure, improve vascular health, and reduce the risk of heart attack. Olive love indeed!

Avocado

Known as the alligator pear in Jamaica, avocados could easily be mistaken for vegetables. (They're a fruit.) But there's no mistaking their cardiovascular benefits. Avocados contain monounsaturated fatty acids, vitamin E, and linoleic and oleic acids. That means they boost good HDL levels and reduce bad LDL levels, which improves cardiovascular health.

They're beloved for other reasons, too. With lots of good stuff for healthy skin, avocados help fight melanoma. And diabetic patients enjoy them since they're a low-sugar, starch-free food.

HOW TO USE

Ditch the butter, cream cheese, and peanut butter! Instead, spread two tablespoons of mashed avocado on your toast and sandwiches. It adds heart-healthy creaminess to puddings and icings, too. Avocado oil is also a great addition to your culinary repertoire. It has a relatively high smoke point compared to other oils (and higher than extra virgin olive oil), so it makes for great sautéing at medium-heat temperatures. It can also be used in sauces and dressings, and topically as a moisturizer.

Apples

Eat an apple a day ... well, make that two. More and more research is revealing that doing so will reduce heart-disease factors like blood cholesterol levels and markers associated with plaque buildup in arteries and inflammation of artery walls. This is all thanks to apples' antioxidants and rich fiber content.

Apples are a great source of antioxidants, including heart-protective vitamin C and polyphenols, which prevent free-radical damage to the heart and arteries. Plus, they contain pectin, which is a soluble fiber that blocks the absorption of cholesterol in the gut and reduces LDL (bad cholesterol) levels. Apples can reduce plaque buildup in the arteries and reduce inflammatory markers, such as C-reactive protein. And as we mentioned earlier, inflammation is a precursor to heart disease.

An apple a day also reduces your risk of respiratory disease, and can help with weight loss, which means the fruit will soon be the apple of your eye, er, heart.

HOW TO USE

Delicious crispy and raw OR baked in the oven with some cinnamon—apples are the perfect snack! Eat them on their own, or cut them up and toss them into salad. You can also incorporate them into desserts, sauces, and main or side dishes. Replace sugar with a chopped-up apple when baking butternut squash to up the sweetness. And apples add the perfect sweetness to an all-green juice!

TIP

The best apples to use when baking are varieties that hold their shape: Cortland, Empire, Granny Smith, Gala, Jonagold, and Golden Delicious. Avoid varieties like Pink Lady and Fuji (which fall apart when baked) and Red Delicious (which tastes much better crunchy and raw).

20. PMS (Please Make it Stop)

Premenstrual syndrome: it's the period (pun intended) when your cool, fun-loving, normal self turns into psycho-chick. For real. But it's totally excusable. Your boobs hurt just running down the stairs, all your clothes immediately become tight, you never know when that zit is about to pop up on your face, and you can barely get out of bed in the morning—coupled with the fact that you couldn't even fall asleep. You may feel tense, irritated, irrational, bloated, crampy, achy, cranky, sad, moody, and hungry for all the wrong foods. Yep—pretty much hell. What's worse is that an estimated three out of four women report having these feelings. It's no wonder men don't understand us.

PMS Facts

The good news? You're not losing your mind when you burst into tears for no apparent reason. Mood swings, fatigue, and depression are common feelings you might experience during PMS. Another number to note? Two hundred. That's the number of different symptoms that have been associated with PMS, and since there isn't enough room to list them all here, the three most commonly reported are feelings of unhappiness, cramps, and mood swings that bring on wicked food cravings. If it's greasy, sugary, salty, fatty, and starchy, it may end up on your plate because the body is trying to compensate for and correct the hormonal gong show. And it totally takes over control. You've lost all sense of reason and it feels as though there's nothing you can do.

But that's not necessarily true. Current thinking suggests that estrogen excess, progesterone deficiencies, vitamin B6 deficiencies, low levels of serotonin, and low calcium could explain PMS. And what you eat a couple of weeks before your period could significantly reduce PMS, or better yet, PCS (psycho-chick syndrome).

TIP

Getting plenty of zzz's and O's can also help reduce irritability and ease cramps during PMS. Sleep helps control mood swings. Orgasms in particular release oxytocin, a chemical that relaxes the uterine wall and eases cramping. Hallelujah.

PMS-Fighting Nutrients
Calcium, Magnesium, and Vitamin D

The symptoms of PMS and of low calcium levels bear a strong similarity. In fact, it's been determined that estrogen regulates calcium metabolism. And since estrogen levels change across the menstrual cycle, calcium absorption also fluctuates. In one study from the Columbia University College of Physicians and Surgeons, women who received 1,200 milligrams of calcium carbonate each day for three menstrual cycles had a 50 percent reduction in PMS symptoms.[108] The equation is easy. Up the intake of calcium, and reduce the cramping and pains associated with PMS.

And while magnesium is one of the top mineral deficiencies at any time of the month, it's especially important to supplement it during PMS because it helps relax nerves and alleviate muscle cramping and headaches.

Finally, consuming vitamin D during PMS is also significant. Vitamin D helps the body absorb calcium—and because calcium helps ease cramping, pairing it with vitamin D can maximize these cramp-curbing benefits. Later, cramps!

TIP

Since PMS is closely linked to estrogen dominance, the same principles apply. See Chapter 7 for more info.

Omega-3 Fatty Acids and GLA

Essential fatty acids (EFAs) are an essential BFF when it comes to PMS. Why? Well, EFAs play important roles in your body's overall health. They're part of every cell, and establish and control cellular metabolism. Omega-3 EFAs not only are great for their anti-inflammatory properties, but also provide energy, maintain body temperature, insulate our nerves, and cushion and protect body tissues. Gamma linolenic acid (GLA) also has amazing anti-inflammatory properties—in particular, its formation of other substances like prostaglandins. These hormone-like prostaglandins are vital chemicals that regulate heartbeat and blood pressure. They also play a role in breaking up cholesterol deposits in the blood. Most important, they help alleviate cramping and backaches during PMS because of their anti-inflammatory properties.

Vitamin B6

B vitamins in general are great for PMS, but B6 in particular is essential in the production of those feel-good neurotransmitters. It helps in the conversion of tryptophan to serotonin, and who doesn't love the high you get off that? Unfortunately, this vitamin is also the first to be depleted during times of tension, so a lack of B6 could seriously lead to more feelings of depression. We know that PMS makes us feel like crap, so you can see why it's so important to keep taking that B6 and keep elevating those serotonin levels. Take 100 milligrams of vitamin B6 a day, combined with other B vitamins, and go to your happy place!

Indole-3-Carbinol

Indole-3-carbinol, or I3C, might not be easy to pronounce, but it's a phytochemical you'll want to incorporate into your diet during PMS. I3C is a strong antioxidant, but most important it helps shift estrogen metabolism to less estrogenic metabolites. Especially during PMS, it helps maintain hormonal balance and can relieve muscle soreness.

Fiber

Fiber is the new black. It does everything from lower cholesterol to normalize blood sugar, which in turn reduces food cravings. It also removes excess estrogen from the body—and that's crucial for helping ease PMS symptoms. If estrogen isn't eliminated properly, it can be reactivated while in the liver and actually re-enter the bloodstream, causing hormonal chaos to ensue. Fiber also helps the body fully utilize progesterone, which if in excess can cause food cravings to rocket. (Here's how it works: to balance the blood-sugar levels fluctuating during PMS, the body releases adrenaline, but if it's not utilized then progesterone isn't used efficiently. Fiber helps to balance this by eliminating it as waste.)

TIP
It's recommended that adults consume 20 to 35 grams of dietary fiber per day.

Nosh on This ... So You Can Squash PMS

What you eat up to two weeks before your period can make a HUGE difference when it comes to PMS. So try to incorporate more PMS-busting foods—and to eliminate PMS-promoting foods, such as dairy, refined carbs, sugars, and alcohols.

Some top PMS-busting foods:

- Cruciferous veggies
- Maca
- Chia seeds
- Sacha inchi seeds
- Hemp seeds
- Bananas
- Cucumbers
- Almonds
- Raw chocolate
- Dark leafy greens
- Apples
- Quinoa
- Oats

Kale

Killer cramps? Curb them with kale. Kale is a dense green leafy vegetable that comes from the cabbage family. Whether it's green or purple, curly or plain-leaved, kale is one of the perfect foods to help during PMS because it contains calcium, magnesium, I3C, and calcium D-glucarate.

Calcium is the simplest and least expensive intervention for PMS; aim for 1,200 milligrams per day to help with cramps. The I3C helps to weaken estrogen levels while the calcium D-glucarate, coupled with the fiber, helps eliminate excess estrogen from your body, making you less estrogenic and significantly reducing the severity of PMS. No more yo-yo hormones for you. In addition, kale is a natural diuretic, helping to eliminate excess water weight!

HOW TO USE

Often relegated as a salad bar garnish, this hearty green has oh-so-much more to offer. Try adding it to a salad filled with other leafy greens. Kale has a crunchier bite and offers a great balance of textures. Or try lightly steaming it, then tossing it with olive oil, black pepper, and sea salt for a side dish that adds color and nutrition. Slice it up with a bunch of other veggies for a delish stir fry. In season in early winter, kale makes a hearty addition to soups or stews. But my all-time fave—and soon to be yours—is kale chips. All you have to do is slice kale leaves into bite-size pieces, removing the stems. Toss in some olive oil, lemon juice, and paprika, and then dehydrate or bake on low. The result: a salty, crunchy substitute for potato chips, loaded with nutrition and none of the guilt!

Halibut

Halibut is your anti-cramping BFF. It's rich in omega-3 fatty acids, which slow down the release of prostaglandins. Prostaglandins regulate pain and inflammation in the body. By managing prostaglandin release with omega-3s, you can reduce headaches as well as pain in the joints, lower back, and abdomen. For these reasons, omega-3s may also reduce breast tenderness, mood changes, and weight gain. And halibut is also a rich source of magnesium, which helps relax nerves and tense muscles and relieve cramping.

HOW TO USE

Forget the standard fish-and-chips fare: halibut's mild flavor lends itself perfectly to grilling and baking without the added saturated fat. Be sure to buy fresh, wild halibut for an optimum nutrition profile. Halibut is great—and at its most nutritious—when baked, steamed, or grilled. Your fish is cooked through when opaque, so don't overcook it, or you'll be looking at a dry, flavorless mess. Halibut pairs well with a variety of herbs: dill, rosemary, and parsley are all great complements. Try experimenting with this omega-3 star by adding it to a sprouted-grain wrap with veggies or tossing it into your favorite soup or pasta.

Quinoa

Pronounced "keen-wa," this is my favorite grain. Although considered a carb, the grain-like crop is closer to being a pseudograin than a real grain, since it's really a seed. (It just looks like a grain, cooks like a grain, tastes like a grain ... so we call it a grain.) Quinoa is known for its high protein content (12 to 18 percent). And unlike common grains, it contains all nine essential amino acids, making it a complete protein. Even better news is that it's easier to digest than meat protein, contains more vitamins and minerals, and has a far lower fat content.

Quinoa is also gluten-free, full of fiber, and contains copious amounts of nutrients, including B vitamins. B vitamins and fiber are crucial for helping balance hormones. B vitamins are essential in the production of serotonin, which helps reduce irritability, depression, and PCS (the aforementioned psycho-chick syndrome). Fiber reduces cravings to binge because it bulks up in the stomach so that you feel fuller longer. This also helps eliminate excess estrogen, balancing hormones and reducing water retention. When estrogen starts to fluctuate, it affects aldosterone, a hormone that affects the way your kidneys hold on to water. This is why you retain more water during PMS. So by noshing on quinoa, your excess water weight starts to normalize and you'll feel zero need to bust out your "fat clothes."

HOW TO USE

I love quinoa so much because it's not only nutri'licious, but also super low maintenance! It takes only 15 minutes to cook, and will last in your fridge for up to five days, making it a quick and easy meal no matter what your time constraints are. Use it as a base for a pasta dish, as a rice substitute, blended into soups or smoothies, added to salads, as a breakfast cereal, or in cookies. Yep, that's right, check out my PMS-busting Chocolate Chip Quinoa Cookies on page 325.

Raw Cashews

Raw cashews are the perfect PMS/PCS snack food. They're crammed with essential vitamins, minerals, and nutrients that help regulate mood, reduce food cravings, and relax muscles. These nuts' most important PMS-busting nutrients include magnesium, vitamin B, vitamin E, and fiber.

Cashews are loaded with magnesium, a powerful nutrient for nervous system function. High levels of magnesium support a relaxed mind and body, which helps alleviate cramping. Magnesium also activates many enzymes required for energy production in the body, which is key when you're fatigued. As B vitamins and magnesium are both involved in serotonin production, they can further help regulate your moods.

What's also great is that they can help keep blood-sugar levels in check, reducing killer cravings and binges. This not only helps regulate energy levels, mood, and cravings, but also can help prevent insulin resistance, type 2 diabetes, and most important, your midsection from bulging over your jeans! Buh-bye PCS and muffin tops, hello hot cool chick!

DID YOU KNOW?

According to studies conducted through the University of Montreal and Université de Yaoundé, cashew-seed extract significantly stimulates blood-sugar absorption by muscle cells.[110]

HOW TO USE

To knock out PMS, reach for raw, unroasted, unsalted cashews. (And no, that doesn't take all the fun out of it!) These little nuts are a rich addition to salads, cereal, and baked goods—but keep in mind that they're also high in fat and calories, so moderation is the way to go. Also, they're not the highest quality of nut. Make sure you get them from a reputable source, as they can have mold content, especially troublesome if you suffer from candida. These days you can also find cashew butter on store shelves, a great alternative to traditional peanut butter. I love using cashews in my guilt-free desserts. Try my Cocoa Mocha Torte or Blueberry Lemon Tart recipes (pages 326 and 328, respectively) to see what I mean. Delici-o-so!

Maca

Maca is definitely a PMS-busting superfood. Its nutrient-dense, hormone-balancing, stress-busting properties will make that time of the month a stroll in the park for you—and everyone around you! Maca is a rich source of I-3-C, which helps change excess bad estrogen into a weaker, beneficial form. And since hormonal imbalances and estrogen dominance typically lead to weight gain, cramping, and mood swings, maca is a must. Plus, its rich fibre content helps to pull the excess estrogen, preventing it from re-circulating. Maca is also rich in calcium and magnesium to help relieve killer cramps.

> ### HOW TO USE
> Discover the many ways to use maca on page 96.

Sacha Inchi Seeds

Omega-3s are key in reducing inflammation, stomach cramping, and regulating mood. Sacha inchi seeds (SaviSeed) are among the richest source, helping you feel fab. Plus, at five grams of fiber per ounce, they will help balance blood-sugar levels, ward off wicked cravings, and keep energy levels stable.

> ### HOW TO USE
> Learn how to incorporate sacha inchi seeds into your diet on page 62.

21. Mentalpause

When it comes to menopause, some women don't witness even the slightest of symptoms (lucky them!), whereas for others the experience is kinda like a horror movie: shrouded in mystery and with a lot of misery involved, but usually working out okay in the end. Well, it's time to pull back the curtain on menopause, because the more you know, the easier it is to fast-forward the misery part!

First off, it's true that you do go a little nuts. Your hormones are raging, your body is changing, and the side effects can be downright weird. Case in point: I was once traveling to Florida for work, and I brought my mother along for a couple of days. The first morning, I woke up and found a crazed, frizzy-haired creature in my room. But it was my mother! "What happened to you?" I gasped. Her normally smooth, perfectly coiffed blond hair had transformed overnight to resemble a really bad, seventies-inspired perm! There was so much frizz and curl that her hair was bigger than her head. But my mom wasn't having it. "You don't understand," she bit back. "It's mentalpause!"

And so a very useful term was born: mentalpause. "Because," my mom explained, "you go mental!"

The Feminine Critique

Periods. You can't live with them. You can't live without them.

With the exception of our Judy Blume–reading years, few women get revved up at the prospect of having a period every month. And yet the "pausing" of the menses (hence "menopause") brings us to tears. Literally!

Still, every woman has to face menopause, typically between the ages of 45 and 55. (Perimenopause is the transition your body makes toward menopause, and it can happen as early as your thirties. Symptoms resemble those of menopause.) When exactly menopause happens is up to your ovaries, which produce the female hormones estrogen and progesterone. These hormones oversee, among other things, your periods. But as you age, your ovaries gradually stop producing eggs while putting out fewer and fewer hormones. Once a complete year passes without your Aunt Flo stopping by, you have officially entered menopause.

Menopause varies between women, with some feeling the full force of its fury and others barely noticing it. (And if you're one of those people who suffer from crazy PMS symptoms, you're likely to experience menopausal symptoms for the same reason, so watch out!) What do I mean? Well, how do hot flashes, mood swings, depression, anxiety, insomnia, and night sweats sound? Okay, how about vaginal dryness and loss of sex drive? That's what I thought. I can hear the horror-flick soundtrack already ...

Heat of the Moment

Is it getting hot in here? Nope, it's just you if you're going through perimenopause or menopause. A hot flash is a feeling of intense heat in the upper part of the body, accompanied by an accelerated heartbeat and a reddening of the chest, neck, and face. The culprit is hormonal: when estrogen levels drop, the brain's hypothalamus—which regulates hormone production—goes into overdrive and increases your internal temperature.

Hot flashes affect more than half of women in perimenopause and about two-thirds of women after menopause. The good news? They usually last no longer than five minutes. The bad news: they can happen for anywhere from a few months to five years!

Hot flashes are the same thing as night sweats, the only difference being when they occur. (Hot flashes happen during the day; night sweats, well, you guessed it, smarty-pants, happen at night.) Unfortunately, "night sweat" isn't an exaggeration. Heavy sweating routinely follows a hot flash, and it can be significant enough to saturate a woman's bedsheets (and if you've got curly hair, look out!).

If you've had a particularly sweaty day (or night), pouring yourself a glass of wine may seem like a good remedy. Uhhh—WRONG! It's precisely that wine (and stress) that can aggravate a hot flash. Alcohol in general, along with coffee and spicy foods, may trigger hot flashes, while stress only makes them worse. Do yourself a favor and take a cold shower instead.

TIP

If cold showers aren't your cup of tea, make yourself a cup of tea! But choose the non-caffeinated, trusted herbal teas, such as peppermint and chamomile, which can calm you down and chill you out (literally).

Estrogenic Herbs: Yay or Nay?

If you've made it this far into the book, you'll know that food and herbs are pretty powerful tools. Powerful enough to change the way you look, the way you feel, and in some cases, the way your endocrine system works.

To that end, there are certain plant-based foods that contain estrogenic compounds called phytoestrogens (or "plant estrogens"). These are made up of isoflavones (found predominantly in soy) and lignans (found in things like flaxseed). Phytoestrogens are weak estrogenic compounds that mimic estrogens in the body (see page 91 on soy), and they're typically recommended as a treatment for menopause symptoms (namely, hot flashes). That's because they bind onto estrogen receptor sites and increase estrogen in the body, theoretically compensating for the lack of estrogen produced by the ovaries.

It sounds simple enough, but phytoestrogens aren't exactly a turnkey solution. In fact, they can cause more harm than good because your hormonal balance is extremely important and extremely picky.

When menopause hits, ovaries stop producing progesterone and estrogen but continue to produce testosterone. Estrogen, however, was never entirely faithful to the ovaries: the adrenal gland and fat cells also produce estrogen and continue to do so even after menopause. And, as you might expect, the more fat you have, the more estrogen your body produces. So while estrogen and progesterone production both decline, progesterone does so faster, and the imbalance of the two is what causes all those lovely side effects we discussed earlier. But the real takeaway is this: your body doesn't necessarily need MORE estrogen. It needs a balance of estrogen and progesterone.

"Pshaw!" you say. "Everyone takes estrogen after menopause. And what's a herb going to do anyway?" Well, in one sense you'd be right. No evidence suggests that phytoestrogen foods or supplements provide any relief for hot flashes/night sweats or other menopausal symptoms. They don't even appear to help lower cholesterol or prevent heart disease, a condition for which postmenopausal women are at increased risk.

HORMONE REPLACEMENT THERAPY

If you think the phytoestrogen fail warrants trying hormone replacement therapy (HRT), studies indicate that excess estrogen increases your risk of breast cancer, while estrogen-only therapy ups the chances of suffering stroke, potentially deadly blood clots, and endometrial cancer, which is a cancer of the uterine lining. A pooled analysis of 51 observational studies showed that hormone therapy with a combination of estrogen and progesterone for five years or longer resulted in a 53 percent increased risk of developing breast cancer and did not protect women from heart disease.[111]

While some long-term studies suggest that supplementing with a weaker form of estrogen might be beneficial, nothing conclusive has been established. And since estrogen dominance is what's likely causing the symptoms in the first place, let's deal with that problem head-on.

Fight the Flashes!

So if herbs and HRT aren't the answer to menopausal symptoms, what is? Here's the shortlist.

Exercise

You know how everyone's always telling you to exercise? Well, if you want to alleviate menopausal symptoms, listen up. Exercise immediately helps reduce estrogen dominance, and in the long term, it helps maintain a fit and healthy body weight. This is important, since fat cells produce estrogen, and reducing their number reduces the amount of estrogen pumping through your body.

Eat Your Veggies

And by "veggies" I mean dark leafy greens and cruciferous vegetables like broccoli, cauliflower, Brussels sprouts, cabbage, turnips, mustard greens, and kale. These are like The Avengers for your health because there's almost nothing they can't tackle. When it comes to menopause, these veggies create a chemical compound called indole-3-carbinol (I3C) when cooked or chewed. This then turns into diindolylmethane in the intestinal tract, which tweaks the metabolism of estrogen so that it becomes a weaker, more beneficial version. The result? You're not nearly so crazy! And, just to make sure these veggies complete the job, their calcium D-glucarate helps eliminate excess toxins and hormones from your body. Their high fiber content, meanwhile, also flushes bad estrogen out. As I said: The Avengers.

Limit Your Vices

I've said it before, and I'll say it again: caffeine and alcohol are NOT your friends during menopause. They, along with cigarette smoking, are mentalpause monsters! High caffeine and alcohol intake aggravate hot flashes, while smoking increases your risk for all sorts of dreadful things like osteoporosis, hip fractures, heart attack, and stroke.

Shun the Spice

Spicy foods are NOT the spice of menopausal life. They may in fact crank up your body's internal thermostat and trigger a hot flash or sweat storm. In other words, steer clear of spicy foods!

Get in the Mood

Put simply, have sex! Even if you're not in the mood—or you feel as dry as the Sahara Desert—bust out the coconut oil, lube up, and have fun. Regularly! (Or at least engage in some foreplay and see what happens.) Besides putting you in a better mood, sex amplifies circulation in the genital area, which helps you maintain your libido ... so you don't *actually* dry up like the Sahara. It's a use-it-or-lose-it scenario, and you really don't want to lose it.

> ### TIP
> Coconut oil makes an edible and pleasurable lubricant for sex.

Meditate, Practice Yoga, and Rest

With hormones out of whack, you may feel overwhelmed or overly emotional, as though you just can't go on or handle what you used to. You're not losing your mind; this is perfectly normal. Hormones are crazy powerful when it comes to your mood, so it's good practice to set aside time in your day to meditate. If that doesn't fit the bill, try enrolling in a breathing or yoga class. Whatever it is that centers you, do it. Even if it's just 10 minutes of breathing and solitude, it will make a world of difference.

Vital Vitamins and Minerals

Menopause may be inevitable, but it's not invincible. In addition to the actions listed above, the following vitamins and minerals pack a powerful punch against menopausal symptoms.

Antioxidant Vitamins C and E

Fat-soluble vitamin E helps regulate hormones and reduce hot flashes and night sweats. Ingest a little vitamin C with your E not only to aid the latter's absorption but also to help mitigate the stress and anxiety associated with menopause. Good sources of vitamin E include almonds and sunflower seeds, while vitamin C is found in foods like red bell peppers and kiwi.

Calcium, Magnesium, and Vitamin D

One look at these bad boys, and you probably think, "Bones." And you're right! All three contribute to bone health, which is particularly important for postmenopausal women.

Since estrogen is integral to the maintenance of strong, healthy bones, its decline in menopause explains why so many postmenopausal women end up with brittle bones. Calcium helps fortify bones, and both magnesium and vitamin D are essential for its absorption. The best, most absorbable sources of all three minerals are dark green, plant-based foods like kale and broccoli. (See Chapter 18 on bones.) In a perfect world you'd eat a great big bowl of them while sitting in the sunshine drinking up all the vitamin D. Hey, make time! Plus, calcium and magnesium help calm your nerves and promote a good night's sleep. Bonus!

B Vitamins

When it comes to menopause, stress is Nemesis No. 1. Nothing exacerbates menopausal symptoms quite like stress, which robs you of energy, clouds your mind, and causes your hormones to go spiraling out of control. Your best nutritional defenses, however, are B vitamins, which provide energy, reduce stress, and boost your mood. (See Chapter 2 on stress and Chapter 5 on depression for more info.)

Fiber

Fiber is your magic pill. It's the card you keep up your sleeve, the trump card you play to win. And that's because it has more good qualities than a Miss America pageant. Fiber helps keep you full on ZERO calories, it keeps you regular, and it sweeps away bad cholesterol, which reduces your risk of cardiovascular disease. Oh, and it also helps eliminate the "bad" estrogen from your body, making you less estrogen dominant. Plus, there's an inverse relationship between fiber and breast cancer: the more fiber consumed daily, the more the risk of breast cancer is reduced.[112]

Here are some of my favorite fiber sources:

RASPBERRIES	1 cup	8 grams
APPLES	1 medium	4.5 grams
BLUEBERRIES	1 cup	3.5 grams
BROCCOLI	1 cup	5 grams
AVOCADO	1	9 grams

(Continued)

BLACK BEANS	1 cup	20 grams
LENTILS	1 cup cooked or ¼ cup dry	15.5 grams
OATS (STEEL CUT)	1 cup cooked or ¼ cup dry	4 grams
QUINOA	1 cup cooked	5 grams
ALMONDS	1 ounce (2 Tbsp)	3.5 grams
SAVI SEEDS	1 ounce (2 Tbsp)	5 grams
CHIA SEEDS	1 ounce (2 Tbsp)	11 grams
VEGA ONE NUTRITIONAL SHAKE	1 scoop	6 grams

Omega-3 Fatty Acids

You may not automatically associate inflammation with menopausal symptoms, but the connection is nonetheless real. Inflammation is associated with all manner of unpleasantness, from hot flashes to osteoporosis, vaginal dryness to joint pain. The best way to fight back is with omega-3 fatty acids, a powerful anti-inflammatory found in foods like oily fish, Savi Seeds, chia seeds, hemp seeds, and walnuts.

But omega-3s do so much more. They help reduce the risk of cardiovascular disease. Fish-oil supplements loaded with omega-3s, for instance, champion the heart and blood vessels by lowering triglyceride levels while increasing the good stuff—HDL.

Omega-3s are also good mood boosters. This is important because there'll certainly be days when you're convinced you're going crazy. Omega-3s will help lessen those feelings, and who can put a price on sanity?

Finally, an Italian study suggests that omega-3s help to significantly reduce the incidence of hot flashes by modulating neurotransmitter function.[113] That alone is worth putting wild salmon on tonight's menu.

What to Eat

Luckily for us, tapping all these menopause-mitigating minerals and vitamins is a matter of natural selection. Of food, that is, not survival. So if mentalpause has you going crazy, here's what you should stock up on.

Kale

Kale has attained celebrity status in the plant kingdom. The ancient Greeks and Romans knew it. Modern nutritionists know it. And, increasingly, the world at large is getting hip to the fact that kale is a pretty amazing food. And for darn good reasons.

Belonging to the cabbage family, this "queen of greens" is low-cal, low-fat, and one of the most nutrient-dense, antioxidant-rich foods. It grows best in a cool climate—chilly weather enhances its sweet taste—so if you live north of the Sunbelt, plant some in your garden (especially the purple variety, it's so pretty)! You won't regret it: kale is rich in a bunch of cancer-fighting flavonoids like lutein and beta carotene, but its highly absorbable calcium, magnesium, vitamin C, fiber, and indole-3-carbinol (I3C) make it especially helpful for menopausal women. You'll remember that calcium and magnesium are important for maintaining bone health after menopause, and that vitamin C helps quell the anxiety that just makes menopause worse. I3C and fiber, meanwhile, help weaken and eliminate estrogen from the body. And because kale helps prevent weight gain, including menopausal weight gain—such are the perks of being low-cal and rich in fiber—it helps stop the vicious cycle of fat cells begetting more estrogen. That, my friends, is what you call a win-win.

HOW TO USE
Kale makes a healthy addition to soups, stews, salads, pizza, and pasta. Or try cooking or sautéing kale all by its pretty self and then drizzling olive oil and lemon juice on top. Kale also makes for some tasty chips AND a nutrient-packed juice. Really, what *can't* this plant do?

TIP
To get the most nutritional bang for your buck, lightly steam kale; or, if eating raw in a salad, massage the kale with lemon, olive oil, and sea salt to make it easier to digest and assimilate.

Peppermint Tea

Of all the mint herbs out there, peppermint is by far the MVP. It has the highest medicinal value of any other mint, thanks to its menthol (which has cooling properties and is the key ingredient for relieving digestive disorders, tension, and insomnia), menthone, and menthyl acetate. It also has calcium, magnesium, and potassium, as well as small amounts of vitamins A and C and folate. Then there's its fancy footwork with essential oils, flavonoids, and phenolic acids, which are what help you digest that big Thanksgiving dinner. Or the dessert buffet at your cousin's wedding. Or your latest postmenopausal binge. Whatever the transgression, the point is that peppermint tea is a digestive lifesaver.

It's also pretty helpful when it comes to menopause. The tea, which is derived from the dried leaves of the peppermint plant (a natural hybrid of spearmint and water mint), can relax you faster than a foot massage. (Well, at least it's a lot cheaper and more accessible.) And when your hormones are raging and your stress is exacerbating all your other unpleasant symptoms, relaxing gets pushed to the top of your priority list.

Peppermint tea can also help relieve hot flashes and slow down an accelerated heartbeat; it's even been shown to improve mood, lethargy, and irritability. So not only will you feel better, those around you will feel better! You can use it to look better, too: peppermint oil is great for dry skin.

HOW TO USE
Obviously you can drink the tea to melt away stress, but you can also add the leaves to salads, meats, and vegetables. Or try placing a warm tea bag on your forehead the next time you have a headache. The leaves can be used to make a versatile oil as well, which can do anything from moisturize to refresh and relax.

Maca

People love maca for a variety of reasons. The indigenous Andeans used this Peruvian plant root and medicinal herb to improve stamina, fertility, energy, and endurance as well as to gain relief from PMS symptoms, menstrual cramps, and tuberculosis. Maca is an adaptogen, meaning it helps restore balance within the entire body system and increase the body's resistance to stress. We love this radish-family plant because it fuels and regulates the endocrine system without containing any hormones itself. It's what we call a giver, not a taker.

And maca really knows how to give. It's rich in potassium and calcium while also containing carbohydrates, fiber, fats, selenium, magnesium, iron, amino acids, and fatty acids. The root of this low-growing herb in particular is an abundant source of protein, iron, minerals, and fiber.

What this means for menopausal women is that it can ameliorate almost every symptom. For starters, maca helps to reduce the hormonal imbalances that cause your body to go haywire. So those hot flashes, night sweats, mood swings, insomnia, fatigue, breast tenderness, vaginal dryness, and diminished libido all become things of the past. It does this by naturally supporting the body's endocrine system. Maca doesn't change blood-hormone levels when ingested; rather, it restores the endocrine system through the hypothalamus–pituitary axis by improving communication between the brain and the pituitary gland as well as the adrenals. This ensures proper hormone balancing and secretion within the body. So basically, it helps ensure that whatever hormone message is required actually gets across. (See page 50 for more on how this works.)

Maca also contains indole-3-carbinols that convert bad (psychotic) estrogen to a weaker, more beneficial form. Plus, maca helps improve mental clarity (so long, brain fog!), increase energy, and lessen the stress effect and depression. It also acts as a natural libido booster, helping to rev up your diminished sex drive. Forget givers and takers. Maca is a lover AND a fighter!

HOW TO USE
Maca can be mixed into your breakfast cereals, blended into your smoothies, or substituted for a portion of the flour in baked goods like cakes and cookies. For cakes, replace a quarter to half of the flour with maca powder.

Chia Seeds

Chia is a Mayan word meaning "strength," and these seeds make for a powerful tool in your quest to conquer (with grace and beauty) menopause.

Ranging in color from white to gray to brown, chia seeds can even out blood-sugar levels and reduce or eliminate the symptoms of high blood pressure, diabetes, and GERD (gastroesophageal reflux disease). But one of their greatest assets is their power to, ahem, move things along. A one-ounce serving of chia seeds has approximately 42 percent of the recommended daily fiber intake (based on a 2,000-calorie diet). All this soluble and insoluble fiber helps to pull toxins (including toxic bad estrogen) from your body, helping to alleviate symptoms. Plus it helps increase the feeling of fullness after eating (meaning you'll need to eat less often) and helps you avoid post-meal blood-sugar crashes.

Chia seeds are chock-full of other good stuff, too. They contain antioxidants and the highest percentage of omega-3 fatty acids (more than 60 percent) of any commercially available source. They also have high levels of protein, calcium, and B vitamins, which help your bones and your brain. And their boron content aids the metabolism of those bone- and muscle-building minerals: calcium, magnesium, manganese, and phosphorus.

As a result, chia seeds keep your brain working at a reasonable clip, your bones strong, and your attitude positive. They may also help reduce hot flashes!

TIP
Two tablespoons of chia seeds provide 11 grams of fiber. That's almost half the daily recommended amount! Add these seeds to your already fiber-rich oatmeal or breakfast smoothie for an easy yet powerful boost.

HOW TO USE
Eat chia seeds on their own as a snack, or blend them into cereals, homemade granola bars, and other dried snack foods. These seeds may be small, but they can absorb up to 20 times their weight in water when used to create the popular "chia gel." You can use them to make easy-peasy jams or add them to smoothies, nut spreads, milkshakes, hot or cold cereals, yogurts, mustard, or anything else you can think of. You can even grind the seeds into "chia flour" and use it in pancakes, waffles, breads, and other baked goods. The seeds are tasteless and odorless, and are easy to store and use.

PART 5

Recipes

Very Berry Mind-Boosting Smoothie

Serves 1

If your memory has been failing you lately, this smoothie is certain to keep your mind razor-sharp! Berries, turmeric, and kale are the winning, brain-boosting trio here, and the banana, berries, and almond milk provide the perfect frothy sweetness. You won't even notice the kale and turmeric in there!

½ cup (125 mL) blueberries, frozen

½ cup (125 mL) blackberries, frozen

1 banana, frozen

1 cup (250 mL) kale

1 tsp (5 mL) turmeric

1½ cups (375 mL) almond milk

½ cup (125 mL) water

Add all ingredients to blender and blend.

SIDE DISH

- Memory boosting
- Anti-inflammatory
- Heart healthy
- Cancer fighting
- Gluten-free
- Dairy-free
- Soy-free

(From top, clockwise)
VegaTini *(page 288)*,
Vega Frappuccino *(page 284)*,
Be-YOU-tifying Cocktail *(page 285)*,
and Very Berry Mind-Boosting
Smoothie *(page 282)*.

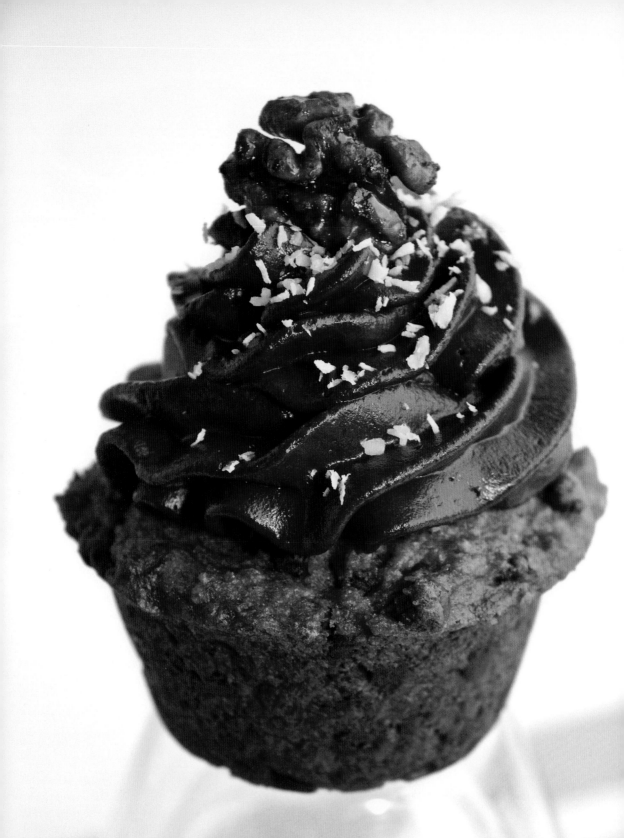

Amaranth, Hazelnut, and Chocolate Chip
Cupcakes *(page 322)*

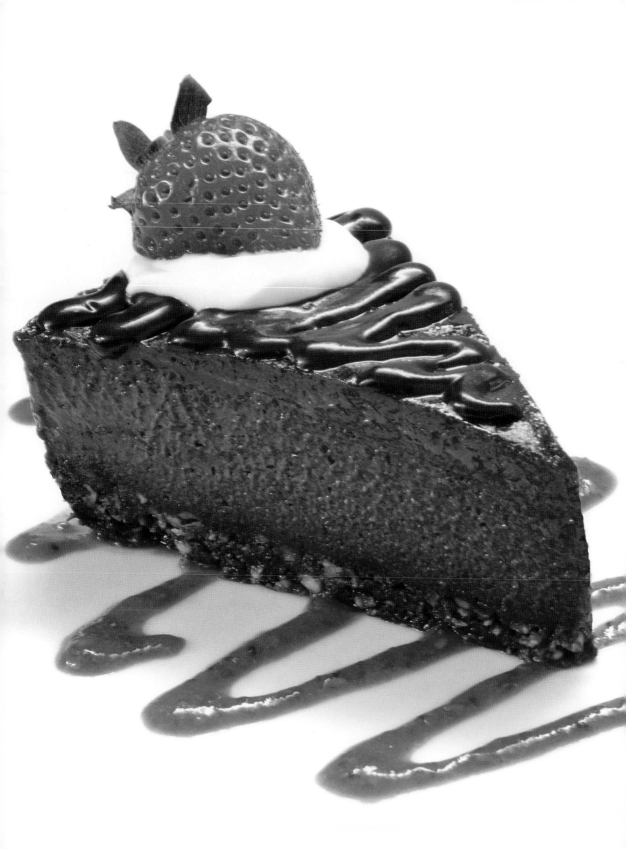

Cocoa Mocha Torte *(page 325)*

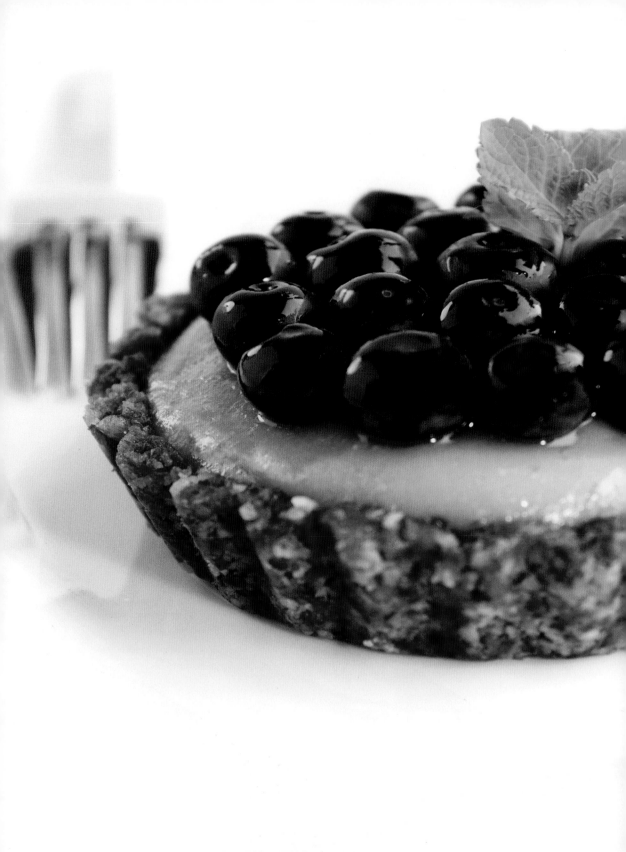

Blueberry Lemon Tart *(page 328)*

Double Chocolate Quinoa Coconut
Haystacks (*page 330*)

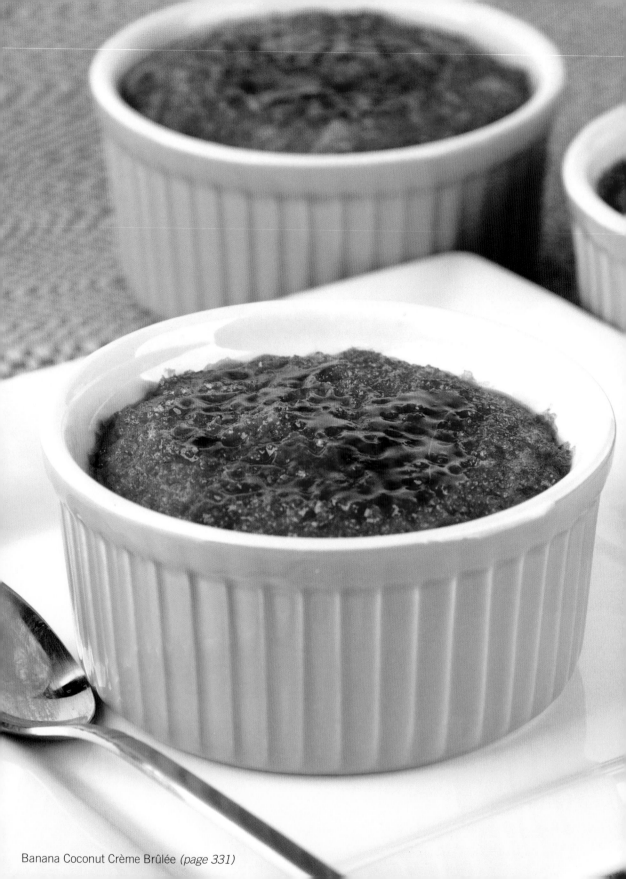

Banana Coconut Crème Brûlée *(page 331)*

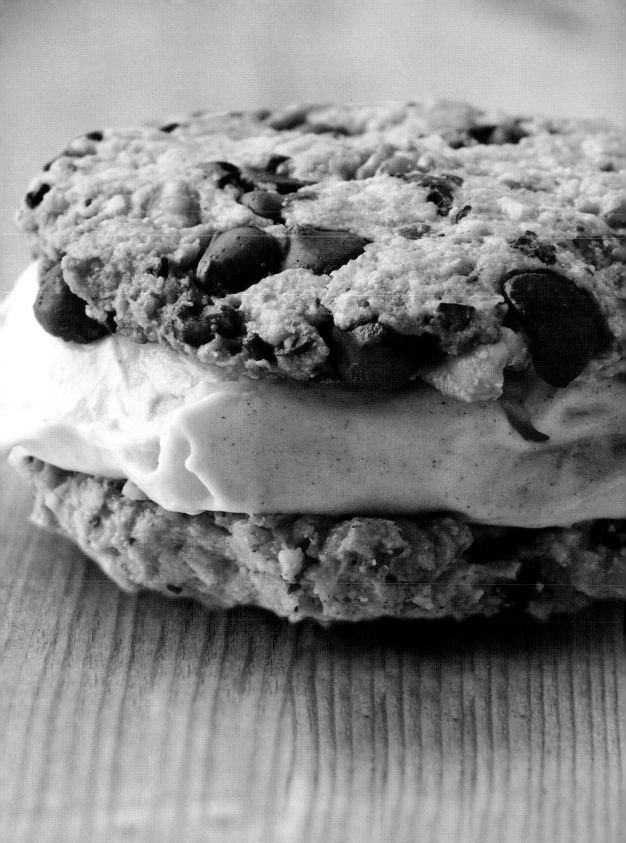

Peggyfied Banana Walnut
Ice Cream Sandwich *(page 334)*

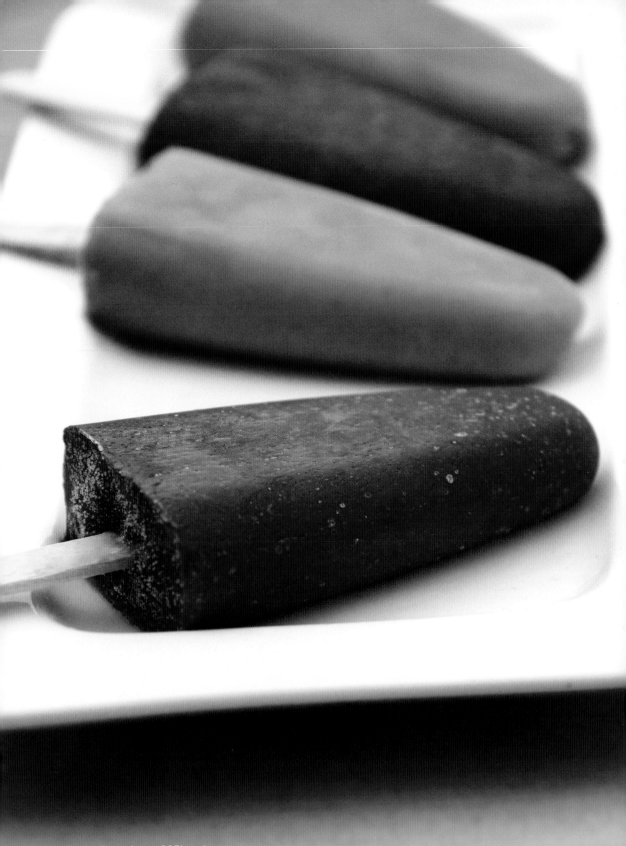

Frozen Fudge Pops *(page 335) and*
Frozen Berry Cherry Pops *(page 336)*

Raspberry Watermelon Mojito

Serves 2

If you're looking for a refreshing summer cocktail, look no further than this delicious mojito. Watermelon not only provides heaps of vitamin C (which can prevent sunstroke), but also is 90 percent water, which makes this the perfect recipe for keeping your body hydrated in the summer heat (or between alcoholic cocktails).

1 cup (250 mL) raspberries
1 cup (250 mL) watermelon, peeled
  and cubed
4 sprigs mint

1 packet Vega hydrator in pomegranate berry
  (optional)
½ lemon, juiced
1 cup (250 mL) mineral water

Add raspberries and watermelon to blender, and blend until smooth and liquid. Add to martini shaker with mint, Vega hydrator (if using), and lemon. Shake, shake, shake. Then fill two glasses halfway, top with mineral water, and enjoy!

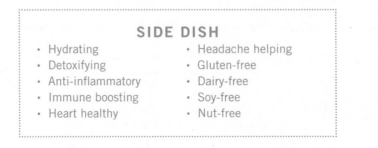

SIDE DISH
- Hydrating
- Detoxifying
- Anti-inflammatory
- Immune boosting
- Heart healthy
- Headache helping
- Gluten-free
- Dairy-free
- Soy-free
- Nut-free

Vega Frappuccino

Serves 1 (or 2 small servings)

You'll never have to wait in line at an overpriced coffee shop again! This icy, frothy frappuccino is loaded with antioxidants, heart-healthy fats, and energy-boosting goodness that will sustain you for hours. The almond butter and frozen banana provide the thick, ice-creamy consistency along with energy-boosting B vitamins. Mesquite imparts a smoky maple sweetness that comes with a hearty dose of antioxidants, while the cinnamon and vanilla add to the sweetness *sans* the sugar.

2 cups (500 mL) vanilla coconut milk

1 scoop Vega One (chocolate)*

1 cup (250 mL) ice

1 large, ripe banana, frozen

1 Tbsp (15 mL) almond butter

1 shot espresso (brewed)

½ tsp (2 mL) cinnamon

½ tsp (2 mL) vanilla

1 tsp (5 mL) mesquite pod meal

Add to blender and blend.

Alternatively, use a chocolate protein powder or 2 heaping tablespoons (30 mL) of cocoa powder.

SIDE DISH

- Energy boosting
- Muffin-top busting
- Blood-sugar balancing
- Antioxidant
- Heart healthy
- Mood boosting
- Gluten-free
- Dairy-free
- Soy-free

Be-YOU-tifying Cocktail
Serves 1

Get amazingly glowing skin from the inside out with this simple and delicious juicy elixir! The coconut water provides immediate hydration and feeds your skin's precious minerals, alongside the rejuvenating and cleansing cucumber and celery. The sweetness of the apple perfectly rounds out the bite of the lemon and ginger. It's a cocktail that might just help you get rid of belly bloat and drop a few pounds, too.

1 stalk celery

¼ cucumber

½ apple

1-inch (2.5 cm) cube fresh peeled ginger

1 cup (250 mL) coconut water

fresh mint leaves

½ lemon, juiced

pinch cayenne pepper

mint for garnish

Add celery, cucumber, apple, ginger, coconut water, mint, and lemon juice to blender. Blend well, adjusting coconut water as necessary. Pour into glass and sprinkle with cayenne. Garnish with fresh mint.

SIDE DISH
- Detoxifying
- Anti-aging
- Skin clearing
- Hydrating
- Weight loss
- Muffin-top busting
- Thunder-thigh thinning
- Energy boosting
- Anti-inflammatory
- Antioxidant
- Gluten-free
- Dairy-free
- Soy-free
- Nut-free

Anti-Belly-Bloating Kombucha Cocktail

Serves 1

Kombucha is a fermented tea with a naturally occurring effervescence, making it the perfect bubbly. Its probiotic and enzymatic properties also make it the ideal bestie for your belly, with the ginger and antioxidant-rich blueberries helping to further soothe tummy troubles. This party drink lets you mingle while keeping your tummy tight!

½ cup (125 mL) blueberries

1 ginger kombucha

1-inch (2.5 cm) piece fresh ginger, peeled

In blender, blend blueberries and ginger and purée until smooth. Pour halfway into champagne flute and top with kombucha (Tonica is my favorite!).

SIDE DISH

- Digestive health
- Anti-inflammatory
- Muffin-top busting
- Antioxidant
- Anti-aging
- Hangover remedy
- Immune boosting
- Gluten-free
- Dairy-free
- Soy-free
- Nut-free

FAB (Fig, Almond, and Banana) Bone-Building Milkshake

Serves 1 (meal size) or 2 (snack size)

The FAB combination is not only incredibly delish, but also amazing for bone health. This thick, frothy shake packs in heaps more digestible calcium and magnesium than a cup of milk. Plus, it tastes as if you're splurging on a rich, indulgent milkshake, but you're not! It's totally guilt-free and will leave you completely satisfied.

1 ripe banana, frozen

¾ cup (175 mL) dried figs, rehydrated in water (so they become plump), or fresh figs

2 cups (500 mL) almond milk

2 Tbsp (30 mL) raw almond butter

Put all ingredients into blender and blend.

SIDE DISH

- Bone health
- Alkalizing
- Mood boosting
- Stress busting
- PMS busting
- Headache prevention
- Libido boosting
- Dairy-free
- Gluten-free
- Soy-free

VegaTini

Serves 1 (meal size) or 2 (snack size)

This is one of the best hangover cocktail remedies: it lets you party like a rock star and still feel great. It helps to rehydrate, replenish precious vitamins and minerals, detox your liver, and reduce the nausea that usually follows a night of indulgence. And even if you didn't drink, this makes an amazing energy-boosting, cleansing shake for anyone, any time of the day!

2½ cups (625 mL) coconut water

1 scoop Vega One in Berry

2-inch (2.5 cm) cube fresh ginger

1 cup (250 mL) frozen strawberries

2 tsp (10 mL) camu camu powder

½ banana, frozen

½ lemon, juiced

Blend all ingredients in a blender.

SIDE DISH

- Cleansing/detoxifying
- Energy boosting
- Immune boosting
- Stress busting
- Heart healthy
- Anti-inflammatory
- Antioxidant
- Alkalizing
- Digestive health
- Anti-cancer
- Dairy-free
- Gluten-free
- Soy-free
- Nut-free

Kombucha Float

Serves 2

There's something nostalgic about an ice cream float. When I was a kid, my mom used to make them for me as a special treat. As an adult, there's no way I could stomach the ice cream–soda combo, so I've rejigged the recipe to make it much healthier and tummy friendly (while making me feel like a five-year-old again).

3 cups (750 mL) kombucha (flavor of choice)   ½ cup peaches, frozen

2 bananas, frozen   ½ tsp (2 mL) cinnamon

In a high-speed blender or food processor, blend frozen bananas, frozen peaches, and cinnamon until well combined and smooth. Scoop out and divide between two glasses. Top with kombucha.

SIDE DISH

- Digestive health
- Flat tummy
- Immune boosting
- Hangover remedy
- Antioxidant

- Dairy-free
- Gluten-free
- Soy-free
- Nut-free

Burn-Baby-Burn Roasted Red Pepper Dip

Serves 4

Ever since I was a child, roasted red peppers have been a staple. My mother and grandmother would roast bushels of peppers when they were in season, then freeze them in jars for use throughout the year. This roasted red pepper dip is one of the ways we'd eat them. It works great as a sandwich spread, a dip for crackers or veggies, blended with feta, and as a sauce for pizza or pasta. Or, as I like to do, eat it on its own with a spoon! It's that good.

6 red bell peppers, roasted and peeled

1 hot chili pepper, roasted and peeled
   (2 if you like it really spicy!)

3 Tbsp (50 mL) extra virgin olive oil

3 cloves garlic, raw

3 Tbsp (50 mL) chopped parsley

½ tsp (2 mL) salt

Add all ingredients to food processer and pulse until well combined.

Serve with cucumber slices, fresh fennel, and yellow bell peppers, along with a grilled sprouted-grain wrap cut into triangles—or use as a yummy, spicy sandwich spread.

SIDE DISH

- Metabolism boosting
- Weight loss
- Immune boosting
- Stress-busting
- Anti-aging
- Skin glowing

- Heart healthy
- Dairy-free
- Gluten-free
- Soy-free
- Nut-free

Hummus

Serves 6

I make this every week—it'll always be found in my fridge! It's such a simple and inexpensive dish, not to mention that it's loaded with fiber and protein. Hummus makes the perfect addition to any meal or snack. It can be eaten with veggies, in a wrap, or even blended into salad dressing for a creamy kick.

2 cups (500 mL) chickpeas, cooked

½ lemon, juiced

1 clove garlic

¼ cup (60 mL) extra virgin olive oil

½ tsp (2 mL) sea salt

1½ tsp (7 mL) cumin, ground

Add all ingredients to food processor or blender and process until smooth and creamy.

Use it as a veggie dip, with pita triangles, in sandwiches and wraps, or add to salad dressing for additional creaminess!

SIDE DISH

- Heart healthy
- Mentalpause busting
- Muffin-top chopping
- Estrogen cleansing
- Energy boosting
- Protein-rich
- Blood-sugar balancing
- Dairy-free
- Gluten-free
- Soy-free
- Nut-free

Raw Greek Dolmadas, Peggyfied (Stuffed Grape Leaves)

Makes about 20 pieces

Dolmadas are a traditional Greek appetizer in which rice, herbs, and sometimes even ground lamb are rolled and hugged between grape leaves. My version provides a tangy twist with jicama—a tuberous root veggie that makes a refreshing, crisp alternative to cooked white rice. This low-calorie, high-fiber substitute contains stress-busting, immune-boosting vitamin C, B vitamins, and minerals, and pairs beautifully with salty Kalamata olives and fresh dill.

2 cups (500 mL) raw jicama

¼ cup (60 mL) pine nuts

⅓ cup (75 mL) + 2 Tbsp (30 mL) extra virgin olive oil

¼ cup (60 mL) freshly squeezed lemon juice

1 green onion, chopped

1 Tbsp (15 mL) chopped fresh mint

1 clove garlic

sea salt and freshly ground white pepper to taste

⅓ cup (75 mL) Kalamata olives

¼ cup (60 mL) chopped fresh dill

1 tsp (2 mL) lemon zest

16 ounces (475 mL) grape leaves

Grate jicama on the coarse side of a box grater. In a high-power blender, blend pine nuts, extra virgin olive oil, lemon juice, green onion, mint, garlic, sea salt, and pepper. Stir enough of the mixture into the jicama to moisten it well.

Reserve some of this mixture for a dip.

Stir in olives, dill, and lemon zest, and mix until well combined.

Rinse the grape leaves with water, then pat dry. Taking one leaf at a time, place it on a clean work surface, vein side up, and cut off stem end. Spoon about 1 Tbsp (15 mL) of jicama filling above the base of the leaf in the middle. Fold up bottom of leaf to cover filling, then fold over each of the sides, and continue rolling.

These can be served raw with reserved dipping sauce. Or place them in a baking dish, drizzle with remaining extra virgin olive oil and lemon, and bake for 10 minutes.

SIDE DISH

- Weight loss
- Anti-aging
- Beautifying
- Antioxidant-rich
- Cleansing/detoxifying
- Heart healthy
- Dairy-free
- Gluten-free
- Soy-free

White Bean and Rosemary Dip

Serves 4

White beans provide an additional take on the traditional hummus. This dip is lower in calories and has great fat-loss potential. Plus, the creamy white beans, extra virgin olive oil, garlic, and rosemary combo can send you on a sensory vaycay right to Tuscany.

1½ cups (375 mL) white kidney beans (one 14-ounce can)

½ lemon, juiced (about 2 tsp/10 mL)

2 Tbsp (30 mL) extra virgin olive oil

1 clove garlic

½ tsp (2 mL) cumin

½ tsp (2 mL) sea salt

pinch cayenne

1 tsp (5 mL) chopped fresh rosemary

Add all ingredients, except rosemary, to food processor, and mix until well combined, scraping down the sides of the processor bowl as necessary.

Transfer to bowl and stir in rosemary.

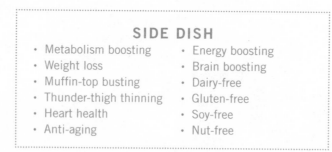

SIDE DISH

- Metabolism boosting
- Weight loss
- Muffin-top busting
- Thunder-thigh thinning
- Heart health
- Anti-aging

- Energy boosting
- Brain boosting
- Dairy-free
- Gluten-free
- Soy-free
- Nut-free

Brain Candied Nuts

Serves 4

Who doesn't love to snack on crunchy nuts? Especially when they're candied! These sweet and spicy morsels are great on their own, but they also add the perfect crunch to salads, veggie side dishes, and thick creamy soups—or (my favorite) oven-baked apples and ice cream.

1 cup (250 mL) walnuts or pecans (or combo
   of the two)

3 Tbsp (50 mL) maple syrup

2 tsp (10 mL) cinnamon

½ tsp (2 mL) cayenne

In a skillet on medium heat, toast nuts until slightly browned, roughly 3 minutes. Then add maple syrup (it will start to sear). Add cinnamon and cayenne right away, stirring until well combined and all the nuts are coated. Remove from heat and transfer nuts to a cooling dish. Let cool completely.

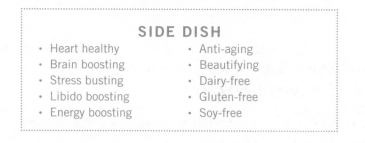

SIDE DISH

- Heart healthy
- Brain boosting
- Stress busting
- Libido boosting
- Energy boosting

- Anti-aging
- Beautifying
- Dairy-free
- Gluten-free
- Soy-free

Mushroom, Chard, and White Bean Crostini

Makes 12 pieces

A perfect little canapé, this crostini not only serves as a favorite party app, but also packs a HUGE nutritional punch. Mushrooms (one of the most powerful immune boosters) pair wonderfully with the steamed chard, creamy white bean dip, and crunchy toast. The kicker? The essence of truffle oil, of course! So while you impress your party guests with flavor and glam, you'll know you're keeping them healthy, too.

1 gluten-free or sprouted-grain loaf from Manna Organics

coconut oil

1 bunch Swiss chard, stemmed and washed

2 cloves garlic, minced

½ pound (225 grams) assorted mushrooms, stemmed (if necessary) and sliced: oyster, shiitake, maitake, chanterelle, cremini

sea salt and freshly ground pepper to taste

White Bean and Rosemary Dip (recipe on page 294)

truffle oil

Heat the oven to 350°F (175°C). Cut the bread into ½-inch (1 cm) slices. Brush both sides lightly with coconut oil and arrange on a baking sheet. Bake, turning once, until golden on both sides, about 15 minutes.

Meanwhile, steam the chard over boiling water just until wilted, about 2 minutes. Remove and, when cool, chop coarsely.

Heat a thin layer of coconut oil in a large skillet over medium-high heat and add the garlic. Cook just until it starts to sizzle, then stir in mushrooms. Stir until they're lightly browned and any liquid they may give off is evaporated, about 6 minutes. Season with salt and pepper.

To assemble, spread the bread with White Bean and Rosemary Dip. Top with chard and mushrooms and drizzle with truffle oil.

Note: When grains are sprouted, much of the gluten is broken down, so it may be tolerable for those with sensitivities. However, if you are celiac, use a gluten-free loaf made from brown rice, millet, amaranth, buckwheat, or quinoa. Food for Life carries a gluten-free brown rice English muffin that works great in this recipe!

SIDE DISH

- Immune boosting
- Heart healthy
- Weight loss
- Anti-cancer
- High fiber
- Dairy-free
- Soy-free
- Nut-free

Immune-Boosting Creamy Crimini Miso Soup

Serves 4

The puréed mushroom and miso combo is not only a creamy, hearty, comforting soup, but also provides a wicked one-two punch in fighting disease and pathogens. Move over chicken noodle, creamy crimini miso is guaranteed to prevent and fight off any cold, flu, and even harmful disease. Kiss belly bloat buh-bye and make room for all those cancer-kicking cells!

2 Tbsp (30 mL) extra virgin olive oil

4½ cups (1.1 L) crimini mushrooms, sliced (about ¾ inch/2 cm)

3 garlic cloves, chopped, plus 1 whole clove

4 cups (1 L) vegetable broth

2 Tbsp (30 mL) yellow miso paste

maitake, shiitake, and white button mushrooms, sliced for crisping (optional)

kelp flakes

truffle oil

Heat the oil in a medium soup pot, then add mushrooms. Sauté until they start to release their moisture, then add chopped garlic and sauté another 30 seconds. Add vegetable broth and miso paste. Bring to a boil, then reduce heat and simmer 5 to 10 minutes.

While the soup is heating, sauté mushroom slices (if using) in a small amount of olive oil until well browned and crisp.

Pour soup into a blender and add whole garlic clove. Blend about 15 to 20 seconds, until no solid pieces remain. Return to pot.

Serve in bowls, topped with a couple shakes of kelp flakes, a drizzle of truffle oil, and the crisped mushrooms.

SIDE DISH

- Immune boosting
- Tumor-growth blocking
- Cold and flu fighting
- Digestive health

- Weight loss
- Beautifying
- Dairy-free
- Gluten-free

- Soy-free
- Nut-free

Veggiful Chili

Serves 8

A big bowl of comfort. This is the perfect meal to satiate even the biggest of eaters. The heartiness of the beans, coupled with chunky veggies in the spicy cumin-infused chili sauce, makes for the ultimate comfort dish. Where's the beef? Trust me, you won't miss it. It's like a hug from the inside out!

3 medium onions, chopped

4 cloves garlic, minced

2 green bell peppers, seeded and chopped

2 red bell peppers, seeded and chopped

2 stalks celery, chopped

2 carrots, chopped

2 Tbsp (30 mL) dried oregano

½ tsp (2 mL) sea salt

½ tsp (2 mL) ground black pepper

2 cups (500 mL) crushed tomatoes

2 tsp (10 mL) ground cumin

2 Tbsp (30 mL) chili powder (or to taste)

2 cups (500 mL) black beans, cooked

2 cups (500 mL) red kidney beans, cooked

Sauté onions until tender in a large pot over medium heat. Add garlic, peppers, celery, and carrots. Season with oregano, salt, and pepper, and sauté until vegetables are cooked through. Add tomatoes, cumin, chili powder, and beans.

Bring to a boil, then reduce heat to low and simmer for 45 minutes.

SIDE DISH

- Heart healthy
- Muffin-top busting
- Thunder-thigh thinning and man-boob busting
- Blood-sugar balancing
- Metabolism boosting
- Mood boosting
- Energy boosting
- Mentalpause banishing
- Dairy-free
- Gluten-free
- Soy-free
- Nut-free

Spicy Chickpea Soup

Serves 8

Add some spice to your life with this hearty soup. The heat and zest of the chipotle bring life to the garbanzo beans (chickpeas), while the turmeric gives your brain and body a heaping boost of goodness.

For the soup:

1 Tbsp (15 mL) extra virgin olive oil

1 small onion, finely chopped

2 cloves garlic, chopped

3 cups (750 mL) cooked chickpeas

2 tsp (10 mL) ground cumin

½ tsp (2 mL) cardamom

½ tsp (2 mL) turmeric

salt and pepper to taste

2 cups (500 mL) vegetable stock

1 chipotle pepper

1 (28-ounce/830 mL) can plum tomatoes

For the toppings:

extra virgin olive oil

chopped fresh chili peppers

sunflower sprouts

kelp granules

hemp seeds

Heat oil in a medium pot over medium heat. Add onions and sauté for 2 to 3 minutes. Add garlic and chickpeas. Season with cumin, cardamom, turmeric, salt, and pepper.

Stir in stock, then chipotle pepper and tomatoes. Simmer 5 to 10 minutes to combine flavors.

Using an immersion blender, partly purée soup (leaving it somewhat chunky). Ladle into bowls and top with any or all of the toppings.

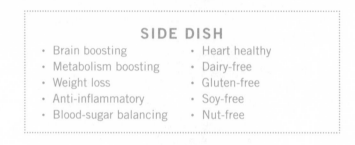

SIDE DISH

- Brain boosting
- Metabolism boosting
- Weight loss
- Anti-inflammatory
- Blood-sugar balancing
- Heart healthy
- Dairy-free
- Gluten-free
- Soy-free
- Nut-free

Kale and Hemp-Seed Salad

Serves 2

Love, love, love this salad. It's super easy to make, and the kale and hemp seeds are the perfect pairing of energy-boosting chlorophyll and superfood goodness. Plus, the creaminess of the avocado adds a dimension of heart-healthy richness.

1 bunch kale

1 avocado, pitted, peeled, and halved,
  + ½ avocado chopped into bite-size cubes

1 tsp (5 mL) salt

2 Tbsp (30 mL) lemon juice

⅓ cup (75 mL) hemp seeds

1 pint (550 mL) cherry tomatoes, halved

1 tsp (5 mL) kelp granules

¼ tsp (1 mL) cayenne pepper (or more
  to taste)

De-stem kale, tear into small pieces, and place in large bowl.

Add avocado, salt, and lemon juice, and massage until the kale is wilted. Add hemp seeds and mix well. Top with chopped avocado and cherry tomatoes. Season lightly with kelp granules and cayenne.

SIDE DISH

- Energy boosting
- Immune boosting
- Brain boosting
- Detoxifying/cleansing
- Muffin-top busting
- Blood-sugar balancing
- Anti-inflammatory
- Bone building
- PMS and mentalpause busting
- Dairy-free
- Gluten-free
- Nut-free
- Soy-free

Grilled Romaine with Sunflower Caesar Dressing

Serves 4

This twist on the traditional Caesar salad will have you asking for more. The grilled, whole romaine head presents beautifully with the pungent, creamy dressing, *sans* the customary egg. The croutons and slivered almonds add a nice crunch to the creaminess, and the kelp lends it all a metabolism-boosting saltiness.

For the grilled romaine:

1 head romaine lettuce

1 Tbsp (15 mL) coconut oil (melted)
   or avocado oil

sea salt and pepper to taste

For the croutons:

2 slices gluten-free brown rice bread

coconut oil, melted

For the dressing:

½ cup (125 mL) extra virgin olive oil

3 Tbsp (50 mL) raw sunflower seeds

2 Tbsp (30 mL) fresh lemon juice

1 Tbsp (15 mL) white balsamic

2 cloves garlic, minced

1 Tbsp (15 mL) Dijon mustard

1 tsp (5 mL) turmeric

For the topping:

slivered almonds

kelp granules

To make the salad, pull off any wilted or brown leaves from the romaine and cut the head in quarters lengthwise. Brush with melted coconut oil or avocado oil and season with sea salt and pepper. Grill a couple of minutes on each side or until wilted.

To make the croutons, brush both sides of the bread with coconut oil. Place on baking sheet and heat on low broiler setting for 2 to 3 minutes per side until golden brown, flipping halfway.

To make the dressing, put all ingredients in a blender and blend until creamy.

To serve, drizzle the dressing over the grilled romaine and then sprinkle kelp granules, slivered almonds, and croutons on top.

SIDE DISH

- Metabolism boosting
- Muffin-top chopping
- Thunder-thigh thinning and man-boob busting
- Energy boosting
- Brain boosting
- Beautifying
- Anti-aging
- Stress busting
- Alkalizing
- Heart healthy
- Blood-sugar balancing
- PMS and mentalpause busting
- Dairy-free
- Soy-free
- Gluten-free

Warm Root-Veggie Salad with Arugula, Sprouts, and Brain Candied Nuts

Serves 4 (snack size) or 2 (meal size)

The sweet earthiness of the beets, pepperiness of the arugula, freshness of the sprouts, and spicy-sweet crunchiness of the walnuts are not only a sensory delight, but can keep your mind razor-sharp as well!

For the salad:

6 medium beets (mix of red, golden, and candy cane)

1 large sweet potato

2 Tbsp (30 mL) coconut oil, melted

3 sprigs rosemary

2 cups (500 mL) arugula

2 cups (500 mL) sprouts (sunflower and purple radish)

For the dressing:

1 Tbsp (15 mL) hemp, chia, or extra virgin olive oil

¼ lemon, juiced

sea salt to taste

For the topping:

Brain Candied Nuts (see recipe on page 295)

To make the veggies, preheat oven to 400°F (200°C). Peel and chop 5 beets (reserving one golden beet) and the sweet potato into 1-inch (2.5 cm) cubes. Toss with coconut oil and fresh rosemary sprigs and line on baking sheet. Roast in oven for about 20 minutes, until veggies cook through.

To make the dressing, peel and thinly slice the remaining (golden) beet using a mandolin or knife. In a bowl, mix the oil, freshly squeezed lemon juice, and sea salt, and whisk with fork. Toss slices of raw beet into mixture to soften, then line on serving plate. Toss remaining dressing with arugula and sprouts. Place on top of raw beets, then top with cooked root veggies and candied nuts and serve.

SIDE DISH

- Weight loss
- Energy boosting
- Brain and memory boosting
- Anti-aging
- Beautifying
- Heart healthy
- Blood-sugar balancing
- Stress busting
- Dairy-free
- Gluten-free
- Soy-free

Cool-Your-Hot-Flash Fennel and Apple Salad

Serves 4

The fresh, crisp, licorice-y fennel aids in digestion and fights mentalpause symptoms while teaming up with hot-flash-fighting Napa cabbage and sweet (but powerful) apple and goji berries. The almonds add an additional stress-busting and libido-boosting crunch.

For the salad:

2 fennel bulbs, trimmed

1 Gala apple

1 cup (250 mL) shredded Napa cabbage

3 Tbsp (50 mL) goji berries

3 Tbsp (50 mL) raw almonds, crushed

For the dressing:

¼ cup (60 mL) extra virgin olive oil

3 Tbsp (50 mL) almonds, blanched and
   soaked

2 Tbsp (30 mL) chopped fresh dill

3 Tbsp (50 mL) lemon juice

sea salt and pepper to taste

1 tsp (5 mL) yacon syrup (or maple syrup
   or coconut sugar)

¼ cup (60 mL) peeled and chopped
   cucumber

Using a mandolin, shred fennel and apple. Add to bowl with shredded cabbage.

To make the dressing, blend all ingredients in high-speed blender until smooth. Add water until desired consistency is reached. Pour dressing over salad, toss, and top with goji berries and raw almonds.

SIDE DISH

- Weight loss
- Banishes menopause
  and PMS symptoms
- Reduces hot flashes
- Thunder-thigh thinning
  and man-boob
  banishing
- Muffin-top chopping
- Metabolism boosting
- Digestive health
- Cleansing/detoxifying
- Dairy-free
- Gluten-free
- Soy-free

Walnut Tacos

Serves 6

Tacos are one of the most perfect meals, with their Mexican flavors and textures—spicy, fresh, crunchy, and creamy—all meshed into one! This version provides a heart-healthy, brain-boosting take by substituting ground walnuts for ground meat. You can also substitute fish, black beans, or whatever your heart desires.

For the chili powder:

2 Tbsp (30 mL) chili powder

1 Tbsp (15 mL) ground cumin

1 ½ tsp (7 mL) ground coriander

1 ½ tsp (7 mL) paprika

1 tsp (5 mL) onion powder

1 tsp (5 mL) garlic powder

½ tsp (2 mL) cayenne

2 tsp (10 mL) salt

For the filling:

2 cups (500 mL) walnuts

2 Tbsp (30 mL) olive oil

For the sauce:

½ cup (125 mL) raw macadamia nuts

1 chipotle pepper

2 Tbsp (30 mL) adobo sauce from peppers

For the taco shell:

1 head Bibb lettuce, leaves separated

Optional toppings:

1 avocado, peeled, pitted

finely diced red onion

diced tomato

sunflower sprouts

shredded red cabbage

cilantro leaves

To make the chili powder, stir all ingredients together in a small bowl. Store in a tightly sealed jar.

To make the taco filling, soak the walnuts in water for about an hour. Drain thoroughly. Process soaked walnuts to the texture of cooked ground beef/turkey. With the processor running, pour in the olive oil. Scrape into a serving bowl and stir in the chili powder.

To make the sauce, blend all ingredients in a high-speed blender until smooth. Scrape into a serving bowl.

To serve, spoon some of the walnut mix onto a lettuce leaf. Then spoon some of the sauce over the walnuts and top with toppings of your choice.

Note: You can use Greek yogurt or soft goat cheese instead of macadamia nuts: using a fork, whisk it with the adobo sauce and a bit of maple syrup for a quick, easy-peasy sauce.

SIDE DISH

- Heart healthy
- Brain boosting
- Energy boosting
- Libido boosting
- Anti-aging
- Beautifying
- Dairy-free
- Gluten-free
- Soy-free

Quinoa Bean Burger

Serves 4

This juicy, "meaty" burger won't have you missin' your meat with its hearty protein- and fiber-rich bean and quinoa duo. Plus, the chili, cumin, and cilantro pack a flavorful punch.

1 cup (250 mL) cooked black beans

½ cup (125 mL) cooked red kidney beans

½ cup (125 mL) red onion, diced

⅓ cup (75 mL) fresh cilantro, stems removed
   and chopped

1 Tbsp (15 mL) extra virgin olive oil

3 garlic cloves, minced

¾ tsp (4 mL) salt

1 Tbsp (15 mL) chili powder

1 Tbsp (15 mL) ground cumin

½ tsp (2 mL) fresh ground black pepper

2 Tbsp (30 mL) ground chia seeds mixed with
   ⅓ cup (75 mL) water

1 cup (250 mL) cooked quinoa

1 cup (250 mL) quinoa flakes (or 100% pure
   rolled oats)

coconut oil

In a food processor, add beans, onion, cilantro, oil, garlic, salt, chili powder, cumin, and pepper. Purée until smooth.

Mix the chia mixture into the bean mixture. Add quinoa and quinoa flakes (or rolled oats) until the mixture is sticky and holds together. Divide mixture into four patties. Grease grill pan with coconut oil and cook about 6 minutes each side.

To serve, garnish with hummus, roasted red pepper dip (see pages 290 and 291 for recipes), tomato, and avocado. Serve on its own, on gluten-free bread, or between two leaves of Bibb lettuce.

SIDE DISH

- Heart healthy
- Weight loss
- Muffin-top busting
- Blood-sugar balancing
- Cleansing/detoxifying
- Stress-busting
- Dairy-free
- Gluten-free
- Nut-free
- Soy-free

Acorn Squash and Quinoa Bowl

Serves 4

Here's a squash-a-roll that not only squashes stress, but also boosts energy and is amazing for your skin. And since we eat with our eyes, this visually appealing, heart-healthy dish is sure to please your entire family.

2 acorn squash

2 Tbsp (15 mL) coconut oil

¼ cup (60 mL) onion, diced

sea salt and pepper to taste

2 cups (500 mL) cooked quinoa

1½ cups (375 mL) chopped fresh spinach

¼ cup (60 mL) chopped dried apricots

¼ cup (60 mL) dried cranberries

⅓ cup (75 mL) chopped toasted pecans

½ cup (125 mL) pomegranate seeds

¼ cup (60 mL) chopped flat-leaf parsley

½ tsp (2 mL) ground cinnamon

2 Tbsp (30 mL) extra virgin olive oil

1 Tbsp (15 mL) lemon juice

2 tsp (10 mL) maple syrup

Preheat oven to 425°F (220°C). Cut squash in half lengthwise, scoop out the seeds, then place the halves cut side down on a baking sheet greased with a tablespoon of coconut oil. Roast until soft, about 30 minutes.

Heat the second tablespoon of coconut oil in a large skillet over medium heat. Add the onions and a pinch of salt and pepper and cook, stirring, until golden, about 15 minutes. Stir in cooked quinoa and add spinach. Remove from heat and cover, just until the spinach wilts, a minute or two.

Add remaining ingredients to the skillet and stir to blend.

Remove squash from the oven. Scoop out part of the flesh, chop, then stir into the quinoa stuffing. Spoon the stuffing into the squash halves and serve.

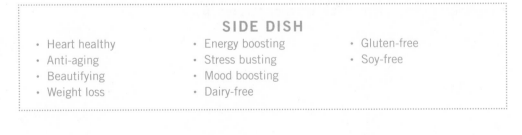

SIDE DISH

- Heart healthy
- Anti-aging
- Beautifying
- Weight loss

- Energy boosting
- Stress busting
- Mood boosting
- Dairy-free

- Gluten-free
- Soy-free

Pasta Imposter: Golden Beet Ravioli

Serves 4

This is a much lighter and much more nutrilicious version of the high-calorie (and often high-fat) traditional ravioli. Raw, thinly sliced golden beets stand in for traditional pasta shells, sandwiching a creamy Kalamata olive and white-bean filling and topped with a fresh, savory, quick-and-easy tomato sauce.

For the ravioli:

2 golden beets

2 Tbsp (30 mL) extra virgin olive oil

2 Tbsp (30 mL) freshly squeezed lemon juice

½ tsp (2 mL) salt

For the filling:

1 cup (250 mL) white beans

½ cup (125 mL) Kalamata olives, pitted

1 Tbsp (15 mL) extra virgin olive oil

For the tomato olive sauce:

(Yield: 1¼ cups/300 mL)

1 Tbsp (15 mL) extra virgin olive oil

1 garlic clove, minced

½ cup (125 mL) crushed tomatoes

5 leaves fresh basil, chopped

2 sprigs fresh oregano, chopped

¼ cup (60 mL) Kalamata olives,
   pitted and chopped

To make the ravioli, peel beets and then slice very thin on a mandolin. Place in large bowl or baking pan and marinate in olive oil, lemon juice, and salt until softened, about 10 minutes.

To make the filling, add white beans to blender or food processor and blend until smooth. Set aside. Then add olives and olive oil to blender (or food processor) and blend into tapenade. Gently fold olive mixture into puréed white beans.

To make the sauce, warm oil in a skillet on low-medium heat. Add garlic, sauté for 2 minutes, then add tomatoes and cook down for about 5 minutes. Then add basil, oregano, and chopped olives.

To assemble, place one beet round on plate, top with filling, then top with second beet round to close into "raviolis." Spoon a dollop of tomato sauce on top. Continue with remaining beets and filling and arrange on serving plate. Garnish with a small fresh basil leaf.

SIDE DISH

- Weight loss
- Muffin-top chopping
- Blood-sugar balancing
- Energy boosting
- Heart healthy
- Anti-aging
- Beautifying
- Detoxifying/cleansing
- Stress busting
- Gluten-free
- Dairy-free
- Nut-free
- Soy-free

Pasta Imposter: Sweet Potato Gnocchi

Serves 4

Sweet potatoes provide a flavorful, high-fiber alternative to traditional gnocchi. Packed with stress-busting B vitamins and calming complex carbohydrates, this dish is the perfect meal to relax with after a long week.

For the gnocchi:

2 large sweet potatoes (about 1½ pounds/
   675 grams), baked until tender

½ tsp (2 mL) salt

1 tsp (5 mL) ground chia seeds stirred
   into 2 Tbsp (30 mL) warm water

1 cup (250 mL) brown rice flour

For the garlic-sage sauce:

3 Tbsp (50 mL) coconut oil

20 small whole sage leaves

3 cloves garlic, minced

For the garnish:

½ cup (125 mL) hazelnuts, toasted
   then chopped

To make the gnocchi, scoop the still-warm sweet potato from the skins into a mixing bowl. Mash very well. Add salt, chia mixture, and enough flour to yield a soft but not sticky dough (start with ¾ cup/175 mL and add the rest if needed). Divide the dough into fourths and roll each into a ½-inch (1.25 cm) log, dusting hands with flour if needed. Cut crosswise into 1-inch (2.5 cm) lengths. Let rest while you make the sauce.

To make the sauce, heat the coconut oil in an 8- or 10-inch (20 or 25 cm) skillet over medium heat. Add sage leaves and fry until crisp and darkened. Remove from oil and place on plate. Add garlic to the oil, stir to make sure all garlic is under the surface, then remove from heat. The heat of the oil will cook the garlic, but keep it from burning. Add sage back into pan.

Bring a large pot of water to a boil. Cook the gnocchi in salted, boiling water for 5 minutes, then lift them out with a spider and place into the skillet of sauce. Toss to coat. Garnish with hazelnuts.

SIDE DISH

- Stress busting
- Blood-sugar balancing
- Heart healthy
- Beautifying
- Anti-aging
- Gluten-free
- Dairy-free
- Soy-free
- Nut-free

Pasta Imposter: Mushroom and Zucchini Fettuccini

Serves 2

Pasta is such a comfort dish for many, but it can be tricky if we're trying to reduce the amount of processed or refined carbs we consume. This pasta imposter comes to the rescue as it whips summer squash into long "fettuccini" noodles using just a potato peeler! Marinated in extra virgin olive oil and tossed with sautéed mushrooms, garlic, and parsley, it makes for a skinny substitution.

1 Tbsp (15 mL) coconut oil

1 cup (250 mL) crimini mushrooms, sliced

1 garlic clove, finely minced, or 1 black (fermented) garlic clove

½ tsp (2 mL) sea salt

4 medium yellow zucchinis

2 Tbsp (30 mL) extra virgin olive oil

1 tsp (5 mL) black pepper

¼ cup (60 mL) flat-leaf Italian parsley, chopped

1 tsp (5 mL) truffle oil

Parmesan cheese (optional)

Heat coconut oil in a large skillet over medium-high heat. Add the mushrooms and garlic and season with ¼ tsp (1 mL) sea salt. Cook, stirring occasionally, until tender, about 5 minutes.

Using a potato peeler, peel the zucchini lengthwise, making zucchini ribbons about the width of fettuccini. Keep going around the entire zucchini and stop just before reaching the seedy core.

Place zucchini noodles in a bowl and toss with oil, remaining ¼ tsp (1 mL) salt, and pepper. Noodles will become soft and pasta-like. Top with mushrooms and parsley and drizzle with truffle oil. Sprinkle with Parmesan (if using).

SIDE DISH

- Weight loss
- Muffin-top chopping
- Thunder-thigh thinning and man-boob busting
- Immune boosting

- Cleansing/detoxifying
- Energy boosting
- Blood-sugar balancing
- Gluten-free
- Soy-free

- Nut-free
- Dairy-free (if Parmesan is omitted)

Peggyfied Pizza Party

Serves 1 to 2

This easy-peasy pizza takes just minutes to make and is extremely satisfying. White beans trick your eyes into seeing mounds of cheese, while the small amount of goat cheese satisfies the palate. The sweetness of the caramelized onions and roasted red peppers balances the saltiness of the olives and sundried tomatoes, and along with the fresh, peppery arugula, it's a perfect pizza party combo!

6 cloves roasted garlic (see note)

1 cup (250 mL) cooked white beans

extra virgin olive oil

1 large gluten-free naan bread

¾ cup (175 ml) tomato sauce, store-bought
   or homemade

¼ cup (60 mL) sautéed onions

¼ cup (60 mL) roasted red peppers,
   cut into strips

¼ cup (60 mL) pitted Kalamata
   olives, chopped

¼ cup (60 mL) sundried tomatoes, sliced

2 ounces crumbled goat cheese (about
   ½ cup/125 mL)

1 cup (250 mL) arugula

1 Tbsp (15 mL) extra virgin olive oil

large pinch dried oregano

Preheat oven to 400°F (200°C).

Put garlic and white beans in food processor. With the processor running, drizzle in just enough olive oil—about 2 Tbsp (30 mL)—to make a creamy mixture.

(Continued)

Spread the naan with tomato sauce, then dot with the roasted garlic–bean mix. Scatter the onions, red peppers, olives, sundried tomatoes, and cheese over the top. Bake until the cheese is melted and lightly browned, about 10 minutes.

Toss the arugula, olive oil, and oregano in small bowl and top the pizza with the dressed arugula.

Note: To roast garlic, cut the top ½ inch (1.25 cm) or so off 2 heads to expose the tips of the cloves. Peel off as much of the "paper" from the heads as you can. Put the heads on a double sheet of aluminum foil and drizzle 1 Tbsp (15 mL) extra virgin olive oil over them. Season with salt and pepper. Wrap the garlic loosely in foil and place directly on the rack of a preheated 375°F (190°C) oven. Roast until the garlic is light brown and the cloves are soft when poked with a paring knife, about 30 minutes. To use, just pull off as many cloves as you need and squeeze the pulp out of the skins.

SIDE DISH

- Energy boosting
- Heart healthy
- Stress busting
- Mood boosting
- Blood-sugar balancing
- Soy-free
- Nut-free
- Gluten-free

Stovetop Kalamata Olive and Tomato Spanish Mackerel

Serves 4

This Mediterranean dish is easy to whip up and uses only one pot on the stove top. Kalamata olives, tomatoes, and Spanish mackerel not only are a trio of Mediterranean goodness, but a secret to beautifying gorgeousness! The abundant dose of healthy fats, vitamin E, and lycopene is the fountain of youth keeping you ageless and looking fabulous!

2 Tbsp (30 mL) extra virgin olive oil

3 cloves garlic, minced

1 (28-ounce/830 mL) can crushed tomatoes

⅓ cup (75 mL) pitted black olives, coarsely chopped

2 Tbsp (30 mL) capers

1 tsp (5 mL) dried oregano

4 (5-ounce/140 gram) Spanish mackerel fillets

sea salt and freshly ground pepper to taste

Heat the oil in an extra-large skillet (one with a lid). Add garlic to the skillet. Add the crushed tomatoes and bring to a simmer. Add olives to the sauce along with capers and oregano; adjust the heat and simmer for 15 minutes.

Slip the fillets into the sauce, spooning some of the sauce on top to cover them. Cover the skillet and simmer until fish is cooked through, about 10 minutes. Season with sea salt and pepper to taste.

Veggie Option: If you want to veggify this dish, try substituting portobello mushrooms for the mackerel. However, they will only take 5 minutes to cook! Thickly sliced zucchini or eggplant are yummy substitutions, too!

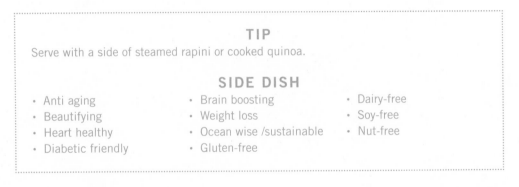

TIP
Serve with a side of steamed rapini or cooked quinoa.

SIDE DISH

- Anti aging
- Beautifying
- Heart healthy
- Diabetic friendly

- Brain boosting
- Weight loss
- Ocean wise /sustainable
- Gluten-free

- Dairy-free
- Soy-free
- Nut-free

Crimini Crusted Black Cod with Truffle Oil and Sunchoke Purée

Serves 4

The crunchy crimini mushroom and miso crust not only provides an immune boost, but rounds out the tenderness and omega-richness of the black cod (also known as sablefish). Plus, it pairs perfectly with the creaminess of the sunchoke purée and hints of truffle. Aside from this sensory explosion of goodness, this dish also keeps your figure fabulous, your heart healthy, and reduces inflammation.

For the cod:

1 cup (250 mL) dried crimini mushrooms

¼ cup (60 mL) avocado oil

1 tsp (5 mL) miso paste

4 (5-ounce/140 gram) black cod fillets

ground pepper to taste

1 lemon, juice and finely grated zest

truffle oil

For the sunchoke purée:

1 medium sunchoke (Jerusalem artichoke), peeled and chopped

2 cloves garlic

¼ tsp (1 mL) ground cumin

sea salt to taste

extra virgin olive oil

To make the cod, use a spice grinder to grind crimini mushrooms into a powder. In a small bowl, whisk avocado oil and miso paste. Brush cod with paste, season with ground pepper, then coat cod with ground mushrooms to form a crust. Bake in oven at 400°F (200°C) for about 10 minutes.

To make the purée, peel, chop, and steam sunchokes for about 10 minutes until soft. Combine with remaining ingredients (except olive oil) in a food processor. Process until finely chopped. While the processor is running, drizzle in enough oil to make a smooth purée, about 1 to 2 Tbsp (15 to 30 mL).

To serve, spread a thick coat of purée along plate, top with the cod, then drizzle with lemon juice and zest and truffle oil.

TIP
If you're completely plant-based, no need to fret! You can substitute tempeh, a fermented soy product, for the cod.

DID YOU KNOW?
Sunchokes, also known as Jerusalem artichokes, are rich in fructooligosaccharide (FOS), a prebiotic fiber that helps balance blood-sugar levels and aids in weight loss.

SIDE DISH

- Heart healthy
- Diabetic friendly
- Anti-inflammatory
- Mood boosting
- Immune boosting

- Anti-aging
- Blood-sugar balancing
- Weight loss
- Ocean wise/sustainable
- Gluten-free

- Dairy-free
- Soy-free
- Nut-free

Maca Chocolate Babycakes with Cherry Cashew Frosting

Makes 24 mini cupcakes or 12 regular-sized ones

A sexy dessert featuring chocolate and maca—an aphrodisiacal combo sure to get you in the mood! Plus, these mini cupcakes are totally moist, fluffy, and decadent. No one would have a clue that they're good for you.

For the cupcakes:

1 Tbsp (15 mL) ground chia seeds

¼ cup (60 mL) warm water

1 ripe banana

2 Tbsp (30 mL) coconut oil

½ cup (125 mL) walnut butter
   (or almond butter)

2 tsp (10 mL) vanilla extract

1 cup (250 mL) almond milk

½ cup (125 mL) coconut sugar

1 cup (250 mL) brown rice flour

½ cup (125 mL) cooked quinoa

3 Tbsp (50 mL) maca powder

⅓ cup (75 mL) cocoa powder

1 tsp (5 mL) baking powder

1 tsp (5 mL) non-aluminum baking soda

½ tsp (2 mL) salt

chopped walnuts

For the cherry cashew frosting:

2 tsp (10 mL) almond extract

2 cups (500 mL) raw cashews

⅓ cup (75 mL) maple syrup

2 cups (500 mL) pitted cherries

3 Tbsp (50 mL) coconut milk or almond milk

To make the cupcakes, preheat oven to 350°F (175°C).

Place ground chia in a small bowl. Add water and mix with a fork. Set aside for gel to form.

Mash banana in a large bowl, then add oil, nut butter, vanilla, and milk and stir to mix. Add the rest of the ingredients and mix until well incorporated.

Grease muffin tins with coconut oil. Drop in batter and bake 25 to 30 minutes, until a toothpick comes out clean.

To make the frosting, add all ingredients to a high-power blender and blend until thick and smooth. Adjust coconut milk as necessary so that mixture is thick enough to hold up as a frosting.

Add frosting to piping bag and frost babycakes (mini cupcakes).

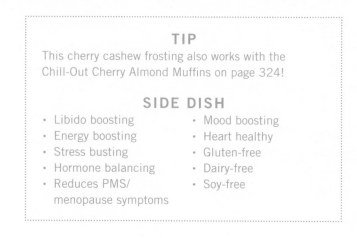

TIP

This cherry cashew frosting also works with the Chill-Out Cherry Almond Muffins on page 324!

SIDE DISH

- Libido boosting
- Energy boosting
- Stress busting
- Hormone balancing
- Reduces PMS/ menopause symptoms
- Mood boosting
- Heart healthy
- Gluten-free
- Dairy-free
- Soy-free

Amaranth, Hazelnut, and Chocolate Chip Cupcakes

Makes 12 (or 24 mini cupcakes)

Amaranth is a pseudo-grain that often gets overlooked. Its nutritional profile is comparable to quinoa and is just as rich in protein and fiber—and it's gluten-free! Because the amaranth seeds are so tiny they work well in baked goods, and taste even better when combined with hazelnuts and chocolate chips in this guilt-free treat!

For the cupcakes:

1 Tbsp (15 mL) ground chia seeds

4 Tbsp (60 mL) warm water

2 Tbsp (30 mL) coconut oil

2 bananas, ripe and mashed

½ cup (125 mL) hazelnut butter

1 Tbsp (15 mL) maple syrup

1 tsp (5 mL) vanilla

½ cup (125 mL) almond or hazelnut milk

¾ cup (175 mL) cooked amaranth

1 cup (250 mL) brown rice flour

2 tsp (10 mL) shredded coconut

1 tsp (5 mL) baking powder

1 tsp (5 mL) non-aluminum baking soda

½ tsp (2 mL) salt

¼ cup (60 mL) mini chocolate chips

¼ cup (60 mL) hazelnuts, toasted, lightly crushed or chopped

For the frosting:

2 very ripe avocados

½ cup (125 mL) maple syrup

¼ cup (60 mL) cocoa powder

2 Tbsp (30 mL) coconut oil

For the topping:

coconut flakes

candied pecans

To make the cupcakes, place ground chia in a small bowl. Add water and mix with a fork. Set aside for gel to form.

Mix oil, banana, hazelnut butter, maple syrup, vanilla, and milk together in a medium bowl. Add the rest of the ingredients and mix until well incorporated. Spoon into muffin tins.

Bake at 350°F (175°C) for 22 minutes.

To make the frosting, cut avocados in half and remove the seeds. Scoop out the flesh into a food processor. Add the maple syrup, cocoa, and coconut oil and blend together until it's all smooth. Refrigerate for 30 minutes before serving.

Once cupcakes have cooled, add frosting to piping bag and pipe onto cupcakes. Sprinkle with coconut flakes and top with candied pecans.

TIP

Swap out ¼ cup (60 mL) of the brown rice flour for Vega One in French Vanilla for an added nutrition boost of protein, chlorophyll, antioxidants, and more!

SIDE DISH

- Heart healthy
- Energy boosting
- Beautifying
- Anti-aging
- Stress busting
- Gluten-free
- Dairy-free
- Soy-free

Chill-Out Cherry Almond Muffins

Makes 12

This calming combination of cherries and almonds is so delish it'll melt your worries away, taking you into a state of pure bliss! Make it in batches and enjoy the zenning effect as you drown out thoughts of crazy work meetings or watch your children run circles around you. Chillax and enjoy!

1 Tbsp (15 mL) ground chia + 4 Tbsp (60 mL) warm water

1 ripe banana

2 Tbsp (30 mL) coconut oil

½ cup (125 mL) walnut butter

1 tsp (5 mL) vanilla extract

1 cup (250 mL) almond milk

1 tsp (5 mL) almond extract

½ cup (125 mL) coconut sugar

1 cup (250 mL) brown rice flour

1 cup (250 mL) 100% pure rolled oats or quinoa flakes

1 tsp (5 mL) baking powder

1 tsp (5 mL) non-aluminum baking soda

½ tsp (2 mL) salt

½ cup (125 mL) slivered almonds

½ cup (125 mL) dried cherries

Place ground chia in a small bowl. Add warm water and mix with a fork. Set aside for gel to form.

Mash banana in a large bowl, then add oil, nut butter, vanilla, and milk, stirring to mix. Add the rest of the ingredients and mix until well incorporated.

Grease large muffin tins with coconut oil. Drop in batter and bake at 350°F (175°C) for 25 to 30 minutes, until toothpick comes out clean.

TIP

For extra stress-busting power, add 3 Tbsp (50 mL) of maca powder to the recipe to help manage cortisol levels.

SIDE DISH

- Stress busting
- Calming
- Heart healthy
- Hormone balancing
- Libido boosting
- Gluten-free
- Dairy-free
- Soy-free

Chocolate Chip Quinoa Cookies

Makes 24 cookies

I've been making these cookies since my investment days—and it's the recipe I use to convert the non-converted to the world of goodness! Everyone LOVES these cookies—especially kids and those who claim to not like healthy or gluten-free eats. They're scrumptious and have a moist, banana bread–like consistency. Try 'em: you'll totally fall in love!

4 large, very ripe bananas

1 tsp (5 mL) vanilla

1 heaping Tbsp (15 mL) almond butter (optional)

½ cup (125 mL) coconut sugar

1 cup (250 mL) quinoa (cooked)

1 cup (250 mL) uncooked quinoa flakes (or 100% pure rolled oats)

1 cup (250 mL) unsweetened, shredded coconut

pinch sea salt

½ cup (125 mL) dark chocolate chips (or nuts, raisins, or other dried fruit)

Preheat oven to 375°F (190°C). In a large mixing bowl, mash bananas with a fork and add vanilla, almond butter (if using), and coconut sugar. Add quinoa, quinoa flakes or oats, coconut, and pinch of salt. Mix until well combined. Stir in chocolate chips and/or raisins.

Line a baking sheet with parchment paper and drop spoonfuls of batter onto sheet. Bake for 25 to 30 minutes. Remove from oven and let cool.

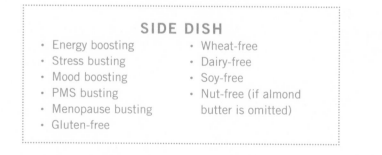

SIDE DISH

- Energy boosting
- Stress busting
- Mood boosting
- PMS busting
- Menopause busting
- Gluten-free

- Wheat-free
- Dairy-free
- Soy-free
- Nut-free (if almond butter is omitted)

Cocoa Mocha Torte

Serves 4 to 8

One word: decadent. It's the only way to describe this rich, velvety, melt-in-your-mouth indulgence. The silky-smooth mousse filling lounges on a chocolate macaroon-like crust. A dollop of tangy raspberry coulis is the icing on the cake, making for a most succulent dessert. And you know what else? It's guilt-free.

For the tart crust:
⅔ cup (150 mL) pecans
⅓ cup (75 mL) hazelnuts
1 cup (250 mL) raisins
1 tsp (5 mL) maple syrup
2 Tbsp (30 mL) coconut,
   unsweetened, shredded
2 Tbsp (30 mL) raw cacao powder

For the filling:
2 cups (500 mL) raw cashews
4 Tbsp (60 mL) cocoa powder
1 shot espresso

½ cup (125 mL) coconut sugar
1 tsp (5 mL) vanilla extract
1 Tbsp (15 mL) ground chia seeds
½ cup (125 mL) water
2 Tbsp (30 mL) psyllium husk (or ground
   chia seeds)

For the raspberry coulis:
1 cup (250 mL) raspberries
1 tsp (5 mL) vanilla extract
1 tsp (2 mL) coconut sugar
1 tsp (5 mL) ground chia

To make the crust, add pecans and hazelnuts to a blender or food processor and blend until ground. Add raisins, and process until finely chopped and the mixture starts to stick together. Then add maple syrup, coconut, and cacao powder and process until combined. Press mixture into two 6-inch (15 cm) springform pans.

To make the filling, add all ingredients (except the psyllium husk) to a high-speed blender and slowly blend, using the plunger to help mix the batter. Modify water to adjust consistency (the batter should be thick). Once blended, add psyllium husk, and blend once more.

Spoon out into springform pans, filling the pans completely. Refrigerate for at least 3 hours.

To make the coulis, use an immersion blender to blend all ingredients until smooth. Pour into a small pitcher.

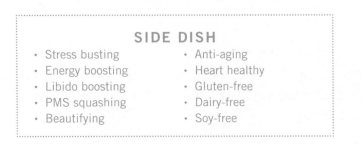

SIDE DISH

- Stress busting
- Energy boosting
- Libido boosting
- PMS squashing
- Beautifying
- Anti-aging
- Heart healthy
- Gluten-free
- Dairy-free
- Soy-free

Blueberry Lemon Tart

Serves 4

This tart is dairy-free, wheat-free, gluten-free, and soy-free. Yet the tangy, lemony cashew-cream filling is packed with vitamin C and protein, aiding in muscle recovery. It's also loaded with antioxidants and minerals, such as magnesium, which help increase bone strength and promote relaxation. And the taste ... absolutely delish.

For the crust:

1 cup (250 mL) raw pecans

1 cup (250 mL) raisins

⅓ cup (75 mL) maple syrup

½ cup (125 mL) coconut water
   (or plain water)

For the filling:

1½ cups (375 mL) raw cashews

1 large lemon, juice and zest

¼ orange, juiced

1 tsp (5 mL) vanilla extract

1 Tbsp (15 mL) ground chia seeds

For the topping:

1 cup (250 mL) + ¼ cup (60 mL)
   wild blueberries

½ tsp (2 mL) vanilla

1 tsp (5 mL) ground chia

To make the crust, measure pecans and raisins into a food processor and process until it becomes a smooth paste. Divide dough into quarters and press into four 6-inch (15 cm) fluted tart pans with removable bottoms. Place in the freezer while you work on the filling.

To make the filling, add all ingredients to a high-power blender and blend until smooth. Pour in more water as needed to make a smooth but thick mixture. Scrape filling into tart shells.

Chill overnight before serving.

To make the topping, add ¼ cup (60 mL) blueberries to food processor with vanilla and ground chia and purée until smooth. Transfer to bowl and stir in remaining cup (250 mL) of whole blueberries. Spoon topping onto tart filling.

SIDE DISH

- Stress busting
- Energy boosting
- PMS squashing
- Beautifying
- Anti-aging
- Heart healthy
- Antioxidant rich
- Gluten-free
- Dairy-free
- Soy-free

Double Chocolate Quinoa Coconut Haystacks

Makes 24 cookies

If you love my Chocolate Chip Quinoa Cookies, and you love chocolate, then you'll LOVE these! The chocolate–coconut combination makes for a decadent treat, while the zinc found in the maple syrup, cocoa, and quinoa can actually help clear acne (and boost libido).

4 large, very ripe bananas

1 tsp (5 mL) vanilla

½ cup (125 mL) maple syrup

1 cup (250 mL) quinoa (cooked)

2 cups (500 mL) unsweetened, shredded coconut

¼ cup (60 mL) cocoa powder

½ cup (125 mL) dark chocolate chips

Preheat oven to 375°F (190°C). In a large mixing bowl, mash bananas with a fork and add vanilla and maple syrup. Add remaining ingredients (except the chocolate chips). Stir until well combined, and then stir in chocolate chips.

Line a baking sheet with parchment paper (or grease the sheet with coconut oil) and drop spoonfuls of batter onto sheet. Bake for about 25 minutes. Remove from oven and let cool.

SIDE DISH

- Energy boosting
- Stress busting
- Libido boosting
- Beautifying
- Immune boosting
- PMS busting
- Menopause busting
- Gluten-free
- Dairy-free
- Soy-free
- Nut-free

Banana Coconut Crème Brûlée

Serves 4

Have a picky dinner guest? Make this! It's sure to please. The vanilla coconut milk imparts a dairy-free richness, while the cashews and mood-boosting bananas add to the smooth, creamy filling. The caramelized coconut sugar makes for a perfect finish. This indulgence is so scrumptious it'll have you (and your guests) licking the ramekins clean!

1½ cups (375 mL) raw cashews

1 cup (250 mL) vanilla coconut milk

1 small ripe banana, whole

⅓ cup (75 mL) coconut sugar plus extra
   for topping

1 tsp (5 mL) vanilla

1 Tbsp (15 mL) coconut oil

1½ tsp (7 mL) ground chia

½ banana, thinly sliced

In a high-speed blender or food processor, combine cashews, coconut milk, banana, coconut sugar, vanilla, and coconut oil until smooth. Add ground chia and continue to blend.

Layer banana slices across bottom of four ramekins. Pour mixture evenly over bananas. Refrigerate for about an hour.

Remove from fridge, then sprinkle coconut sugar to completely cover the top of each ramekin. Place ramekins on a baking sheet and put in the oven with the broiler set to high for just a few minutes, caramelizing the sugar until it's bubbling and golden. You can also use a blowtorch, but with coconut sugar, it doesn't work as well (raw cane sugar can also work).

Refrigerate for an hour before serving.

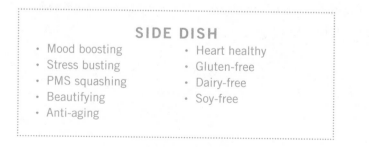

SIDE DISH

- Mood boosting
- Stress busting
- PMS squashing
- Beautifying
- Anti-aging
- Heart healthy
- Gluten-free
- Dairy-free
- Soy-free

Almond Butter Chocolate Chip Cookies

Makes 25 cookies

These cookies trump milk when it comes to bone health. Almonds (in the form of almond but-ter) are an excellent source of calcium *and* magnesium, making for the perfect bone-building balance. Plus, they're extremely alkalizing—a key factor in preserving healthy bones. The cacao nibs provide another dose of magnesium (they're one of its highest plant-based sources). The walnuts add a delicious crunch while the raisins and chocolate chips add to the sweetness.

1 cup (250 mL) raw almond butter

2 Tbsp (30 mL) ground chia (mixed with
   ⅓ cup/75 mL water)

½ tsp (2 mL) cinnamon

½ cup (125 mL) coconut sugar

pinch sea salt

1 cup (250 mL) 100% rolled oats

1 cup (250 mL) coconut flakes, unsweetened

¼ cup (60 mL) raisins

¼ cup (60 mL) cacao nibs

¼ cup (60 mL) chocolate chips

⅓ cup (75 mL) walnuts, chopped/crushed

Note: You can substitute tahini (or even hazelnut butter) for the almond butter. Tahini is one of the highest sources of calcium: it has approximately seven times more calcium than a cup of milk!

Preheat oven to 350°F (175°C).

In a large bowl, mix almond butter, chia mixture, cinnamon, coconut sugar, and sea salt until well combined, then mix in remaining ingredients. You may want to get in there with your hands to make sure everything's well combined and a dough-like consistency is formed.

Roll into golf-size balls in your hands, then press flat on a cookie sheet lined with parchment paper or greased with coconut oil. Smooth the tops and form into rounds.

Bake until golden, about 20 minutes. Let cool completely before eating.

SIDE DISH

- Bone building
- Energy boosting
- Stress busting
- Beautifying

- Heart healthy
- Dairy-free
- Soy-free
- Gluten-free*

* To make this gluten-free, be sure to get 100% pure oats and chocolate chips to ensure there's no cross-contamination or addition of wheat products.

Peggyfied Banana Walnut Ice Cream Sandwich

Serves 4

Yum, yum in your tum. This is SOOO good! Life doesn't get much better than an ice cream sandwich—especially when it's totally healthy and guilt-free. The taste is so surreal. Frozen bananas blend up into a smooth, creamy ice cream, with hints of maple, walnuts, vanilla, and cinnamon. Then the cold, soft, scrumptious goodness is sandwiched between two large, insanely delish almond chocolate chip cookies ... heaven!

For the banana walnut ice cream:

4 very ripe bananas, frozen

seeds from 1 vanilla bean pod

½ tsp (2 mL) ground cinnamon

¼ cup (60 mL) crushed walnuts

1 Tbsp (15 mL) maple syrup

For the cookies:

Use the Almond Butter Chocolate Chip Cookies recipe (page 332), but form into larger balls and press flat into 4-inch (10 cm) discs

To make the ice cream, blend frozen bananas, vanilla seeds, and cinnamon. Transfer to a container and stir in walnuts and maple syrup. Keep in the freezer until needed.

To make the ice cream sandwich, place one cookie on plate upside down, flat side facing up. Using an ice cream scoop, place one scoop of banana walnut ice cream on top of cookie, then press down using other cookie, forming a sandwich.

SIDE DISH

- Mood boosting (warning: may cause ridiculous levels of happiness)
- Stress busting
- Chill-out factor
- PMS busting
- Energy boosting
- Bone building
- Alkalizing
- Blood-sugar balancing
- Gluten-free
- Soy-free
- Dairy-free

Frozen Fudge Pops

Serves 6

You won't buy store-bought fudge popsicles again after you try these! The avocado (which, really, you won't taste) provides the heart-healthy, beautifying creamy richness that's masked by the chocolatey goodness. Perfect for kids, and the adult kid-at-heart.

1 very ripe avocado
1¾ cups (425 mL) vanilla coconut milk
¼ cup (60 mL) + 1 Tbsp (15 mL)
   cocoa powder

½ cup (125 mL) coconut sugar
   (or maple syrup)
2 tsp (10 mL) vanilla extract
2 tsp (10 mL) coconut oil
½ tsp (2 mL) salt

Scoop out avocado flesh into a food processor. Add remaining ingredients and process until smooth. Pour the filling into popsicle molds. Freeze for 30 minutes, then insert popsicle sticks and continue freezing overnight (or at least 3 hours).

SIDE DISH

- Heart healthy
- Beautifying
- Anti-aging
- Energy boosting
- Blood-sugar balancing
- Gluten-free
- Soy-free
- Dairy-free
- Nut-free

Frozen Berry Cherry Pops

Serves 6

Next time you're out enjoying the sunshine, be sure to nosh on this frozen treat. Its raspberries and cherries are the perfect things to cool you down: both are a great source of vitamin C, which helps prevent heatstroke, plus they're super rich in antioxidants, which keep your skin healthy and protect it from UV damage. A beautifying popsicle? Yes, please!

2 cups (500 mL) pitted cherries

1 cup (250 mL) raspberries

½ cup (125 mL) coconut milk

1 Tbsp (15 mL) raw honey

1 banana

Add all ingredients to blender and blend until smooth. Pour the filling into popsicle molds. Freeze for 30 minutes, then insert popsicle stick and continue freezing overnight (or at least 3 hours).

SIDE DISH

- Brain boosting
- Antioxidant
- Anti-inflammatory
- Energy boosting
- Stress busting
- Mood boosting
- Beautifying
- Gluten-free
- Dairy-free
- Soy-free
- Nut-free

Resources

All-in-One Health Supplements

VEGA

Plant-based supplements and foods

When I'm traveling or on the go, I know I can easily get my nutrition needs covered with Vega. And I cannot stress enough how in love I am with Vega One, their all-in-one nutritional shake. This has been my breakfast staple for years no matter where I am! It's kind of like an insurance policy to ensure that all your daily nutritional needs are covered (French Vanilla is my favorite!). I'm also a big fan of the Vega Chlorella (I am convinced this is where all my energy comes from), Vega Maca, Vega Savi Seeds, and their energizing smoothies.

www.myvega.com

Beauty and Natural Care Products

CRAWFORD STREET SKINCARE

www.crawfordskincare.com

DR. HAUSCHKA

www.drhauschka.com

GREEN BEAVER

www.greenbeaver.com

HUGO NATURALS

www.hugonaturals.com

MYCHELLE
This skincare line is one of my favorites. It's one of the cleanest, has amazing ingredients (the packaging explains which foods they come from), and is very effective and affordable! Plus, the cute, small packaging makes it great for travel.
www.mychelle.com

Food and Drink

COCONUT BLISS
The best tasting coconut milk ice cream—cherry amaretto is my favorite flavor!
www.coconutbliss.com

COCONUT SECRET
Coconut nectar, coconut flour
www.coconutsecret.com

COCOS PURE
Coconut water
www.cocospure.com

ECOIDEAS
Coconut palm sugar
www.ecoideas.com

FOOD FOR LIFE BAKING COMPANY
Sprouted-grain bread, gluten-free bread, gluten-free tortillas, and pizza crusts
www.foodforlife.com

GIDDY YOYO
Chocolate
www.giddyyoyo.com

GOGO QUINOA
www.gogoquinoa.com

GREEN AND BLACK'S
Organic chocolate and cocoa
www.greenandblacks.com

KALIKORI
Olive oil
www.kalikorioliveoil.com

LIVE ORGANIC FOOD BAR
Raw snacks
www.livefoodbar.com

LIVING NUTZ
Soaked, sprouted, dehydrated nuts
www.livingnutz.com

MANNA ORGANICS
Sprouted-grain loaf
www.mannaorganicbakery.com

MANITOBA HARVEST
Hemp products
www.manitobaharvest.com

NATURE'S EARTHLY CHOICE
Quinoa, hemp, chia, Chia Goodness Cereal
www.earthlychoice.com

NAVITAS NATURALS
Superfoods such as yacon syrup, mesquite pod, golden berries, and gogi berries
www.navitasnaturals.com

NOURISH TEA
Traditional medicinals and a wide variety of herbal and healing teas
www.nourishtea.ca

ORGANIC TRADITIONS
Camu camu powder, gogi berries, holy basil, cacao nibs, and other superfoods
www.organictraditions.com

PRANA
Chia seeds, nuts, snacks
www.pranana.com

SARAFINO
Olive oil
www.sarafino.com

SEA TANGLE NOODLE COMPANY
Kelp noodles
www.kelpnoodles.com

SILVER LEAF
Olive oil
www.stevesproduce-organics.com

SO DELICIOUS
Coconut milk
www.sodelicious.com

SPICE MARKET
The best gluten-free pizza I've ever tried!
www.spicemarket.ca

SUNFOOD
Raw foods and superfoods
www.sunfood.com

TONICA
Kombucha
www.tonicakombucha.com

UPAYA NATURALS
Raw foods, nuts, cacao, snacks, supplements, kitchen appliances
www.upayanaturals.com

VEGA
Plant-based nutritional bars, snacks, and oils
You know what my favorite Vega all-in-one nutritional shake is? It also comes in a bar, wrapped in chocolate, and contains the same dose of nutrients. Yes, please! Chocolate almond is my favorite. Vega is also the home to Savi Seeds (sacha inchi seeds), antioxidant EFA oil blend, and plant-based nutritional bars such as the whole food energy bar and vibrancy bars.
www.myvega.com

Sports Nutrition
VEGA SPORT
Plant-based sports nutrition
For all you active types (or even types that just need more energy), Vega's Sport line provides plant-based performance nutrition. Its pre-workout energizer does just that, but is also a great coffee substitute for a healthy energy boost. I love to drink Vega's electrolyte hydrator during a workout or as a calorie-free way to drink more water. And its performance protein and bars are great for recovery.
www.vegasport.com

Supplements
AOR
Nutritional supplements such as B-complex, rhodiola, vitamin D
www.aor.com

ASCENTA HEALTH
Fish oils
www.ascentahealth.com

DOUGLAS LABS
Relora, which is amazing for stress
www.douglaslabs.com

E3 LIVE
AFA blue-green algae
www.e3live.com

GENESIS TODAY
A vast array of superfood supplements and superfood juices
www.genesistoday.com

GENUINE HEALTH
Fast Joint Care + natural eggshell membrane
www.genuinehealth.com

JAMIESON
NEM (Natural Eggshell Membrane)
www.jamiesonvitamins.com

LIVRELIEF
Pain relief cream
www.livrelief.com

METAGENICS
Nutritional supplements such as probiotics, vitamin D drops
www.metagenics.com

NATURAL FACTORS

Glucosamine sulfate & NEM (natural eggshell membrane)

www.naturalfactors.com

NEW CHAPTER

Vitamins, superfoods, probiotics, zyflamend (for inflammation)

www.newchapter.com

PURE HEALTH

Superfood supplements, such as green coffee extract, capucacu, and garcinia cambogia (for weight loss), as well as gogi and mangosteen

www.purehealth100.com

SBT SEABUCKTHORN

For skin and heart health

www.seabuckthorn.com

ST. FRANCIS HERB FARM

Supplements such as passionflower and valerian

www.stfrancisherbfarm.com

TRAUMEEL

Homeopathic pain relief

www.traumeel.ca and www.heelusa.com

References

Akhondzadeh, B. A., Moshiri, E., Noorbala, A. A., Jamshidi, A. H., Abbasi, S. H., & Akhondzadeh, S. (2007). Comparison of petal of *Crocus sativus* L. and fluoxetine in the treatment of depressed outpatients: A pilot double-blind randomized trial. *Progress in Neuro-Psychopharmacology & Biological Psychiatry, 31*(2), 439–442.

Akhondzadeh, S., Fallah-Pour, H., Afkham, K., Jamshidi, A.-H., & Khalighi-Cigaroudi, F. (2004). Comparison of *Crocus sativus* L. and imipramine in the treatment of mild to moderate depression: a pilot double-blind randomized trial. *BMC Complementary and Alternative Medicine, 4*(1), 12.

Akhondzadeh, S., Naghavi, H. R., Vazirian, M., Shayeganpour, A., Rashidi, H., & Khani, M. (2001). Passionflower in the treatment of generalized anxiety: A pilot double-blind randomized controlled trial with oxazepam. *Journal of Clinical Pharmacy and Therapeutics, 26*(5), 363–367.

Auborn, K. (2003). Indole-3-carbinol is a negative regulator of estrogen. *Journal of Nutrition, 133,* 2470S–2475S.

Basu, A., Sanchez, K., Leyva, M. J., Wu, M., Betts, N. M., Aston, C. E., & Lyons, T. J. (2010). Green tea supplementation affects body weight, lipids, and lipid peroxidation in obese subjects with metabolic syndrome. *Journal of the American College of Nutrition, 29*(1), 31–40.

Bent, S., Padula, A., Moore, D., Patterson, M., & Mehling, W. (2006). Valerian for sleep: A systematic review and meta-analysis. *American Journal of Medicine, 119*(12), 1005–1012.

Bhattacharyya, D., Sur, T. K., Jana, U., & Debnath, P. K. (2008). Controlled programmed trial of *Ocimum sanctum* leaf on generalized anxiety disorders. *Nepal Medical College Journal, 10*(3), 176–179.

Blask, D., Dauchy, R. T., & Sauer, L. (2005). Putting cancer to sleep at night: The neuroendocrine/circadian melatonin signal. *Endocrine, 27*(2), 179–188.

British Nutrition Foundations. (2001). *Mood and food.* Retrieved from http://www.britishnutrition.org.uk/home.asp?siteId=43&sectionId=1436&subSubSectionId=1420&subSectionId=336&parentSection=302&which=5

Brown, M. (2009). *Evening primrose oil—for the active lifestyle.* Retrieved from http://www.hhnews.com/epo.htm

Burkhardt, S., Tan, D. X., Manchester, L. C., Hardeland, R., & Reiter, R. J. (2001). Detection and quantification of the antioxidant melatonin in Montmorency and Balaton tart cherries (*Prunus cerasus*). *Journal of Agricultural and Food Chemistry, 49*(10), 4898–4902.

Chen, S., Oh, S.-R., Phung, S., Hur, G., Ye, J. J., Kwok, S. L., et al. (2006). Anti-aromatase activity of phytochemicals in white button mushrooms (*Agaricus bisporus*). *Cancer Research, 66*(24), 12026–12034.

Chopra, D. (1995). *Perfect digestion: The complete mind-body programme for overcoming disorders.* New York: Crown Publishing.

Chow, N., Fretz, M., Hamburger, M., & Butterweck, V. (2011). Telemetry as a tool to measure sedative effects of a valerian root extract and its single constituents in mice. *Planta medica, 77*(8), 795–803.

Connolly, D. A., McHugh, M. P., Padilla-Zakour, O. I., Carlson, L., & Sayers, S. P. (2006). Efficacy of a tart cherry juice blend in preventing the symptoms of muscle damage. *British Journal of Sports Medicine, 40*(8), 679–683.

Costa, G. (2010). Lavoro a turni e rischio di cancro della mammella. *Giornale italiano di medicina del lavoro ed ergonomia, 32*(4), 454–457.

DeNoon, D. (2005). *Drink more diet soda, gain more weight?: Overweight risk soars 41% with each daily can of diet soft drink.* Retrieved from http://www.webmd.com/diet/news/20050613/drink-more-diet-soda-gain-more-weight

Dilworth, L. L., Omoruyi, F. O., Simon, O. R., Morrison, E. Y., & Asemota, H. N. (2005). The effect of phytic acid on the levels of blood glucose and some enzymes of carbohydrate and lipid metabolism. *The West Indian Medical Journal, 54*(2), 102–106.

Docherty, J. P., Sack, D. A., Roffman, M., Finch, M., & Komorowski, J. R. (2005). A double-blind, placebo-controlled, exploratory trial of chromium picolinate in atypical depression: Effect on carbohydrate craving. *Journal of Psychiatric Practice, 11*(5), 302–314.

Duan, P., & Wang, Z. M. (2002). [Clinical study on effect of *Astragalus* in efficacy enhancing and toxicity reducing of chemotherapy in patients of malignant tumor]. *Zhongguo Zhong xi yi jie he za zhi Zhongguo Zhongxiyi jiehe zazhi, 22*(7), 515–517.

Erickson, R. (2010). *Good foods to alleviate menstrual cramps.* Retrieved from http://www.livestrong.com/article/94790-good-foods-alleviate-menstrual-cramps

Federation of American Societies for Experimental Biology. (2010). *Honey as an antibiotic: Scientists identify a secret ingredient in honey that kills bacteria.* Retrieved from http://www.sciencedaily.com/releases/2010/06/100630111037.htm#

Feily, A., & Namazi, M. R. (2009). Aloe vera in dermatology: A brief review. *Giornale italiano di dermatologia e venereologia : Organo ufficiale, 144*(1), 85–91.

Grimes, M. (2009). *Licorice treats peptic ulcers and Helicobacter pylori infection.* Retrieved from http://www.naturalnews.com/026711_ulcers_licorice_peptic.html

Hlebowicz, J., Darwiche, G., Bjorgell, O., & Almer, L. (2007). Effect of apple cider vinegar on delayed gastric emptying in patients with type 1 diabetes mellitus: A pilot study. *BMC Gastroenterology, 7*, 46.

Howatson, G., McHugh, M. P., Hill, J. A., Brouner, J., Jewell, A. P., van Someren, K. A., et al. (2010). Influence of tart cherry juice on indices of recovery following marathon running. *Scandinavian Journal of Medicine & Science in Sports, 20*(6), 843–852.

Jazayeri, S., Tehrani-Doost, M., Keshavarz, S. A., Hosseini, M., Djazayery, A., Amini, H., et al. (2008). Comparison of therapeutic effects of omega-3 fatty acid eicosapentaenoic acid and fluoxetine, separately and in combination, in major depressive disorder. *Australian and New Zealand Journal of Psychiatry, 42*(3), 192–198.

Kang, S. Y., Seeram, N. P., Nair, M. G., & Bourquin, L. D. (2003). Tart cherry anthocyanins inhibit tumor development in Apc(Min) mice and reduce proliferation of human colon cancer cells. *Cancer Letters, 194*(1), 13–19.

Khan, A., Safdar, M., Ali, K. M. M., Khattak, K. N., & Anderson, R. A. (2003). Cinnamon improves glucose and lipids of people with type 2 diabetes. *Diabetes Care, 26*(12), 3215–3218.

Kuehl, K. S., Perrier, E. T., Elliot, D. L., & Chesnutt, J. C. (2010). Efficacy of tart cherry juice in reducing muscle pain during running: A randomized controlled trial. *Journal of the International Society of Sports Nutrition, 7*, 17.

Larkworthy, W., & Holgate, P. F. (1975). Deglycyrrhizinized liquorice in the treatment of chronic duodenal ulcer: A retrospective endoscopic survey of 32 patients. *The Practitioner, 215*(1290), 787–792.

Lewith, G. T., Godfrey, A. D., & Prescott, P. (2005). A single-blinded, randomized pilot study evaluating the aroma of *Lavandula augustifolia* as a treatment for mild insomnia. *Journal of Alternative and Complementary Medicine*, 11(4), 631–637.

Li, X. M., Ma, Y. L., & Liu, X. J. (2007). Effect of the *Lycium barbarum* polysaccharides on age-related oxidative stress in aged mice. *Journal of Ethnopharmacology*, 111(3), 504–511.

Lin, P. Y., & Su, K. P. (2007). A meta-analytic review of double-blind, placebo-controlled trials of antidepressant efficacy of omega-3 fatty acids. *Journal of Clinical Psychiatry*, 68(7), 1056–1061.

Ludvik, B., Neuffer, B., & Pacini, G. (2004). Efficacy of *Ipomoea batatas* (Caiapo) on diabetes control in type 2 diabetic subjects treated with diet. *Diabetes Care*, 27(2), 436–440.

Ma, T. (2011). *What does fiber do to help ease PMS?* Retrieved from http://ezinearticles.com/?What-Does-Fiber-Do-To-Help-Ease-PMS?&id=1010265

Maenthaisong, R., Chaiyakunapruk, N., Niruntraporn, S., & Kongkaew, C. (2007). The efficacy of aloe vera used for burn wound healing: A systematic review. *Burns: Journal of the International Society for Burn Injuries*, 33(6), 713–718.

Martin, J., Wang, Z. Q., Zhang, X. H., Wachtel, D., Volaufova, J., Matthews D. E., & Cefalu, W. T. (2006). Chromium picolinate supplementation attenuates body weight gain and increases insulin sensitivity in subjects with type 2 diabetes. *Diabetes Care*, 29(8), 1826–1832.

Murray, M. T. (1995). *The healing power of herbs: The enlightened person's guide to the wonders of medicinal plants.* Rocklin, CA: Prima Pub.

Noorbala, A., Akhondzadeh, S., Tahmacebipour, N., & Jamshidi, A. (2005). Hydro-alcoholic extract of L. versus fluoxetine in the treatment of mild to moderate depression: A double-blind, randomized pilot trial. *Journal of Ethnopharmacology*, 97(2), 281–284.

Oi, Y., Imafuku, M., Shishido, C., Kominato, Y., Nishimura, S., & Iwai, K. (2001). Garlic supplementation increases testicular testosterone and decreases plasma corticosterone in rats fed a high protein diet. *Journal of Nutrition*, 131(8), 2150–2156.

Ozgoli, G., Goli, M., & Simbar, M. (2009). Effects of ginger capsules on pregnancy, nausea, and vomiting. *Journal of Alternative and Complementary Medicine*, 15(3), 243–246.

Patel, S. R., Malhotra, A., White, D. P., Gottlieb, D. J., & Hu, F. B. (2006). Association between reduced sleep and weight gain in women. *American Journal of Epidemiology*, 164(10), 947–954.

Pawlosky, R. (2001). Physiological compartmental analysis of alpha-linolenic acid metabolism in adult humans. *Journal of Lipid Research*, 42, 1257–1265.

Pigeon, W. R., Carr, M., Gorman, C., & Perlis, M. L. (2010). Effects of a tart cherry juice beverage on the sleep of older adults with insomnia: A pilot study. *Journal of Medicinal Food*, 13(3), 579–583.

Pongrojpaw, D., Somprasit, C., & Chanthasenanont, A. (2007). A randomized comparison of ginger and dimenhydrinate in the treatment of nausea and vomiting in pregnancy. *Journal of the Medical Association of Thailand*, 90(9), 1703–1709.

Psychology Today. (2003). *Vitamin C: Stress buster.* Retrieved from http://www.psychologytoday.com/articles/200304/vitamin-c-stress-buster

Qi, F., Li, A., Inagaki, Y., Gao, J., Li, J., Kokudo, N., et al. (2010). Chinese herbal medicines as adjuvant treatment during chemo- or radio-therapy for cancer. *Bioscience Trends*, 4(6), 297–307.

Ried, K., Sullivan, T., Fakler, P., Frank, O. R., & Stocks, N. P. (2010). Does chocolate reduce blood pressure? A meta-analysis. *BMC Medicine*, 8(1), 39.

Sansom, W. (2005). *New analysis suggests 'diet soda paradox'—Less sugar, more weight.* Retrieved from http://www.uthscsa.edu/hscnews/singleformat2.asp?newID=1539

Sephton, S., & Spiegel, D. (2003). Circadian disruption in cancer: A neuroendocrine-immune pathway from stress to disease? *Brain, Behavior, and Immunity*, 17(5), 321–328.

Shepherd, C. (2003). *Evening primrose oil: Lifting the curse of PMS*. Retrieved from http://www.evening-primrose-oil. com/pms.html

Snitker, S., Fujishima, Y., Shen, H., Ott, S., Pi-Sunyer, X., Furuhata, Y., et al. (2009). Effects of novel capsinoid treatment on fatness and energy metabolism in humans: Possible pharmacogenetic implications. *The American Journal of Clinical Nutrition, 89*(1), 45–50.

Somerfield, S. D. (1991). Honey and healing. *Journal of the Royal Society of Medicine, 84*(3), 179.

Srinivasan, V., Spence, D. W., Pandi-Perumal, S. R., Trakht, I., & Cardinali, D. P. (2008). Therapeutic actions of melatonin in cancer: Possible mechanisms. *Integrative Cancer Therapies, 7*(3), 189–203.

Stoll, A., Emanuel Severus, W., Freeman, M., Rueter, S., Zboyan, H., Diamond, E., et al. (1999). Omega 3 fatty acids in bipolar disorder: A preliminary double-blind, placebo-controlled trial. *Archives of General Psychiatry, 56*(5), 407–412.

Swithers, S. E., & Davidson, T. L. (2008). A role for sweet taste: Calorie predictive relations in energy regulation by rats. *Behavioral Neuroscience, 122*(1), 161–173.

Takikawa, M. (2010). Dietary anthocyanin-rich bilberry extract ameliorates hyperglycemia and insulin sensitivity via activation of amp-activated protein kinase in diabetic mice. *Journal of Nutrition, 140*(3), 527.

Traustadottir, T., Davies, S. S., Stock, A. A., Su, Y., Heward, C. B., Roberts, L., & Harman, S. M. (2009). Tart cherry juice decreases oxidative stress in healthy older men and women. *Journal of Nutrition, 139*(10), 1896–1900.

Turner, N. (2011). *Four keys to kick PMS*. Retrieved from http://www.truestarhealth.com/members/archives. asp?content=14ml3p1a97

Wang, Y., Han, T., Zhu, Y., Zheng, C. J., Ming, Q. L., Rahman, K., & Qin, L. P. (2010). Antidepressant properties of bioactive fractions from the extract of *Crocus sativus L. Journal of Natural Medicines, 64*(1), 24–30.

Wurtman, J. (2010). *The antidepressant diet*. Retrieved from http://www.psychologytoday.com/blog/ the-antidepressant-diet/201008/you-can-prevent-pms-destroying-your-diet

Zhang, Y., Vareed, S. K., & Nair, M. G. (2005). Human tumor cell growth inhibition by nontoxic anthocyanidins, the pigments in fruits and vegetables. *Life Sciences, 76*(13), 1465–1472.

Endnotes

1   http://psycnet.apa.org/index.cfm?fa=buy.optionToBuy&id=2003-01140-012

2   http://books.google.ca/books/about/A_New_Approach_to_Degenerative_Disease_a.html?id=opJlXwAACAAJ&redir_esc=y

3   www.ncbi.nlm.nih.gov/pubmed/18326600

4   www.ncbi.nlm.nih.gov/pubmed/11590482

5   www.ncbi.nlm.nih.gov/pubmed/19253862

6   www.ncbi.nlm.nih.gov/pubmed/20584271

7   http://nutraxin.com.tr/pdf/PassifloraIncarnata/Passiflora_02.pdf

8   www.ncbi.nlm.nih.gov/pubmed/12511112

9   http://care.diabetesjournals.org/content/27/2/436.long

10   www.ncbi.nlm.nih.gov/pubmed/16454147

11   www.ncbi.nlm.nih.gov/pubmed/16914506

12   http://jnci.oxfordjournals.org/content/93/20/1557.short

13   http://cancerres.aacrjournals.org/content/66/20/9789.short

14   www.sciencedaily.com/releases/2010/10/101004211637.htm

15   www.sciencedirect.com/science/article/pii/S0899900712000809

16   www.ncbi.nlm.nih.gov/pubmed/20438325

17   www.jissn.com/content/7/1/17

18   www.ncbi.nlm.nih.gov/pubmed/16131287

19   www.ivillage.com/married-sex-survey/6-b-165966

20   www.smellandtaste.org/_/index.cfm?action=research.sexual

21   http://jn.nutrition.org/content/131/8/2150.full

22   Philpott, W., & Kalita, D. (1980). *Brain Allergies*. New Canaan, CT: Keats Publishing.

23   www.mattitolonen.fi/files/pdf/APA_2006.pdf
     http://archpsyc.jamanetwork.com/article.aspx?articleid=204999#qundefined

24   www.ncbi.nlm.nih.gov/pubmed/21903025
     www.mattitolonen.fi/files/pdf/APA_2006.pdf

25   www.sciencedirect.com/science/article/pii/S0278584606004040

26   http://onlinelibrary.wiley.com/doi/10.1002/ptr.1647/abstract

27   www.ncbi.nlm.nih.gov/pubmed/1873372?dopt=Abstract&holding=f1000,f1000m,isrctn

28   http://psychcentral.com/news/2008/03/12/stress-affects-learning-and-memory/2031.html

29   www.bmj.com/content/339/bmj.b2462

30   www.ncbi.nlm.nih.gov/pubmed/22473784

31   Kaplan, B. J. (1988, October). The relevance of food for children's cognitive and behavioural
      health. *Canadian Journal of Behavioural Science*, 20(4), 359–373. doi: 10.1037/h0079936

32   www.ncbi.nlm.nih.gov/pubmed/10821328

33   http://rsw.sagepub.com/content/4/3/349.short

34   http://nnr.sagepub.com/content/2/3/123.short

35   www.sciencedaily.com/releases/2008/08/080804165312.htm

36   http://epirev.oxfordjournals.org/content/29/1/62.full.pdf+html

37   www.ncbi.nlm.nih.gov/pubmed/20524996

38   http://ihsite.com/user/Raquel%20Martin%20Soy%20Doc.pdf

39   http://ehp.niehs.nih.gov/2013/01/1205826/

40   http://jco.ascopubs.org/content/early/2012/05/18/JCO.2011.37.9792.abstract

41   www.ncbi.nlm.nih.gov/pubmed/19048616

42   www.ncbi.nlm.nih.gov/pubmed/20595643

43   www.ncbi.nlm.nih.gov/pubmed/19056576

44   http://onlinelibrary.wiley.com/store/10.1111/j.1750-3841.2007.00535.x/asset/j.1750-3841.
      2007.00535.x.pdf?v=1&t=hcsgqkgz&s=243c3e10730169c543dd597ba9370e06731dc3d6

45   www.ncbi.nlm.nih.gov/pubmed/19571169
      www.jacn.org/content/24/suppl_6/537S.full

46   http://ajcn.nutrition.org/content/early/2010/09/01/ajcn.2010.29355.short

47   www.sciencedirect.com/science/article/pii/S0261561409000302

48   http://care.diabetesjournals.org/content/26/12/3215.short

49   www.jissn.com/content/3/2/45

50   www.ncbi.nlm.nih.gov/pubmed/20089785

51   http://journals.lww.com/practicalpsychiatry/
      Abstract/2005/09000/A_Double_Blind,_Placebo_Controlled,_Exploratory.4.aspx

52   www.ncbi.nlm.nih.gov/pmc/articles/PMC2933390/

53   Zhang, H., et al. (2008). Risk factors for sebaceous gland diseases and their relationship to gas-
      trointestinal dysfunction in Han adolescents. *Journal of Dermatology*, 35, 555–561.
      www.ncbi.nlm.nih.gov/pubmed/18837699

54   www.ncbi.nlm.nih.gov/pubmed/18194824
      www.ncbi.nlm.nih.gov/pubmed/20361171

55   www.ncbi.nlm.nih.gov/pubmed/3207614

56   www.ncbi.nlm.nih.gov/pmc/articles/PMC1297205

57   www.fasebj.org/content/24/7/2576.full

58   http://archderm.jamanetwork.com/article.aspx?articleid=512013
      www.sciencedirect.com/science/article/pii/S1085562905000283

59   www.ncbi.nlm.nih.gov/pubmed/17957907

60   www.ncbi.nlm.nih.gov/pmc/articles/PMC2916885/?tool=pubmed

61   www.ncbi.nlm.nih.gov/pubmed/17513409

62   www.ncbi.nlm.nih.gov/pubmed/20921274

63   Jensen, Gitte S., et al. (2000, January). Consumption of Aphanizomenonflos-aquae has rapid effects on the circulation and function of immune cells in humans: A novel approach to nutritional mobilization of the immune system. *Journal of the American Nutraceutical Association*, 2(3).

64   Weidong Lu, M. B., et al. (2007). Acupuncture for chemotherapy-induced leukopenia: Exploratory meta-analysis of randomized controlled trials. *Journal of the Society for Integrative Oncology*, 5(1), 1–10.

65   www.cmu.edu/news/stories/archives/2012/april/april2_stressdisease.html

66   www.ncbi.nlm.nih.gov/pubmed/22176840

     www.uidaho.edu/research/fundingagencies/seedgrant/fy2011proposals/vella www.ncbi.nlm.nih.gov/pubmed/21836102

     http://cebp.aacrjournals.org/content/19/11/2691.full

67   http://medicalxpress.com/news/2012-10-sedentary-behavior-primary.html

68   www.umm.edu/altmed/articles/omega-3-000316.htm

     www.jacn.org/content/21/6/495.full

69   www.jacn.org/content/21/6/495.full

70   Tilwe, G. H., et al. (2001). Efficacy and tolerability of oral enzyme therapy as compared to diclofenac in active osteoarthrosis of knee joint: An open randomized controlled clinical trial. *Journal of the Association of Physicians of India*, 49, 617–621.

71   www.sciencedaily.com/releases/2012/02/120223103920.htm

72   http://dx.doi.org/10.4049/%u200Bjimmunol.1102412

73   www.sciencedaily.com/releases/2010/03/100317112055.htm

74   www.sciencedaily.com/releases/2009/02/090204172437.htm

75   www.ncbi.nlm.nih.gov/pubmed/18006902

76   www.ncbi.nlm.nih.gov/pubmed/7922442

     www.ncbi.nlm.nih.gov/pubmed/16842224

77   http://pubs.acs.org/doi/abs/10.1021/np050327j

     www.sciencedirect.com/science/article/pii/S0944711305000371

     www.sciencedirect.com/science/article/pii/030438359503913H

78   www.sciencedirect.com/science/article/pii/030698778990162X

     www.sciencedirect.com/science/article/pii/030698779290059L

     www.sciencedirect.com/science/article/pii/S1567576908002270

     http://online.liebertpub.com/doi/abs/10.1089/jmf.2005.8.125

79   www.springerlink.com/content/8u2hq45g49q07171

     www.tandfonline.com/doi/abs/10.1300/J237v07n02_02

80   www.ncbi.nlm.nih.gov/pubmed/20943052

     http://140.121.155.217/seminar/M97320043-3.pdf

     http://cat.inist.fr/?aModele=afficheN&cpsidt=3103805)

81   www.sciencedirect.com/science/article/pii/S0306987706000867

     http://informahealthcare.com/doi/abs/10.1080/10520290701791839

     http://ukpmc.ac.uk/abstract/MED/19418416

82   http://onlinelibrary.wiley.com/doi/10.1002/ibd.21320/full

     www.ncbi.nlm.nih.gov/pubmed/22894886

83 www.choosecherries.com/pdfs/cherries_FINAL_Red_Report.pdf

84 www.sciencedirect.com/science/article/pii/S0166432803004650
http://online.liebertpub.com/doi/abs/10.1089/jmf.2008.0270
http://onlinelibrary.wiley.com/doi/10.1111/j.1600-0838.2009.01005.x/abstract

85 www.jimmunol.org/content/170/8/4335.short
http://jn.nutrition.org/content/131/7/2034.short

86 Chalmers, J. (1970). Geographic variations of senile osteoporosis. *Journal of Bone and Joint Surgery*, 52B, 667.

87 www.ncbi.nlm.nih.gov/pubmed/17269852

88 Bolland, M. J., et al. (2011). Calcium supplements with or without vitamin D and risk of cardiovascular events: Reanalysis of the Women's Health Initiative limited access dataset and meta-analysis. *BMJ*, 342 (April): d2040 DOI: 10.1136/bmj.d2040

89 Johnson, N., et al. (1970). Effect of level of protein intake on urinary and fecal calcium and calcium retention. *Journal of Nutrition*, 100, 1425.
Allen, L., et al. (1979). Protein-induced hypercalcuria: A longer-term study. *American Journal of Clinical Nutrition*, 32, 741.

90 www.ncbi.nlm.nih.gov/pmc/articles/PMC3031450

91 Case-control study of risk factors for hip fractures in the elderly. (1994). *American Journal of Epidemiology*, 139(5).

92 http://online.liebertpub.com/doi/abs/10.1089/jwh.1997.6.49

93 Feskanich, D., Willett, W. C., Stampfer, M. J., & Colditz, G. A. (1997). Milk, dietary calcium, and bone fractures in women: A 12-year prospective study. *American Journal of Public Health*, 87, 992–997.

94 http://europepmc.org/abstract/MED/10439632

95 http://ajcn.nutrition.org/content/80/3/715.abstract

96 www.sciencedirect.com/science/article/pii/S0952327803000632

97 www.nejm.org/doi/full/10.1056/NEJM199709043371003).

98 www.heartandstroke.bc.ca/site/c.kpIPKXOyFmG/b.3644453/k.3454/Statistics.htm

99 www.startwithyourheart.com/resources/508SWYH_BurdenofCVDinNCJuly2010.pdf

100 Vogelzangs, N., Beekman, A. T. F., Milaneschi, Y., Bandinelli, S., Ferrucci, L., & Penninx, B. (2010). Urinary cortisol and six-year risk of all-cause and cardiovascular mortality. *Journal of Clinical Endocrinology & Metabolism*, doi: 10.1210/jc.2010-0192

101 http://jama.jamanetwork.com/article.aspx?articleid=192034#qundefined
Archer, S. L., Liu, K., Dyer, A. R., et al. (1998). Relationship between changes in dietary sucrose and high density lipoprotein cholesterol: The CARDIA Study. Coronary Artery Risk Development in Young Adults. *Annals of Epidemiology*, 8, 433–438.
Ernst, N., Fisher, M., Smith, W., et al. (1980). The association of plasma high-density lipoprotein cholesterol with dietary intake and alcohol consumption. The Lipid Research Clinics Prevalence Study. *Circulation*, 62, 41–52.
Liu, S., Willett, W. C., Stampfer, M. J., et al. (2000). A prospective study of dietary glycemic load, carbohydrate intake, and risk of coronary heart disease in US women. *American Journal of Clinical Nutrition*, 71, 1455–1461.

102 http://circ.ahajournals.org/cgi/content/meeting_abstract/124/21_MeetingAbstracts/A14667?sid=6929860a-dd87-4c1a-b544-c2de026fd650

103 www.sciencedaily.com/releases/2012/07/120716131325.htm

104 www.ncbi.nlm.nih.gov/pubmed/8209876?dopt=Abstract
     http://ods.od.nih.gov/factsheets/VitaminE-HealthProfessional
105 http://jn.nutrition.org/content/136/3/741S.full
106 http://agris.fao.org/agris-search/search/display.do?f=1988/US/US88292.xml;US883246288
     http://ukpmc.ac.uk/abstract/MED/12052487
     www.sciencedirect.com/science/article/pii/S0891584998002664
     http://jama.jamanetwork.com/article.aspx?articleid=382213
107 www.gastroamrosenberg.ch/upload/prj1/publikationen/ajm%202002%20n%203%20fatty%20mta.pdf
     http://ukpmc.ac.uk/abstract/MED/18757090
     www.biomedcentral.com/1471-2261/6/38
     http://onlinelibrary.wiley.com/doi/10.1046/j.1365-2796.1996.410753000.x/abstract
108 www.jacn.org/content/19/2/220.long
109 www.ncbi.nlm.nih.gov/pubmed/9731851
110 www.sciencedaily.com/releases/2010/07/100714104101.htm
111 http://jama.jamanetwork.com/article.aspx?articleid=196803
112 http://ajcn.nutrition.org/content/97/2/344.abstract
113 www.ncbi.nlm.nih.gov/pubmed/15917152

Index

asparagus, 53–54
aspartame, 86
astragalus, 200–201
atherosclerosis, 240
autoimmune diseases, 211
avocado, 164, 173, 256–57

B

banana, 164, 173
   and coconut crème brûlée, 331
   and walnut ice cream sandwich, 334
B-cells, role in healing, 193
beans and quinoa burgers, 308
beets, 78, 79
   golden, ravioli, 310–11
bentonite clay, 146
berries, 146, 156
   blueberry and lemon tart, 328–29
   frozen, cherry popsicles, 336
   smoothie, mind-boosting, 282
beta carotene, 119, 171, 199
beta glucans, 196–97
Be-YOU-tifying Cocktail, 285
bilberries, 108
biotin. See vitamin B7
bisphenol-A, 92–93
blackheads, 131
bloating, 180–84
blood clots, 240, 249
blood glucose/sugar
   and Brazil nuts, 66
   imbalances, and emotions, 27, 57
   and insulin, 103, 104–5
   levels, and sugar consumption, 71, 85, 87, 134
   nutrients for controlling, 120, 261
   stabilizing, 19, 20, 23, 24, 25, 31, 34–35,
      62, 66, 79, 88, 105, 106, 107, 108, 109,
      126, 187, 199, 255, 265, 266, 277
   and stress, 26, 34–35
   and sugar, 104–5
   and tryptophan, 57
blood pressure
   effect of cortisol, 27
   effect of salt, 247
   measuring, 239–40

   reducing, 101, 243, 246, 248, 250, 251, 254,
      255, 256, 261
   risks of high, 240, 247
   and sex life, 47
   and sleep deprivation, 40
   and stress, 26, 32, 246
blood-sugar balance recipes, 284, 291, 299–304,
      308, 310–16, 318–19, 334, 335
blueberries, wild, 80
blueberry and lemon tart, 328–29
body scrubs, 146–47
bone health recipes, 287, 301, 332–34
bones
   calcium and, 224–26
   components of, 222–23
   and exercise, 229
   food and nutrients for healthy, 225–26, 232–37
   health, and acid-alkaline balance, 228–29
   and hormonal balance, 230–31
   loss, causes of, 231–32
   osteoporosis, 223
   protein and, 226–27
   purpose, 222
BPA. See bisphenol-A
brain, 12–13, 70, 71–81
brain booster recipes, 294, 295, 300–304, 306–7,
      317, 336
Brazil nuts, 65–66
breath freshener, 107, 167
breathing, and stress, 38
broccoli, 79, 80, 94–95, 237
bromaline, 212. See also pineapple
burgers: quinoa bean, 308
butter replacements, 24
B vitamins, 17–18, 60, 73, 81, 94, 273. See also
    vitamin B12

C

cacao, 32, 33
caffeine, 28, 40, 57, 145, 271
cake: cocoa mocha torte, 326–27
calcium, 17, 30, 102, 224–26, 229, 232, 235–37,
      249, 250, 260, 272
calcium D-glucarate, 93
camu camu berries, 123

canapés: mushroom, chard, and white bean
crostini, 296–97
cancer, and melatonin production, 40–41
cancer prevention recipes, 288, 296–98
capsicum, 220
carbohydrates, 27, 34–35, 46, 72, 247
cardiovascular health. *See* heart health
carotenoids, 119
cashews, 264–65
catechins, 95–96
cayenne pepper, 100–102
cellulite, 144–46
CGF, 19
chamomile, 43–44, 159
cherries, tart, 42, 218–19
cherry
    almond muffins, 324
    and berry popsicles, 336
chia seeds, 107–8, 255–56, 277–78
chickpeas
    hummus, 291
    spicy soup, 300
chili: veggie, 299
chlorella, 18–20, 216–17
Chlorella Growth Factor, 19
chlorophyll, 18, 20
chocolate, 28, 32–33
    chip and almond butter cookies, 332–33
    chip quinoa cookies, 325
    cocoa mocha torte, 326–27
    frozen fudge popsicles, 335
    and maca cupcakes, 320–21
    quinoa coconut haystacks, 330
cholesterol
    causes of high, 242, 247
    high, and erectile dysfunction, 49
    lowering, 46, 52, 62, 95, 101, 106, 107, 124,
        126, 185, 197, 243, 246, 248, 251, 252, 253,
        255, 257, 261, 273
    purpose of, 241
    sources, 242
    and trans fats, 245
    types, 241
choline, 79
Chopra, Deepak, 185

chromium, 108, 109, 110
chrysin, 33–34, 44
cinnamon, 106–7
circulatory system, 101, 145
citric acid, 155
clams, 22–23
cocoa butter, 149–50
coconut, 23–25, 155
    chocolate quinoa haystacks, 330
coconut oil, 126–27, 140, 149, 163, 164
coconut palm sugar, 87
cod, black, crimini crusted, 318–19
co-enzyme Q10, 248–49
coffee, 156
Cohen, Dr. Sheldon, 207
colds, and inflammation, 207
collagen, 117–18
cookies
    almond butter chocolate chip, 332–33
    chocolate chip quinoa, 325
    chocolate quinoa coconut haystacks, 330
copper, 121, 172
cortisol, 26, 27, 34, 71, 133, 230–31
cravings, food, 27–28
crème brûlée, banana coconut, 331
crostini, mushroom, chard, and white bean,
    296–97
cucumber juice, 159
cupcakes
    amaranth, hazelnut, and chocolate chip,
        322–23
    maca chocolate, 320–21
cupuacu, 128–29
curcumin, 75, 213

D
dairy
    alternatives, 25
    non-heme iron in, 16
    and skin health, 134–35
    as source of calcium, 226–27
dairy-free recipes, 282–85, 287–88, 290–314,
    317–36
dehydration, 23, 24, 27
dementia, 75

beverages to improve, 285, 288

and chlorophyll, 18, 19

effect of sex life on, 47

foods and nutrients to strengthen, 193–203

functions of, 192–93

recipes for boosting, 283, 290, 296–98, 301, 314, 318–19, 330

and stress, 207

and sunflower sprouts, 20

immunoglobulin A (IgA), 47

indigestion, 40, 44

Indole-3-carbinol, 93, 96, 261

inflammation

    acute, 192, 205–6

    atherosclerosis, 240

    brain, and memory decline, 72

    causes, 71, 205, 206–11

    chronic, 192, 205–6

    and disease, 206

    foods to treat, 75, 101, 214–19

    herbal/homeopathic treatments, 219–20

    and immune system, 192

    and menopause, 274

    and omega-6 fatty acids, 59

    and toxins, 135

    treatments for, 211–14

inflammatory bowel disease, 75

infrared sauna, 145

insomnia, 34, 37, 42–46. *See also* sleep

insulin

    and blood glucose, 104–5

    and carbohydrates, 46

    resistance, 103, 104–5

    role in weight gain, 104

    sweet potato effect on, 35

iodine

    importance of, 99

    kelp as source, 100

    in sea vegetables, 21–22

    sources, 21–22, 100, 137

    and soy, 92

    and thyroid function, 21–22, 99

IQ, 72, 73

iron

    absorption, 16–17

in AFA, 199

in clams, 22–23

deficiency, 15–16

as energy booster, 15–16

foods with, 16–17

and hair care, 171–72

heme, 16

non-heme, 16

sources, 172

and vitamin C, 16

J

jojoba oil, 150, 163

journal, 38

K

kale, 235–36, 262–63, 275

    and hemp seed salad, 301

kelp, 22, 100

kimchi, 141

kombucha, 189–90

    cocktail, 286

    float, 289

L

lactic acid, 155

L-arginine, 49, 54

lavender, 141

lavender oil, 45, 141, 142, 160

LDL, 101, 106, 241, 249, 252, 257

legumes, 17

lemon balm, 45

lemons, 142, 156, 160, 174

lemon water, 93–94

libido, 47, 48, 50–51. *See also* sex

libido boosting recipes, 287, 295, 306–7, 320–21, 324, 326–27, 330

licorice, 186

licorice oil, 141–42

lip gloss, home-made, 165–66

liver, 93–94

low-density lipoprotein. *See* LDL

L-tyrosine, 55

lutein, 94, 119, 210, 275

lycopene, 119

peppermint, 188

peppermint tea, 275–76

pesticides, 92

pH. See acid-alkaline balance

phenylethylamine, 199

Philpott, Dr. William, 57

phospholipids, 73

phthalates, 92–93

phytates, 17

phytoestrogens, 91–92

phytosterols, 52

pies and tarts: blueberry lemon tart, 328–29

pimples, 131–32

pineapple, 217–18. See also bromaline

pituitary gland, 98–99

pizza, 315–16

PMS (premenstrual syndrome), 259–66

PMS relief recipes, 287, 301–3, 305, 320–21, 325–31, 334

polyphenolic antioxidants, 119–20, 128

polysaccharides, 127

polyunsaturated fats, 126

popsicles
frozen berry cherry, 336
frozen fudge, 335

potassium, 250

potatoes, 210

probiotics, 25, 136, 189, 195–96

protein
and bone loss, 226–27
digestion of, 183
and food combining, 183
and hair growth, 170
sources, 19, 62–63, 107, 170, 227
and weight loss, 102

protein-rich foods, recipe, 291

pumpkin, 164

pumpkin seeds, 52

PVC. See phthalates

Q

quinoa, 81, 264
and acorn squash bowl, 309
bean burgers, 308

chocolate chip cookies, 325

chocolate coconut haystacks, 330

R

raspberry coulis, 326–27

ravioli, golden beet, 310–11

red blood cells, 18, 20

Relora, 37

resveratrol, 120

rheumatoid arthritis, 75, 128, 207, 211, 213, 214, 216

RNA, 19

roasted red pepper dip, 290

romaine, grilled, Caesar salad, 302–3

romaine lettuce, 109–10

rosemary, 77

rosewater, 160

S

sacha inchi seeds, 62–64

saffron, 64–65

salads
dressings, 302–3, 304, 305
fennel and apple, 305
grilled romaine Caesar, 302–3
kale and hemp seed, 301
warm vegetable, 304

salmon, 217, 237

salt/sodium, 27, 247, 250

saturated fats, 48, 126, 149, 244, 245

sauces
raspberry coulis, 326–27
tomato olive, 310–11

saunas, 145

scrubs. See body scrubs

sea-buckthorn oil, 150, 162–63, 252–54

sea salt, 156

sea vegetables, 21–22

selenium, 50, 54, 65, 120

serotonin, 27, 45, 57, 58, 60, 86

sesame seeds, 235

sex, 33–34, 47, 48–55, 271

shea nut butter, 149

silica, 121–22, 171, 234

skin
    acne causes, 132–35
    beneficial effects of DMAE on, 72
    body scrubs, 146–47
    dry brushing of, 145
    exfoliating, 153–54
    improving look of, 145–52
    moisturizing, 147–52
skin care, 117–29, 130–43, 158. *See also* facial care
    recipes, 285
skin care products, 112–14, 147, 151–52, 157
sleep, 38, 39–46
smoking, 246–47
smoothies. *See also* milkshakes
    beautifying cocktail, 285
    berry mind-boosting, 282
    frappuccino, 284
    kombucha float, 289
snacks: candied nuts, 295
soups
    crimini miso, 298
    spicy chickpea, 300
soy, 91–92
soy-free recipes, 282–85, 287–88, 290–336
spinach, 66–67
starch, digestion of, 183
stevia, 87
stomach, 180–84
strawberries, 156
stress, 26–38, 71, 133, 186, 200, 206–7,
    230–31, 246
stress control recipes, 287–88, 290, 295,
    302–4, 308–13, 315–16, 320–34, 336
sugar, 28, 57, 71–72, 78, 84–88, 104, 134,
    155, 242, 247
sunchoke purée, 318–19
sunflower lecithin, 76–77
sunflower sprouts, 20–21
sweating, 145, 185
sweet potato, 34–35, 139–40
    gnocchi, 312–13

T

tacos: walnut, 306–7
tannins, 17

tartaric acid, 155
tart cherries, 42
T-cells, 193
tea tree oil, 142
testosterone, 48, 54, 132, 172–73
thyroid, 21–22, 65, 95, 98–99, 100–102
tomato
    mackerel, and olives, 317
    and olive sauce, 310–11
tomatoes, and inflammation, 210
toners, facial, 159–61
tooth whitener, home-made, 167
toxins, 135, 145, 146, 185
trans fats, 245
traumeel, 220
triglycerides, 49, 61, 241, 242, 247, 255, 274
tryptophan, 45–46, 57, 58, 62–63, 76, 79
turmeric, 75–76, 213, 214–15
tyrosine, 15, 21, 48–49

U

ursolic acid, 31

V

valerian root, 43
Vega Frappuccino, 284
VegaTini, 288
vegetable
    chili, 299
    salad, warm, 304
vegetables, 183, 210, 270–71.
        See also sea vegetables
vitamin A, 35, 118–19, 137, 171, 195
vitamin B1, 66
vitamin B2, 35–36
vitamin B3, 49, 54, 60, 73
vitamin B5, 35, 73
vitamin B6, 29, 35, 46, 49, 60, 261
vitamin B7, 170–71
vitamin B9, 73
vitamin B12, 17–18, 23, 60, 73, 202
vitamin C
    benefits, 117–18, 195
    effect on immune system, 195
    and hair care, 171

vitamin C (*continued*)
    for heart health, 248
    and iron, 16
    and memory, 74
    for menopause symptoms, 272
    and skin care, 117–18
    sources, 30, 35, 74, 118, 171, 195, 272
    and stress, 30
    and weight control, 41
vitamin D
    benefits, 193–94
    for bone health, 233
    and calcium, 233
    effect on immune system, 193–94
    for inflammation, 213
    for menopause symptoms, 272
    for premenstrual syndrome, 260
    sources, 194
    supplements, 233
    and weight control, 102
vitamin E
    benefits, 195
    effect on immune system, 195
    and hair care, 171
    for heart health, 248
    for menopause symptoms, 272
    and sexual function, 50
    and skin care, 118, 137
    sources, 36, 53–54, 66, 118, 137, 171, 272
vitamin K, 79, 214, 233–34
vitamins
    in chlorella, 20
    in chocolate, 32
    and stress, 29–30
    and sugar, 71–72
    in sunflower sprouts, 20

W
wakame, 22
walnuts, 54–55, 80, 81, 140
    and banana ice cream sandwich, 334
    tacos, 306–7
water, 23, 146, 163
weight control, 27, 37, 40, 41, 84–87, 89–91, 92, 94, 96–97, 98–99, 100–101, 102, 104, 105–10
weight control recipes, 284–85, 290–94, 296–305, 308–11, 314, 317–19
wheat free recipes, 299, 310–11, 325
white beans
    and mushroom and chard crostini, 296–97
    and rosemary dip, 294
whiteheads, 131

Y
yacon syrup, 88, 105–6
yerba maté, 102
yoga, 271–72
yogurt, 25, 164, 173

Z
zinc
    in AFA, 199
    in almonds, 36
    benefits, 120, 136, 201–2
    and hair loss, 172–73
    and libido, 48
    and memory, 74
    in miso, 201–2
    role in erectile dysfunction, 52
    and skin care, 120–21, 136
    sources, 48, 74, 121, 137, 173
    and testosterone production, 48, 54
    in walnuts, 55
zucchini and mushroom fettuccini, 314